Handbook of Herbal Medicine

Handbook of Herbal Medicine

Editor: Charlotte Cherrill

STATES
ACADEMIC PRESS
www.statesacademicpress.com

www.statesacademicpress.com

STATES
ACADEMIC PRESS

Cataloging-in-Publication Data

Handbook of herbal medicine / edited by Charlotte Cherrill.
p. cm.
Includes bibliographical references and index.
ISBN 978-1-63989-796-4
1. Herbs--Therapeutic use. 2. Medicine, Botanic. 3. Materia medica, Vegetable.
4. Medicinal plants. 5. Botany, Medical. I. Cherrill, Charlotte.
RM666.H33 H36 2023
615.321--dc23

States Academic Press,
109 South 5th Street,
Brooklyn, NY 11249, USA

ISBN 978-1-63989-796-4 (Hardback)

Contents

Preface

The world is advancing at a fast pace like never before. Therefore, the need is to keep up with the latest developments. This book was an idea that came to fruition when the specialists in the area realized the need to coordinate together and document essential themes in the subject. That's when I was requested to be the editor. Editing this book has been an honour as it brings together diverse authors researching on different streams of the field. The book collates essential materials contributed by veterans in the area which can be utilized by students and researchers alike.

Herbal medicine refers to the study of medicinal plants and other natural resources, which are the foundation of traditional medicine. It also involves the use of minerals, fungal and bee products, some animal parts, and shells. Plants synthesize various chemical compounds, which serve a variety of functions such as defense against diseases, insects, fungi, and herbivorous mammals. Many phytochemicals have been found in plants with established or potential biological activity. A single plant may synthesize a vast range of phytochemicals. There are four main biochemical classes of compounds found in plants, which include polyphenols, alkaloids, terpenes and glycosides. This book provides significant information to help develop a good understanding of herbal medicine. It presents researches and studies performed by experts across the globe. This book will prove to be immensely beneficial to students and researchers in this field.

Each chapter is a sole-standing publication that reflects each author´s interpretation. Thus, the book displays a multi-facetted picture of our current understanding of application, resources and aspects of the field. I would like to thank the contributors of this book and my family for their endless support.

Editor

1

Phomaketide A Inhibits Lymphangiogenesis in Human Lymphatic Endothelial Cells

Huai-Ching Tai [1,2,†], Tzong-Huei Lee [3], Chih-Hsin Tang [4,5,6], Lei-Po Chen [7,8,†], Wei-Cheng Chen [7,8], Ming-Shian Lee [3], Pei-Chi Chen [9], Chih-Yang Lin [9], Chih-Wen Chi [10], Yu-Jen Chen [10,11], Cheng-Ta Lai [12], Shiou-Sheng Chen [13,14], Kuang-Wen Liao [8,15,16], Chien-Hsing Lee [17,18,*] and Shih-Wei Wang [9,19,*]

1 School of Medicine, Fu-Jen Catholic University, New Taipei City 242, Taiwan; taihuai48@hotmail.com
2 Department of Urology, Fu-Jen Catholic University Hospital, New Taipei City 242, Taiwan
3 Institute of Fisheries Science, National Taiwan University, Taipei 106, Taiwan; thlee1@ntu.edu.tw (T.-H.L.); d301101010@tmu.edu.tw (M.-S.L.)
4 Chinese Medicine Research Center, China Medical University, Taichung 404, Taiwan; chtang@mail.cmu.edu.tw
5 Department of Pharmacology, School of Medicine, China Medical University, Taichung 404, Taiwan
6 Department of Biotechnology, College of Health Science, Asia University, Taichung 413, Taiwan
7 Department of Orthopaedics, MacKay Memorial Hospital, Taipei 104, Taiwan; robert82ccc@gmail.com (L.-P.C.); wchena7648@gmail.com (W.-C.C.)
8 Ph.D. Degree Program of Biomedical Science and Engineering, National Chiao Tung University, Hsinchu 300, Taiwan; liaonms@pchome.com.tw
9 Department of Medicine, Mackay Medical College, New Taipei City 252, Taiwan; 1622689043new@gmail.com (P.-C.C.); p123400@hotmail.com (C.-Y.L.)
10 Department of Medical Research, MacKay Memorial Hospital, New Taipei City 251, Taiwan; d48906003@yahoo.com.tw (C.-W.C.); chenmdphd@gmail.com (Y.-J.C.)
11 Department of Radiation Oncology, MacKay Memorial Hospital, Taipei 104, Taiwan
12 Division of Colon and Rectal Surgery, Department of Surgery, MacKay Memorial Hospital, Taipei 104, Taiwan; laichengta@gmail.com
13 Division of Urology, Taipei City Hospital HepingFuyou Branch, Taipei 100, Taiwan; DAB67@tpech.gov.tw
14 Commission for General Education, National United University, Miaoli 360, Taiwan
15 Institute of Molecular Medicine and Bioengineering, National Chiao Tung University, Hsinchu 300, Taiwan
16 Department of Biotechnology and Bioindustry Sciences, National Cheng Kung University, Tainan 300, Taiwan
17 Department of Pharmacology, Graduate Institute of Medicine, College of Medicine, Kaohsiung Medical University, Kaohsiung 807, Taiwan
18 Department of Medical Research, Kaohsiung Medical University Hospital, Kaohsiung 807, Taiwan
19 Graduate Institute of Natural Products, College of Pharmacy, Kaohsiung Medical University, Kaohsiung 807, Taiwan
* Correspondence: chlee0818@gmail.com (C.-H.L.); shihwei@mmc.edu.tw (S.-W.W.)

† These authors contributed equally to this work.

Abstract: Lymphangiogenesis is an important biological process associated with cancer metastasis. The development of new drugs that block lymphangiogenesis represents a promising therapeutic strategy. Marine fungus-derived compound phomaketide A, isolated from the fermented broth of *Phoma* sp. NTOU4195, has been reported to exhibit anti-angiogenic and anti-inflammatory effects. However, its anti-lymphangiogenic activity has not been clarified to date. In this study, we showed that phomaketide A inhibited cell growth, migration, and tube formation of lymphatic endothelial cells (LECs) without an evidence of cytotoxicity. Mechanistic investigations revealed that phomaketide A reduced LECs-induced lymphangiogenesis via vascular endothelial growth factor receptor-3 (VEGFR-3), protein kinase Cδ (PKCδ), and endothelial nitric oxide synthase (eNOS) signalings. Furthermore, human proteome array analysis indicated that phomaketide A significantly enhanced the protein levels of various protease inhibitors, including cystatin A, serpin B6, tissue factor pathway inhibitor (TFPI), and tissue inhibitor matrix metalloproteinase 1 (TIMP-1). Importantly, phomaketide A impeded tumor growth and lymphangiogenesis by decreasing the expression of LYVE-1, a specific marker for lymphatic vessels, in tumor xenograft animal model. These results suggest that phomaketide A may impair lymphangiogenesis by suppressing VEGFR-3, PKCδ, and eNOS signaling cascades, while simultaneously activating protease inhibitors in human LECs. We document for the first time that phomaketide A inhibits lymphangiogenesis both *in vitro* and *in vivo*, which suggests that this natural product could potentially treat cancer metastasis.

Keywords: phomaketide A; lymphangiogenesis; lymphatic endothelial cells; vascular endothelial growth factor receptor-3

---

1. Introduction

Cancer metastasis enables cancer cells to spread from the primary tumor and establish themselves in other tissues. Lymphatic circulation is a common route for cancer metastasis [1], with the thin walls and few tight junctions in the lymphatic vessels offering good permeability. Moreover, the lack of basal lamina and associated pericytes, means that lymphatic capillaries have an easy opening for the uptake of macromolecular cancer cells into the lymphatic vessels [2,3]. Lymphangiogenesis, the process by which new lymphatic vessels grow out of pre-existing vessels, enables lymphatic endothelial cells (LECs) to proliferate and migrate through lymphatic vessels surrounding the tumors [4,5]. Lymphangiogenic factors, including vascular endothelial growth factor (VEGF)-C or D, predominantly bind to VEGF receptor-3 (VEGFR-3), and promote several downstream signaling pathways for regulating lymphangiogenesis [6–8]. During the lymphangiogenic process, LEC survival, proliferation, migration and tube formation depends upon the activation of the VEGF-C/VEGFR-3 axis [9]. In various experimental tumor models, overexpression of VEGF-C can induce lymphangiogenesis and disseminate metastatic tumor cells to lymph nodes [10], and the use of neutralizing antibodies against VEGF-C and VEGFR-3 can prevent tumor lymphangiogenesis and lymphatic metastasis [11]. Thus, selective targeting of VEGFR-3-dependent lymphangiogenesis can potentially block cancer progression and metastasis.

Marine bacteria, microalgae and fungi have proven to be a rich source of bioactive metabolites possessing biological and pharmacological properties with enormous therapeutic potential [12]. We have previously demonstrated that phomaketide A, isolated from the marine endophytic fungal strain *Phoma* sp. NTOU4195, exerts anti-angiogenic and anti-inflammatory effects [13]. However, no data exist as to the effects of phomaketide A on tumor lymphangiogenesis. We therefore explored the *in vitro* and *in vivo* anti-lymphangiogenic effects and mechanisms of phomaketide A.

2. Results

2.1. Anti-Lymphangiogeneic Effects of Phomaketide A on Human LECs

To examine the growth-inhibitory effects of phomaketide A (Figure 1A), we treated human LECs with various concentrations of phomaketide A. Figure 1B illustrates how phomaketide A inhibited LECs growth in a concentration-dependent manner ($IC_{50} = 3.7 \pm 0.6$ μM). The lymphangiogenesis inhibitor, rapamycin, served as a positive control [14]. Next, the results of a tube formation assay showed that phomaketide A significantly reduced LECs tube formation (Figure 2A). Since the migratory ability of endothelial cells is another essential characteristic of lymphangiogenesis [15], we therefore evaluated the effect of phomaketide A on LECs migration. We found that phomaketide A markedly reduced the numbers of LECs that migrated through the Transwell inserts (Figure 2B).

Moreover, there were no discernable increase on the levels of lactate dehydrogenase (LDH) with either dose of phomaketide A as compared with untreated human LECs (controls) (Figure 2D). Thus, phomaketide A appears to exert anti-lymphangiogenic effects without any evidence of cytotoxicity in human LECs.

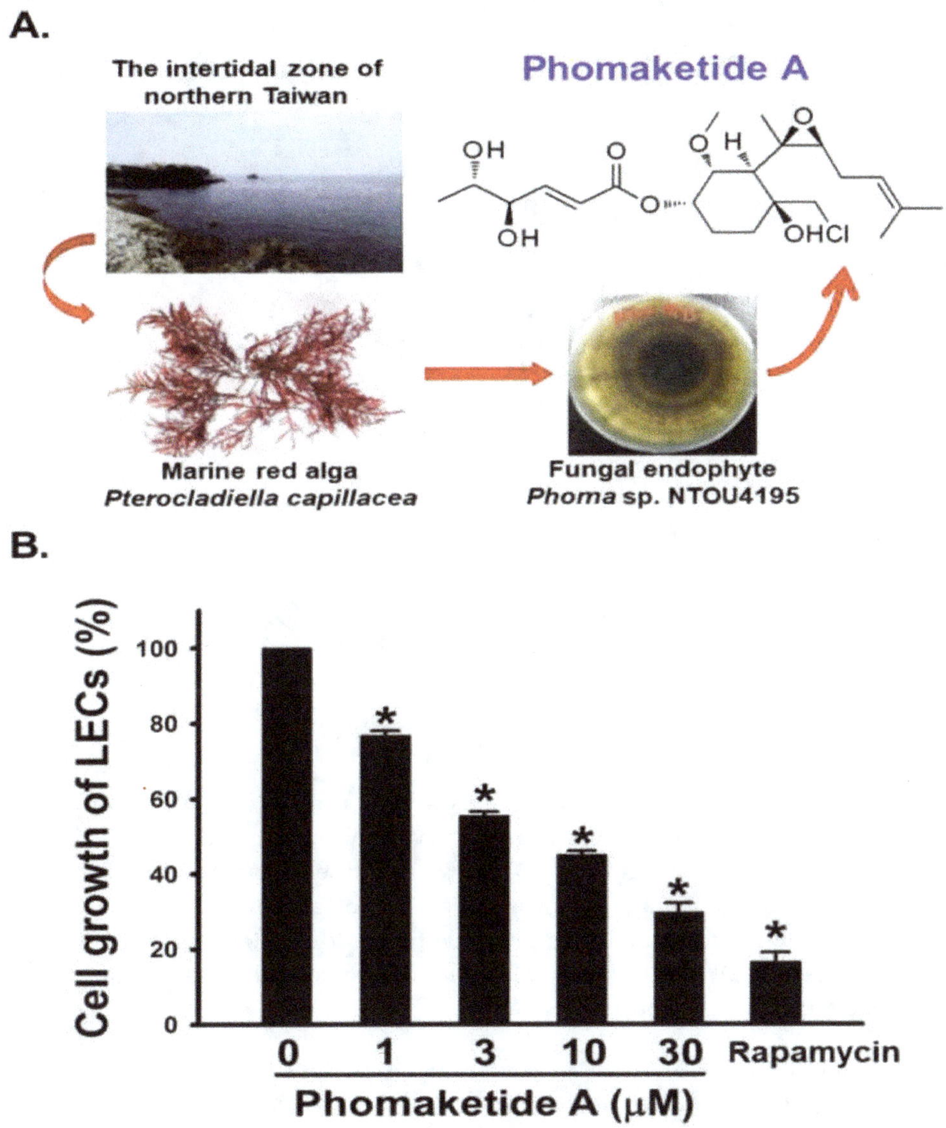

Figure 1. Effects of phomaketide A on cell growth of human lymphatic endothelial cells (LECs). (**A**) Phomaketide A was identified from the fermented broth and mycelium of *Phoma* sp. NTOU4195 isolated from the marine red alga *Pterocladiella capillacea* harvested along the north coast of Taiwan. (**B**) Cells were treated with various concentrations of phomaketide A and rapamycin (10 μM) for 48 h, and anti-lymphangiogenic activity was explored in a cell growth assay (N = 3). Data are expressed as the mean ± SEM. * $p < 0.05$ compared with the control group.

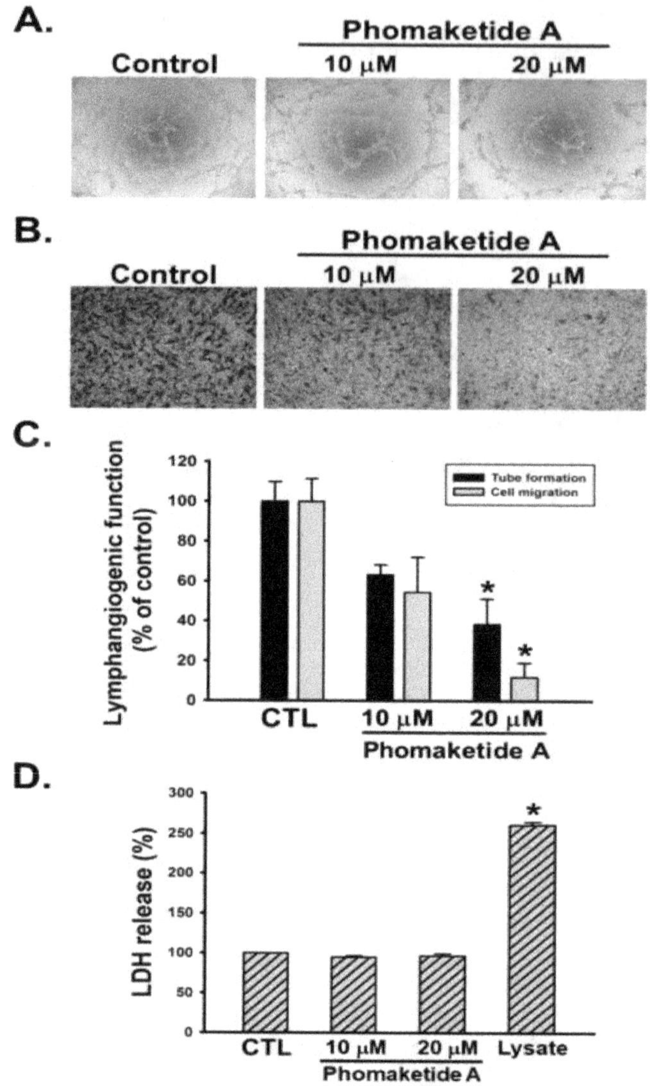

Figure 2. Effects of phomaketide A on human LECs tube formation, migration, and cytotoxicity. Cells were treated with the indicated concentrations of phomaketide A for 8 h. Capillary-like structure formation (**A**) and cell migration (**B**) were examined by tube formation and Transwell assays, respectively (N = 4–6). (**C**) ImageJ software was used to validate the lymphangiogenic functions of phomaketide A. (**D**) Cells were treated with phomaketide A for 24 h, then cytotoxicity was evaluated by lactate dehydrogenase (LDH) assay (N = 3). Data are expressed as the mean ± SEM. * $p < 0.05$ compared with the control (CTL) group.

2.2. Phomaketide A Inhibits the VEGFR-3 and PKCδ Signaling Pathway in Human LECs

To elucidate the mechanisms employed by phomaketide A to regulate lymphangiogenesis, we explored its effects upon VEGFR-3 in LECs. Figure 3A,B illustrate the significant suppression by phomaketide A upon the phosphorylation of VEGFR-3. We also investigated the effects of phomaketide A upon the signal transduction downstream of VEGFR-3. The results indicated that phomaketide A dramatically decreased the phosphorylation of PKCδ, but did not affect the phosphorylated levels of Akt, Erk, or FAK in the LECs (Figure 3C,D). Our results demonstrate that phomaketide A reduces lymphangiogenesis through VEGFR-3 and PKCδ-dependent pathways in human LECs.

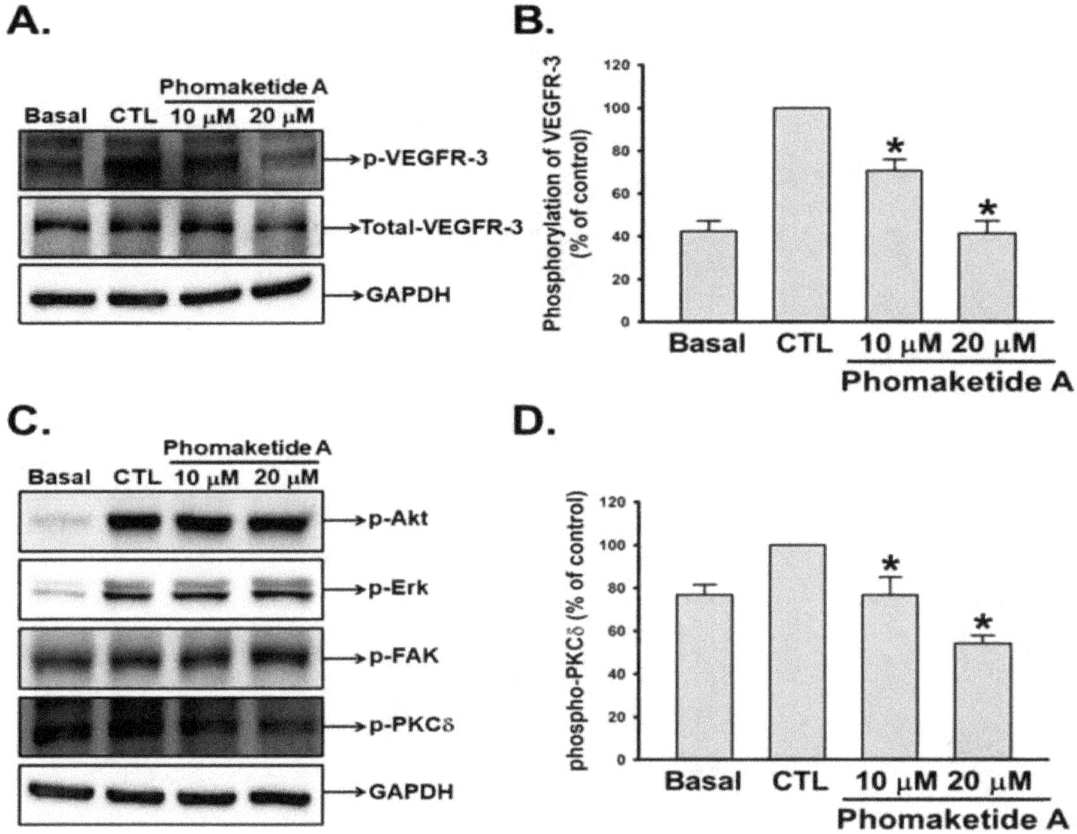

Figure 3. Modulation of phomaketide A on VEGFR-3 and downstream signaling pathways in human LECs. (**A** and **C**) Quiescent LECs were treated with or without EGM-2MV medium in the absence (CTL) or presence of phomaketide A for 5–10 min. The phosphorylation of VEGFR-3, Akt, Erk, FAK, and PKCδ were determined by Western blot analysis (N = 5–7). The quantitative densitometry of the relative levels of phosphorylated VEGFR-3 and PKCδ were measured by Image-Pro Plus processing software (**B** and **D**). Data are expressed as the mean ± SEM. * $p < 0.05$ compared with the control (CTL) group.

2.3. *Phomaketide A Impedes eNOS Activation in Human LECs*

Recent studies have documented that integrin α9, integrin β1, and endothelial nitric oxide synthase (eNOS) were associated with VEGFR-3-mediated lymphangiogenesis [8,16,17]. We therefore investigated whether phomaketide A inhibits LECs-induced lymphangiogenesis via these molecular signals. We found that phomaketide A significantly suppressed the phosphorylation and expression of eNOS but did not impair the protein levels of integrin α9 and β1 (Figure 4A,B). Activation of nuclear factor-κB (NF-κB) and overexpression of Id-1 (inhibitor of differentiation/DNA binding) are critical for multiple physiological and pathological processes, including lymphangiogenesis [17–19]. Here, we found that phomaketide A did not alter the phosphorylation of p65 or IκBα, nor the expression of Id-1 in LECs. We suggest that the eNOS signaling pathway is involved in phomaketide A-induced anti-lymphangiogenic effects in human LECs.

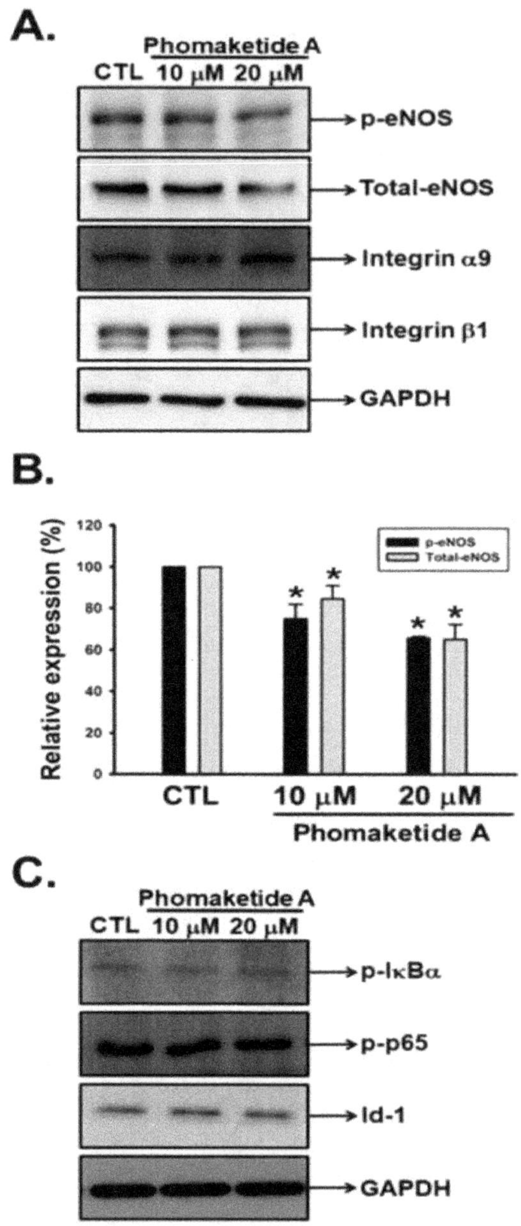

Figure 4. Effects of phomaketide A on pro-lymphangiogenic signals and transcription factors in human LECs. (**A** and **C**) Cells were treated with the indicated concentrations of phomaketide A for 8 h, and the indicated phosphorylated and total proteins were determined by Western blot analysis (N = 4–6). Image-Pro Plus processing software quantified the relative level of protein (**B**). Data are expressed as the mean ± SEM. * $p < 0.05$ compared with the control (CTL) group.

2.4. Phomaketide A Increases the Expression Profile of Protease Inhibitors in Human LECs

Proteolytic activities of cells are coordinately regulated by proteases and protease inhibitors in a coordinated fashion for the degradation of the extracellular matrix (ECM). Analysis of protease and/or protease inhibitor expression profiles is essential to determine how they affect normal cellular function and dysregulate LECs lymphangiogenesis [20]. Using human proteome arrays, we found that phomaketide A did not affect the relative expression of 35 human proteases (Supplementary Figure 1). However, phomaketide A substantially increased the levels of protein expression of several human protease inhibitors in LECs (Figure 5A); the four most significantly upregulated protease inhibitors were cystatin A, serpin B6, tissue factor pathway inhibitor (TFPI), and tissue inhibitor matrix metalloproteinase 1 (TIMP-1) (Figure 5B). These results indicate that phomaketide A may inhibit lymphangiogenesis via the upregulation of cystatin A, serpin B6, TFPI, and TIMP-1 in LECs.

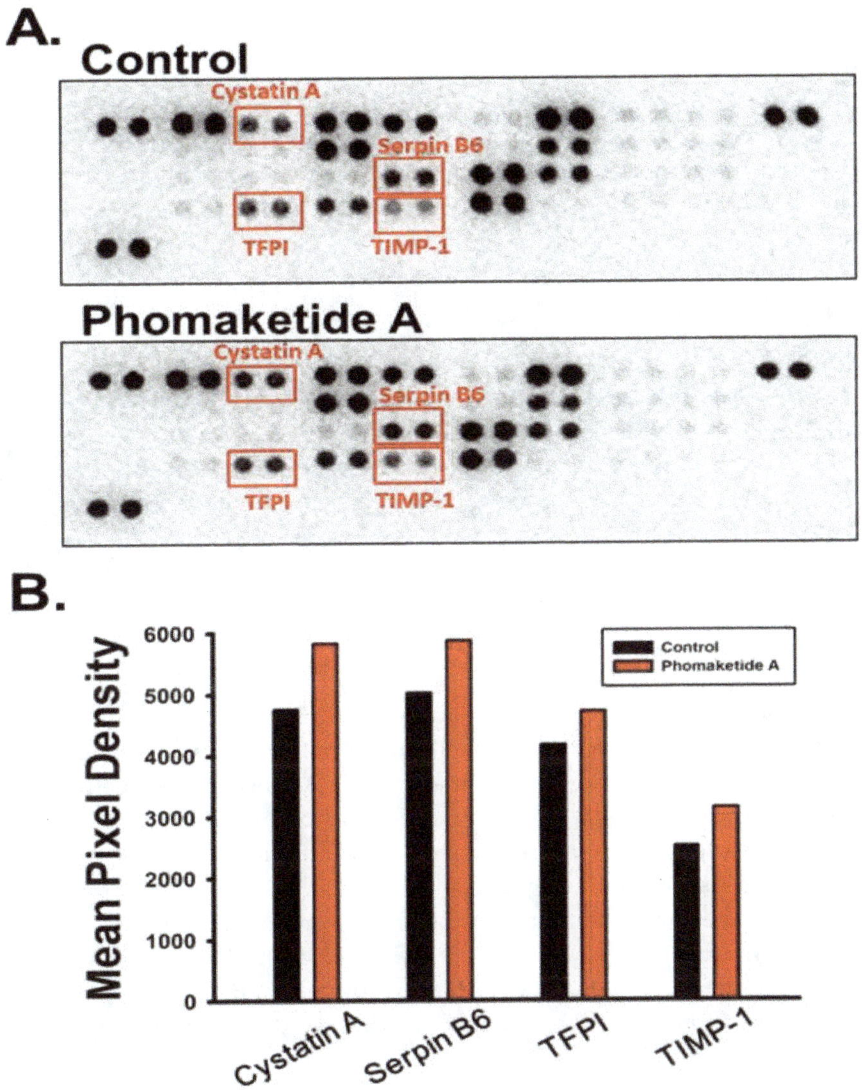

Figure 5. Effects of phomaketide A on protease inhibitor expression profiles in human LECs. (**A**) LECs were treated with phomaketide A (20 μM) for 8 h, then total cell lysates were collected. Significant changes in protein spots detected by human protease inhibitor array are indicated. (**B**) Profiles of mean spot pixel densities for upregulated protease inhibitors were analyzed using ImageJ software.

2.5. Phomaketide A Impairs Tumor Lymphangiogenesis in the A549 Xenograft Model

To validate *in vivo* significance of the cellular observations, we determined the effect of phomaketide A on tumor xenograft growth. As shown in Figure 6A, phomaketide A repressed A549 tumor growth via a remarkable reduction of bioluminescence activity. Furthermore, we found that phomaketide A dramatically decreased the tumor volume and weight of A549 xenografts (Figure 6B,C). Immunohistochemical analysis revealed that the expression of LYVE-1, the key specific marker for lymphatic vessels [21], was obviously decreased by phomaketide A (Figure 6D). Based on these findings, we propose that phomaketide A blocks *in vivo* tumor progression by suppressing lymphangiogenesis.

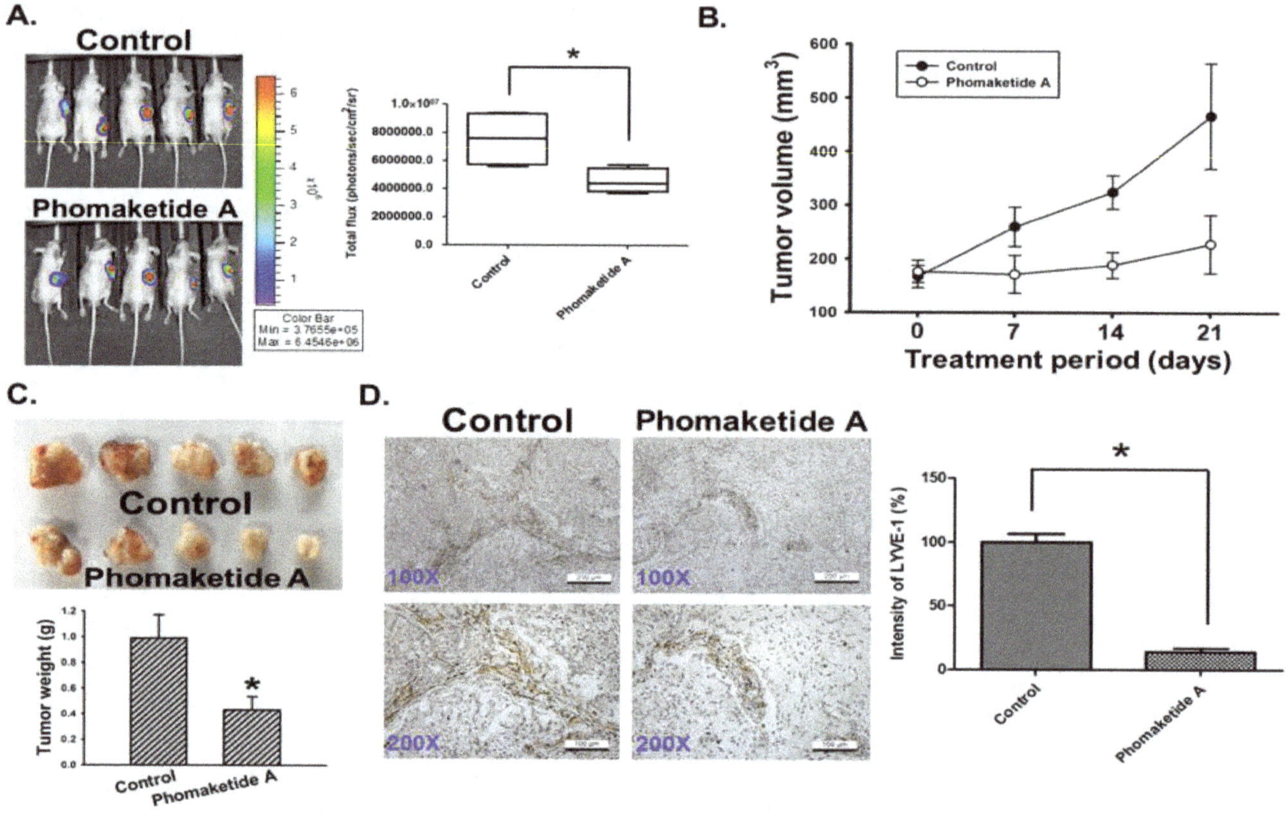

Figure 6. Effects of phomaketide A on tumor-associated lymphangiogenesis. (**A**) A549-Leu cells were injected into flank sites of nude mice for 4 weeks. Then, animals (five mice/group) were given vehicle (control) and phomaketide A (20 mg/kg) by i.p. injection for 3 consecutive weeks. The tumor size was monitored by bioluminescence imaging. Representative IVIS images of tumor growth and quantitative analysis of imaging signal intensity was seen on day 21. (**B**) Treatment period was indicated (days 0–21), and tumor volume was measured manually every week. (**C**) A549 tumor samples from animals were obtained and weighted at the end of the treatment. (**D**) The xenograft tumors were excised and stained with lymphatic vessel marker LYVE-1 by IHC analysis (N = 4). Representative images of LYVE-1 expression in tumor specimens are seen. The quantification of LYVE-1 expression was analyzed using ImageJ software. Data are expressed as the mean ± SEM. *, $p < 0.05$ compared with the control group.

3. Discussion

Several studies have shown that marine-derived compounds possess biological activity and pharmacological effect in cancer models with little or no side effects [22–24]. To our knowledge, this is the first study illustrating the anti-lymphangiogenesis property of phomaketide A. Marine organisms are the cradle for many excellent pharmaceutical products, particularly in anti-lymphangiogenesis. For example, fucoidan from *Undaria pinnatifida* sporophylls exerts anti-metastasis and anti-lymphangiogenesis activities by reducing HIF-1α/VEGF-C resulting in attenuation of the PI3K/Akt/mTOR signaling pathways [25]. In addition, toluquinol, isolated from the culture broth of the marine fungus *Penicillium* sp. HL-85-ALS5-R004, has been reported to suppress lymphangiogenesis by down-regulating the VEGF-C/VEGFR-3 cascade [26]. A recent study has shown that tuberazines C obtained from Taiwanese zoanthid *Palythoa tuberculosa* displayed the anti-lymphangiogenesis effect through the suppression of cell growth and tube formation in human LECs [14]. Here, we discover that phomaketide A, isolated from the marine endophytic fungal strain *Phoma* sp. NTOU4195 [13], possesses the anti-lymphangiogenic function against human LECs. Marine-derived natural product phomaketide A has the potential to impede tumor-associated lymphangiogenesis and metastasis.

VEGFR-3 has been reported to play an important role in lymphangiogenesis and tumor invasion through the lymphatics [27]. On stimulation by its ligand VEGF-C, VEGFR-3 was phosphorylated which promotes the proliferation and migration of LECs resulting in lymphangiogenesis [9]. Previous studies showed that Ki23057 inhibits phosphorylation of VEGFR-3 against the lymphangiogenesis of gastric cancer [27]. In the current study, we demonstrated that phomaketide A significantly inhibited the phosphorylation of VEGFR-3 in human LECs. Moreover, PKC δ is associated with the phosphorylation of VEGFR-3 in endothelial cells [28]. Our results found that phomaketide A also induced the reduction of PKCδ phosphorylation. PKCδ mediated by VEGFR-3 phosphorylation underlying phomaketide A treatment deserves further investigation. In addition, eNOS is involved in VEGF-C-induced lymphangiogenesis and plays a vital role in lymphatic metastasis [8]. Doxycycline can decrease eNOS phosphorylation to inhibit LECs proliferation [29]. Pro-inflammatory cytokines, IL-20 and IL-33, also activate the phosphorylation of eNOS to promote the proliferation, migration and tube formation of LECs [30,31]. In the current study, phomaketide A suppressed the phosphorylation and expression of eNOS in LECs, confirming the importance of eNOS in LECs-regulated lymphangiogenic processes.

Proteolytic processing of VEGF-C regulates lymphatic vessel growth for activating LECs lymphangiogenesis [32,33], whereas lymphatic vessel outgrowth is reduced by protease inhibitor [34]. Several studies demonstrate that serine proteinase inhibitor (serpin) functioned as a lymphangiogenesis inhibitor to suppress the lymphatic metastasis of cancer and the LECs proliferation and migration [35–37]. The expression of tissue inhibitor of metalloproteinase-2 (TIMP-2) is lower or negative in patients with lymph node metastasis [38]. Furthermore, matrix metalloproteinases inhibitors are well recognized to impair lymphangiogenesis [39]. Our results showed that anti-lymphangiogenic effects of phomaketide A were associated with the induction of protease inhibitors such as cystatin A, serpin B6, TFPI and TIMP-1. Meanwhile, several studies have demonstrated that promotion of these protease inhibitors can induce anti-angiogenic effects [40–43]. Our previous report reveals that phomaketide A is a novel angiogenesis inhibitor [13]. Phomaketide A is a potential dual-effect agent that could be used for cancer treatment through the inhibition of angiogenesis and lymphangiogenesis.

In conclusion, this report discloses a novel mechanism by which phomaketide A reduces LECs lymphangiogenesis *in vitro* and *in vivo*. We demonstrate that phomaketide A antagonizes lymphangiogenesis by decreasing VEGFR-3 and its downstream PKCδ and eNOS signaling pathways, as well as increasing protease inhibitors in human LECs (Figure 7). Our previous study demonstrates promising *in vitro* effects with phomaketide A in human EPCs. In this study, we show that phomaketide A also exerts anti-lymphangiogenic effect in LECs (IC_{50}, 3.7 $\pm$ 0.6 μM), and profoundly inhibit the proliferation of A549 lung cancer cells, with an IC_{50} value of 3.0 $\pm$ 0.3 μM (Supplementary Figure S2). We therefore suggest that phomaketide A acts selective and potent inhibitory effects upon endothelial cells and A549 cancer cells. Phomaketide A can coordinately induce anti-angiogenic, anti-lymphangiogenic, and anti-cancer effects in A549 tumor microenvironment, resulting in the inhibition of *in vivo* tumor progression. The detailed anti-cancer effects and mechanisms of phomaketide A in A549 cancer cells should be further investigated. LECs have been proposed to dictate tumor lymphangiogenesis and metastasis in microenvironment. Our findings suggest that phomaketide A may serve as a lead candidate for further development for novel lymphangiogenesis inhibitors to block cancer progression and metastasis.

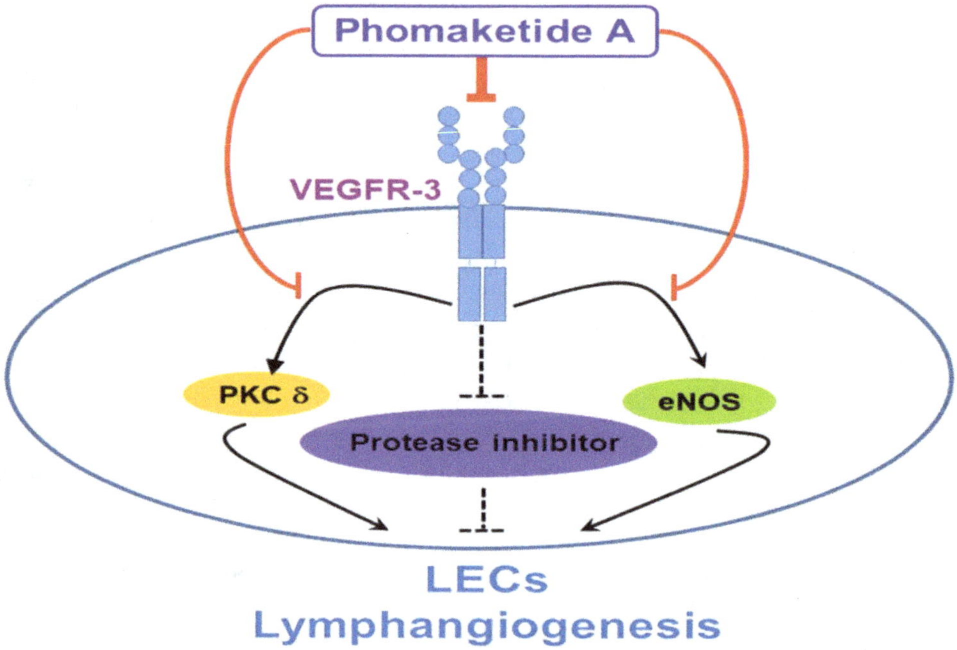

Figure 7. Schema of phomaketide A-induced anti-lymphangiogenic mechanism in human LECs. This study reveals phomaketide A as a promising anti-lymphangiogenic agent. Phomaketide A may inhibit lymphangiogenesis by decreasing VEGFR-3 and its downstream PKCδ and eNOS signaling pathways, as well as increasing protease inhibitors in human LECs.

4. Materials and Methods

4.1. Materials

Phomaketide A was isolated from the fermentation broth and mycelium of the endophytic fungal strain *Phoma* sp. NTOU4195 as previously described [13]. Rapamycin was purchased from Cayman Chemical (Ann Arbor, MI, USA). The compounds were dissolved in dimethyl sulfoxide (DMSO) at 20 mM as a stock solution for all assays. DMSO was used as the vehicle control in the experiments. DMSO and other chemical agents were obtained from Sigma-Aldrich (St. Louis, MO, USA). Rabbit polyclonal antibody specific for phospho-VEGFR-3 (Tyr1230/1231) was purchased from Cell Application (San Diego, CA, USA). Rabbit monoclonal antibodies specific for phospho-Akt (Ser473), phospho-ERK (Thr202/Tyr204), phospho-FAK (Tyr397), phospho-PKCδ (Thr505), phospho-eNOS (Ser1177), eNOS, Integrin β1, VEGFR-3, and GAPDH were purchased from Cell Signaling Technologies (Boston, MA, USA). Rabbit monoclonal antibodies specific for Integrin α9, phospho-p65 (Ser536) and phospho-IκBα (Ser32) were purchased from Abcam (Cambridge, MA, USA). Rabbit polyclonal antibody specific for Id-1 was purchased from Santa Cruz Biotechnology (Santa Cruz, CA, USA). Gibco-BRL life technologies (Grand Island, NY, USA) supplied Dulbecco's modified Eagle's medium (DMEM), fetal bovine serum (FBS), and all other cell culture reagents. Matrigel was obtained from BD Biosciences (Bedford, MA, USA).

4.2. Cell Culture

The human lymphatic endothelial cells (LECs) were purchased from Lonza (Walkersville, MD, USA). LECs were cultured in EGM-2MV medium consisting of EBM-2 basal medium and SingleQuots kit (Lonza). A549 cell line was purchased from American Type Culture Collection (Manassas, Virginia, USA). To establish the luciferase-tagged A549 cells (A549-Leu cells), pLenti PGK Blast V5-LUC (w528-1) for expression of the firefly luciferase was purchased from the Addgene (Plasmid #19166; Watertown, MA, USA). Lentiviruses were prepared according to standard protocols. For transduction, 3×10^5 A549 cells were seeded in a 6-well plate and the lentivirus was added (multiplicity of infection =

10) in medium containing polybrene (8 μg/mL). The culture medium was changed after 24 h. The cells were incubated with 5 μg/mL blasticidin for 48 h for stable clone selection. The surviving cells were selected, and clonal cell populations were expanded as A549-Luc cell line. A549-Leu cells were maintained in DMEM, supplemented with 10% fetal bovine serum (FBS). The cells culture conditions are recorded in our previous paper [14].

4.3. Cell Growth Assay

LECs were cultured in 96-well plates at a density of 5×10^3 cells in each well. Overnight, the culture medium was replaced with fresh EGM-2MV medium in the presence of either vehicle (DMSO) or phomaketide A for 48 h treatment. The assay on cell growth of LECs was determined by the method based on our previous study [14].

4.4. Capillary Tube Formation Assay

The capillary tube formation assay was performed on Matrigel-coated 96-well plates. LECs were seeded at a density of 2×10^4 cells per well and incubated in EGM-2MV medium and the indicated concentration of tested compounds, for 8 h at 37 °C. The detection and quantification of LECs tube formation were examined according to previously described procedures [14].

4.5. Cell Migration Assay

The cell migration assay was conducted in Transwell inserts (Corning, NY, USA) with 2.5×10^4 of LECs per well seeded onto the upper chamber with EBM-2 basal medium. The upper chamber was transferred and incubated in the bottom chamber with EGM-2MV medium and the indicated concentration of tested compounds was for 8 h. Cell migration was determined according to our previous protocol [44].

4.6. Cytotoxicity Assay

LECs (5×10^3 cells/well) were seeded onto 96-well plates and incubated with EGM-2MV medium in the presence of a vehicle (DMSO) or phomaketide A for 8 h of treatment. Release of lactate dehydrogenase (LDH) into the medium was measured using a cytotoxicity assay kit (Promega, Madison, WI, USA) according to an established protocol [14].

4.7. Western Blot Analysis

After the treatment of LECs, the reaction was terminated by the addition of lysis buffer containing a protease inhibitor cocktail (Roche, Mannheim, Germany). Total cell lysates were electrophoresed using SDS-PAGE and subsequently transferred to polyvinylidene difluoride membranes. After blocking the blots with 4% bovine serum albumin, they were treated with primary antibody and then peroxidase-conjugated secondary antibody. The blots were visualized using enhanced chemiluminescence and monitored using the UVP Biospectrum system (UVP, Upland, CA, USA).

4.8. Proteome Profile Arrays

Human protease and protease inhibitor antibody arrays (R&D Systems, Minneapolis, MN, USA) were used to analyze the expression profiles of protease and protease inhibitor according to the manufacturer's instructions. UVP Biospectrum system was used to detect chemiluminescent signals, which were further analyzed using ImageJ software.

4.9. In Vivo Tumor Xenograft Model

All animal procedures were performed according to approved protocols issued by the China Medical University (Taichung, Taiwan) Institutional Animal Care and Use Committees. Male nude mice (4-week of age) were used in the subcutaneous xenograft model. A549-Leu cells (2×10^6 cells) were resuspended in 0.1 mL of 50% serum-free medium and 50% Matrigel, and injected into the right flank of each animal. Four weeks after A549-Leu cells injection, the mice were randomized into experimental and control groups according to bioluminescence imaging from the Xenogen IVIS imaging system 200 (PerkinElmer, MA, USA). Then, the mice were treated with phomaketide A (20 mg/kg) or the vehicle control every other day by intraperitoneal (i.p.) administration (five mice per group). After the treatment, the animals were sacrificed, and the tumor specimens were resected for immunohistochemical (IHC) analysis.

4.10. IHC Analysis

The tumor tissues were placed on glass slides, rehydrated and incubated in 3% hydrogen peroxide to block the endogenous peroxidase activity. After trypsinization, nonspecific antibody-binding sites were blocked using 3% bovine serum albumin in PBS. IHC analysis was carried out to determine the expression of lymphangiogenic marker according to the standard protocol [45].

4.11. Statistical Analysis

Data points represent the mean $\pm$ standard error of mean (SEM). Statistical analyses of data were done with one-way ANOVA followed by Student's t-test. The difference is significant if the p value is < 0.05.

Author Contributions: S.-W.W., C.-H.T., and Y.-J.C. designed and conceived the study. T.-H.L. and M.-S.L. isolated and purified the phomaketide A. H.-C.T., L.-P.C., P.-C.C. and C.-Y.L. performed the experimental work and drew the diagrams. C.-W.C., C.-T.L., and S.-S.C. analyzed and interpreted the data. H.-C.T., K.-W.L., C.-H.L. and S.-W.W. wrote and revised the manuscript, W.-C.C. validated the manuscript. All authors read and approved the final manuscript.

Acknowledgments: We thank Iona J. MacDonald for her English language editing of this manuscript.

References

1. Paduch, R. The role of lymphangiogenesis and angiogenesis in tumor metastasis. *Cell. Oncol. (Dordr.)* **2016**, *39*, 397–410. [CrossRef] [PubMed]
2. Tammela, T.; Alitalo, K. Lymphangiogenesis: Molecular mechanisms and future promise. *Cell* **2010**, *140*, 460–476. [CrossRef] [PubMed]
3. Alderfer, L.; Wei, A.; Hanjaya-Putra, D. Lymphatic Tissue Engineering and Regeneration. *J. Biol. Eng.* **2018**, *12*, 32. [CrossRef] [PubMed]
4. Kataru, R.P.; Kim, H.; Jang, C.; Choi, D.K.; Koh, B.I.; Kim, M.; Gollamudi, S.; Kim, Y.K.; Lee, S.H.; Koh, G.Y. T lymphocytes negatively regulate lymph node lymphatic vessel formation. *Immunity* **2011**, *34*, 96–107. [CrossRef]
5. Yeo, K.P.; Angeli, V. Bidirectional Crosstalk between Lymphatic Endothelial Cell and T Cell and Its Implications in Tumor Immunity. *Front. Immunol.* **2017**, *8*, 83. [CrossRef]
6. Stacker, S.A.; Williams, S.P.; Karnezis, T.; Shayan, R.; Fox, S.B.; Achen, M.G. Lymphangiogenesis and lymphatic vessel remodelling in cancer. *Nat. Rev. Cancer* **2014**, *14*, 159–172. [CrossRef] [PubMed]
7. Vaahtomeri, K.; Karaman, S.; Makinen, T.; Alitalo, K. Lymphangiogenesis guidance by paracrine and pericellular factors. *Genes Dev.* **2017**, *31*, 1615–1634. [CrossRef]
8. Lahdenranta, J.; Hagendoorn, J.; Padera, T.P.; Hoshida, T.; Nelson, G.; Kashiwagi, S.; Jain, R.K.; Fukumura, D. Endothelial nitric oxide synthase mediates lymphangiogenesis and lymphatic metastasis. *Cancer Res.* **2009**, *69*, 2801–2808. [CrossRef] [PubMed]
9. Makinen, T.; Veikkola, T.; Mustjoki, S.; Karpanen, T.; Catimel, B.; Nice, E.C.; Wise, L.; Mercer, A.; Kowalski, H.; Kerjaschki, D.; et al. Isolated lymphatic endothelial cells transduce growth, survival and migratory signals via the VEGF-C/D receptor VEGFR-3. *EMBO J.* **2001**, *20*, 4762–4773. [CrossRef] [PubMed]

10. Alam, A.; Blanc, I.; Gueguen-Dorbes, G.; Duclos, O.; Bonnin, J.; Barron, P.; Laplace, M.C.; Morin, G.; Gaujarengues, F.; Dol, F.; et al. SAR131675, a potent and selective VEGFR-3-TK inhibitor with antilymphangiogenic, antitumoral, and antimetastatic activities. *Mol. Cancer Ther.* **2012**, *11*, 1637–1649. [CrossRef] [PubMed]
11. Norrmen, C.; Tammela, T.; Petrova, T.V.; Alitalo, K. Biological basis of therapeutic lymphangiogenesis. *Circulation* **2011**, *123*, 1335–1351. [CrossRef]
12. Rateb, M.E.; Ebel, R. Secondary metabolites of fungi from marine habitats. *Nat. Prod. Rep.* **2011**, *28*, 290–344. [CrossRef] [PubMed]
13. Lee, M.S.; Wang, S.W.; Wang, G.J.; Pang, K.L.; Lee, C.K.; Kuo, Y.H.; Cha, H.J.; Lin, R.K.; Lee, T.H. Angiogenesis Inhibitors and Anti-Inflammatory Agents from Phoma sp. NTOU4195. *J. Nat. Prod.* **2016**, *79*, 2983–2990. [CrossRef] [PubMed]
14. Chen, S.R.; Wang, S.W.; Su, C.J.; Hu, H.C.; Yang, Y.L.; Hsieh, C.T.; Peng, C.C.; Chang, F.R.; Cheng, Y.B. Anti-Lymphangiogenesis Components from Zoanthid Palythoa tuberculosa. *Mar. Drugs* **2018**, *16*, 47. [CrossRef] [PubMed]
15. Prangsaengtong, O.; Athikomkulchai, S.; Xu, J.; Koizumi, K.; Inujima, A.; Shibahara, N.; Shimada, Y.; Tadtong, S.; Awale, S. Chrysin Inhibits Lymphangiogenesis in Vitro. *Biol. Pharm. Bull.* **2016**, *39*, 466–472. [CrossRef]
16. Urner, S.; Planas-Paz, L.; Hilger, L.S.; Henning, C.; Branopolski, A.; Kelly-Goss, M.; Stanczuk, L.; Pitter, B.; Montanez, E.; Peirce, S.M.; et al. Identification of ILK as a critical regulator of VEGFR3 signalling and lymphatic vascular growth. *EMBO J.* **2019**, *38*, e99322. [CrossRef]
17. Flister, M.J.; Wilber, A.; Hall, K.L.; Iwata, C.; Miyazono, K.; Nisato, R.E.; Pepper, M.S.; Zawieja, D.C.; Ran, S. Inflammation induces lymphangiogenesis through up-regulation of VEGFR-3 mediated by NF-kappaB and Prox1. *Blood* **2010**, *115*, 418–429. [CrossRef]
18. Dong, Z.; Wei, F.; Zhou, C.; Sumida, T.; Hamakawa, H.; Hu, Y.; Liu, S. Silencing Id-1 inhibits lymphangiogenesis through down-regulation of VEGF-C in oral squamous cell carcinoma. *Oral Oncol.* **2011**, *47*, 27–32. [CrossRef]
19. Si, C.F.; Guo, J.Q.; Yang, Y.M.; Zhang, N.; Pan, C.R.; Zhang, Q.H.; Zhang, T.G.; Zhou, C.J. Nuclear and cytoplasmic Id-1 expression patterns play different roles in angiogenesis and lymphangiogenesis in gastric carcinoma. *Ann. Diagn. Pathol.* **2011**, *15*, 46–51. [CrossRef]
20. Leppanen, V.M.; Tvorogov, D.; Kisko, K.; Prota, A.E.; Jeltsch, M.; Anisimov, A.; Markovic-Mueller, S.; Stuttfeld, E.; Goldie, K.N.; Ballmer-Hofer, K.; et al. Structural and mechanistic insights into VEGF receptor 3 ligand binding and activation. *Proc. Natl. Acad. Sci. USA* **2013**, *110*, 12960–12965. [CrossRef] [PubMed]
21. Banerji, S.; Ni, J.; Wang, S.X.; Clasper, S.; Su, J.; Tammi, R.; Jones, M.; Jackson, D.G. LYVE-1, a new homologue of the CD44 glycoprotein, is a lymph-specific receptor for hyaluronan. *J. Cell Biol.* **1999**, *144*, 789–801. [CrossRef] [PubMed]
22. Castro-Carvalho, B.; Ramos, A.A.; Prata-Sena, M.; Malhao, F.; Moreira, M.; Gargiulo, D.; Dethoup, T.; Buttachon, S.; Kijjoa, A.; Rocha, E. Marine-derived Fungi Extracts Enhance the Cytotoxic Activity of Doxorubicin in Nonsmall Cell Lung Cancer Cells A459. *Pharmacogn. Res.* **2017**, *9* (Suppl. S1), S92–S98.
23. Aspeslagh, S.; Stein, M.; Bahleda, R.; Hollebecque, A.; Salles, G.; Gyan, E.; Fudio, S.; Extremera, S.; Alfaro, V.; Soto-Matos, A.; et al. Phase I dose-escalation study of plitidepsin in combination with sorafenib or gemcitabine in patients with refractory solid tumors or lymphomas. *Anticancer Drugs* **2017**, *28*, 341–349. [CrossRef] [PubMed]
24. Yu, C.I.; Chen, C.Y.; Liu, W.; Chang, P.C.; Huang, C.W.; Han, K.F.; Lin, I.P.; Lin, M.Y.; Lee, C.H. Sandensolide Induces Oxidative Stress-Mediated Apoptosis in Oral Cancer Cells and in Zebrafish Xenograft Model. *Mar. Drugs* **2018**, *16*, 387. [CrossRef] [PubMed]
25. Teng, H.; Yang, Y.; Wei, H.; Liu, Z.; Liu, Z.; Ma, Y.; Gao, Z.; Hou, L.; Zou, X. Fucoidan Suppresses Hypoxia-Induced Lymphangiogenesis and Lymphatic Metastasis in Mouse Hepatocarcinoma. *Mar. Drugs* **2015**, *13*, 3514–3530. [CrossRef]
26. Garcia-Caballero, M.; Blacher, S.; Paupert, J.; Quesada, A.R.; Medina, M.A.; Noel, A. Novel application assigned to toluquinol: Inhibition of lymphangiogenesis by interfering with VEGF-C/VEGFR-3 signalling pathway. *Br. J. Pharmacol.* **2016**, *173*, 1966–1987. [CrossRef]

27. Yashiro, M.; Shinto, O.; Nakamura, K.; Tendo, M.; Matsuoka, T.; Matsuzaki, T.; Kaizaki, R.; Ohira, M.; Miwa, A.; Hirakawa, K. Effects of VEGFR-3 phosphorylation inhibitor on lymph node metastasis in an orthotopic diffuse-type gastric carcinoma model. *Br. J. Cancer* **2009**, *101*, 1100–1106. [CrossRef]
28. Wang, J.F.; Zhang, X.; Groopman, J.E. Activation of vascular endothelial growth factor receptor-3 and its downstream signaling promote cell survival under oxidative stress. *J. Biol. Chem.* **2004**, *279*, 27088–27097. [CrossRef]
29. Han, L.; Su, W.; Huang, J.; Zhou, J.; Qiu, S.; Liang, D. Doxycycline inhibits inflammation-induced lymphangiogenesis in mouse cornea by multiple mechanisms. *PLoS ONE* **2014**, *9*, e108931. [CrossRef]
30. Han, L.; Zhang, M.; Liang, X.; Jia, X.; Jia, J.; Zhao, M.; Fan, Y. Interleukin-33 promotes inflammation-induced lymphangiogenesis via ST2/TRAF6-mediated Akt/eNOS/NO signalling pathway. *Sci. Rep.* **2017**, *7*, 10602. [CrossRef]
31. Hammer, T.; Tritsaris, K.; Hubschmann, M.V.; Gibson, J.; Nisato, R.E.; Pepper, M.S.; Dissing, S. IL-20 activates human lymphatic endothelial cells causing cell signalling and tube formation. *Microvasc. Res.* **2009**, *78*, 25–32. [CrossRef]
32. Jeltsch, M.; Jha, S.K.; Tvorogov, D.; Anisimov, A.; Leppanen, V.M.; Holopainen, T.; Kivela, R.; Ortega, S.; Karpanen, T.; Alitalo, K. CCBE1 enhances lymphangiogenesis via A disintegrin and metalloprotease with thrombospondin motifs-3-mediated vascular endothelial growth factor-C activation. *Circulation* **2014**, *129*, 1962–1971. [CrossRef]
33. Bui, H.M.; Enis, D.; Robciuc, M.R.; Nurmi, H.J.; Cohen, J.; Chen, M.; Yang, Y.; Dhillon, V.; Johnson, K.; Zhang, H.; et al. Proteolytic activation defines distinct lymphangiogenic mechanisms for VEGFC and VEGFD. *J. Clin. Investig.* **2016**, *126*, 2167–2180. [CrossRef]
34. Detry, B.; Bruyere, F.; Erpicum, C.; Paupert, J.; Lamaye, F.; Maillard, C.; Lenoir, B.; Foidart, J.M.; Thiry, M.; Noel, A. Digging deeper into lymphatic vessel formation in vitro and in vivo. *BMC Cell Biol.* **2011**, *12*, 29. [CrossRef]
35. Ma, C.; Luo, C.; Yin, H.; Zhang, Y.; Xiong, W.; Zhang, T.; Gao, T.; Wang, X.; Che, D.; Fang, Z.; et al. Kallistatin inhibits lymphangiogenesis and lymphatic metastasis of gastric cancer by downregulating VEGF-C expression and secretion. *Gastric Cancer* **2018**, *21*, 617–631. [CrossRef] [PubMed]
36. Ma, C.; Yin, H.; Zhong, J.; Zhang, Y.; Luo, C.; Che, D.; Fang, Z.; Li, L.; Qin, S.; Liang, J.; et al. Kallistatin exerts anti-lymphangiogenic effects by inhibiting lymphatic endothelial cell proliferation, migration and tube formation. *Int. J. Oncol.* **2017**, *50*, 2000–2010. [CrossRef] [PubMed]
37. Liu, Z.; Shi, Y.; Meng, W.; Liu, Y.; Yang, K.; Wu, S.; Peng, Z. Expression and localization of maspin in cervical cancer and its role in tumor progression and lymphangiogenesis. *Arch. Gynecol. Obstet.* **2014**, *289*, 373–382. [CrossRef]
38. Yang, X.; Zhai, N.; Sun, M.; Zhao, Z.; Yang, J.; Chen, K.; Zhang, H. Influence of lymphatic endothelial cells on proliferation and invasiveness of esophageal carcinoma cells in vitro and lymphangiogenesis in vivo. *Med. Oncol.* **2015**, *32*, 222. [CrossRef]
39. Bruyere, F.; Melen-Lamalle, L.; Blacher, S.; Roland, G.; Thiry, M.; Moons, L.; Frankenne, F.; Carmeliet, P.; Alitalo, K.; Libert, C.; et al. Modeling lymphangiogenesis in a three-dimensional culture system. *Nat. Methods* **2008**, *5*, 431–437. [CrossRef]
40. Li, W.; Ding, F.; Zhang, L.; Liu, Z.; Wu, Y.; Luo, A.; Wu, M.; Wang, M.; Zhan, Q.; Liu, Z. Overexpression of stefin A in human esophageal squamous cell carcinoma cells inhibits tumor cell growth, angiogenesis, invasion, and metastasis. *Clin. Cancer Res.* **2005**, *11*, 8753–8762. [CrossRef]
41. Benarafa, C.; Remold-O'Donnell, E. The ovalbumin serpins revisited: Perspective from the chicken genome of clade B serpin evolution in vertebrates. *Proc. Natl. Acad. Sci. USA* **2005**, *102*, 11367–11372. [CrossRef]
42. Zhai, L.L.; Wu, Y.; Huang, D.W.; Tang, Z.G. Increased matrix metalloproteinase-2 expression and reduced tissue factor pathway inhibitor-2 expression correlate with angiogenesis and early postoperative recurrence of pancreatic carcinoma. *Am. J. Transl. Res.* **2015**, *7*, 2412–2422.
43. Abraham, V.; Cao, G.; Parambath, A.; Lawal, F.; Handumrongkul, C.; Debs, R.; DeLisser, H.M. Involvement of TIMP-1 in PECAM-1-mediated tumor dissemination. *Int. J. Oncol.* **2018**, *53*, 488–502. [CrossRef]
44. Chen, W.C.; Chung, C.H.; Lu, Y.C.; Wu, M.H.; Chou, P.H.; Yen, J.Y.; Lai, Y.W.; Wang, G.S.; Liu, S.C.; Cheng, J.K.;

et al. BMP-2 induces angiogenesis by provoking integrin alpha6 expression in human endothelial progenitor cells. *Biochem. Pharmacol.* **2018**, *150*, 256–266. [CrossRef]

45. Su, C.M.; Tang, C.H.; Chi, M.J.; Lin, C.Y.; Fong, Y.C.; Liu, Y.C.; Chen, W.C.; Wang, S.W. Resistin facilitates VEGF-C-associated lymphangiogenesis by inhibiting miR-186 in human chondrosarcoma cells. *Biochem. Pharmacol.* **2018**, *154*, 234–242. [CrossRef]

2

Effects of Aqueous Extract of Three Cultivars of Banana *(Musa acuminata)* Fruit Peel on Kidney and Liver Function Indices in Wistar Rats

Chidi Edenta [1], Stanley I. R. Okoduwa [2,3,*] and Oche Okpe [4]

1 Department of Biochemistry, Renaissance University, Ugbawka, Enugu State 402212, Nigeria; chidiedenta@gmail.com

2 Directorate of Research and Development, Nigerian Institute of Leather and Science Technology, Zaria, Kaduna State 810221, Nigeria

3 Infohealth Awareness Unit, SIRONigeria Global Limited, Abuja, Federal Capital Territory 900288, Nigeria

4 Department of Biochemistry, Federal University of Agriculture, Makurdi, Benue State 970101, Nigeria; ocheking10@gmail.com

* Correspondence: siroplc@yahoo.com or stanley@sironigeria.com

Academic Editor: James D. Adams

Abstract: Background: *Musa acuminata* fruit peels are used in the northern part of Nigeria for the treatment of hypertension and other cardiovascular related diseases. The effects of aqueous extracts of ripped fruit peel of three cultivars of *Musa acuminata* (*Saro, Ominni* and *Oranta*) on the hepatic and renal parameters of normal rats were examined. **Methods:** Fruit peel aqueous extracts (FPAE) of the 3 cultivars of Bananas (100 mg/kg b.w.) were administered by oral intubation (that is through esophageal cannula) to normal rats (140–180 g) for a period of 28 days. Blood samples were collected for determination of plasma aspartate amino transferase (AST), alanine amino transferase (ALT), alkaline phosphatase ALK-P), total protein, albumin, creatinine as well as urea. **Results:** From the results obtained, there were no significant ($p < 0.05$) changes in the ALK-P, AST, ALT, total protein and albumin among the experimental rats administered FPAE of the 3 cultivars of *Musa acuminata* when compared with the normal control group. There was a significant ($p < 0.05$) increase in the level of serum creatinine (in mg/dL) (1.53 $\pm$ 0.23) when compared to the normal control (0.72 $\pm$ 0.15), *Ominni* (0.92 $\pm$ 0.39) and *Oranta* (0.74 $\pm$ 0.22). Similarly, there was a significant ($p < 0.05$) increase in the level of serum urea (in mg/dL) of *Saro* (41.56 $\pm$ 4.68) when compared to the normal control (26.05 $\pm$ 0.73), *Ommini* (28.44 $\pm$ 2.43) and *Oranta* (26.10 $\pm$ 2.94). **Conclusion:** The findings reveal the *Saro* cultivar of *Musa acuminata* to be nephrotoxic and not a good potential drug candidate among the cultivars studied hence should be discouraged in the treatment of hypertension and other cardiovascular related diseases.

Keywords: banana; *Musa sapientum*; hepatotoxicity; nephrotoxicity; wistar rat; rats

1. Introduction

The liver plays a central role in the metabolism of drug, xenobiotics, protein synthesis and in maintaining biological equilibrium in organisms [1]. Although the liver is the target for most xenobiotics, the kidney usually shares in the burden of xenobiotic exposure, and the two organs carry out most of the biotransformation of xenobiotics [2]. Herbal drugs play a role in the management of various liver disorders, most of which speed up the natural healing processes of the liver [3]. Since ancient times, people have been exploring nature, particularly plants, in search of new drugs, and this has resulted in the use of a large number of medicinal plants with curative properties to treat various diseases [4]. The popularity and availability of the traditional remedies have generated concerns regarding the safety, efficacy and the responsibility of practitioners using traditional remedies [1]. Banana is one such plant that has gained popularity in treatment of various ailment.

Banana, generally known as *Musa sapientum*, is a familiar tropical fruit in the world. It originated mainly from intra- and inter-specific hybridizations between two wild diploid species, *M. acuminata* Colla ('A' genome) and *M. Balbisiana* Colla ('B' genome) [5]. Banana is a treelike perennial herb that grows 5–9 m in height, with a tuberous rhizome and a hard, long pseudo-stem. The inflorescence is big, with a reddish-brown bract, and is eaten as a vegetable. The ripe fruits are sweet, juicy and full of seeds, and the peel is thick [6,7]. Banana is the most popular fruit in industrialized countries. It is cultivated in over 130 countries as the second-most produced fruit after citrus [8,9]. It contributes approximately 17% of the world's total fruit production [8]. It is one of a good number of consumed fruits in tropical and subtropical regions of the world [10]. The scientific names of most cultivated bananas are *Musa acuminata*, *Musa balbisiana*, and *Musa* × *paradisiaca* for the hybrid *Musa acuminata* × *M. balbisiana*, depending on their genomic constitution. The old scientific name *Musa sapientum* is no longer used. The classification of cultivated bananas has long been a problematic issue for taxonomists. Bananas were originally placed into two species based only on their uses as food: *Musa sapientum* for dessert bananas and *Musa paradisiaca* for plantains. Series of papers published from 1947 onwards showed that *Musa sapientum* and *Musa paradisiaca* were actually cultivars, and were descendants of two wild seed-producing species, *Musa acuminata* and *Musa balbisiana*. In Nigeria, some of the most common edible banana cultivars include *Musa paradisiaca*, *Musa acuminata* (Cavendish banana) (MAC), and *Musa acuminata* (Red Dacca) (MAR) [11]. The cultivated varieties can present different genomic combinations: AA, AB, AAA, AAB, ABB, AAAA, AAAB, AABB and ABBB, diploids, triploids and tetraploids [5,12]. South-western Nigeria often blends the dried *Musa* spp. peels with the yam flour, as part of their stable foods [7].

The peels of bananas, constitute up to 35% of the ripe fruit, and are regarded as household and industrial food waste, being discarded in large quantities [13]. Taking a piece of banana peel and placing it on a wart, with the yellow side out, can be a natural alternative for killing off a wart; rubbing the affected area of a mosquito bite with the inside of a banana skin reduces swelling and irritation [14]. The peels of ripe bananas can be used to make a poultice for wounds, which is wrapped around an injury to reduce pain or swelling [15]. Banana tree has an important local and traditional value for treating anemic people. They are regarded as healthy food for children from around six months of age, because it does not produce cramps or diarrhea [16]. The ripe fruits/or pseudo-stems of bananas are used to treat diarrhea. The juice from *Musa* spp., is used to treat abdominal pain [16,17]. Unripe banana peels are used as a food source in scientific research, owing to their chemical composition, which was first described by [18]. Bioactive compounds such as alkaloids, anthocyanins, flavonoids, glycosides, phlobatannins, tannins, and terpenoids have been reported in banana peels, and these compounds have been shown to exert various biological and pharmacological effects (antibacterial, antihypertensive, antidiabetic, and anti-inflammatory activities) [16]. For the purpose of this research work, only three of the genomic combinations of *Musa acuminata* were used, which are the ones distributed within Nigeria. The cultivars are AA, AAB and ABB. Locally they are called "*Saro*", "*Paranta/Oranta*" and "*Amina/Ominni*" respectively [12].

Musa acuminata fruit peels are used in the northern part of Nigeria for the treatment of hypertension and other cardiovascular related diseases [5]. Despite that several scientific studies that have validated the folkloric uses of different parts of the *banana*, there is no study in the open scientific literature that has provided scientific evidence for the claimed use of the peel of *Musa acuminata* in the management of cardiovascular related diseases. Additionally, no research has been done to determine the effects of its fruit peels on hepatic and renal parameters in rats. Therefore, this study was aimed at evaluating the effects of aqueous extract of three cultivars of *Musa acuminata* fruit peel on kidney and liver function indices in wistar rats.

2. Materials and Methods

2.1. Plant Sample Collection and Identification

The ripe banana fruit peels of the species (cultivars) *Saro, Oranta* and *Ominni* were collected from their natural habitat within Samaru (located on latitude: 11°9′55.3″ N and longitude: 7°39′5.84″ E), Zaria area of Kaduna State, Nigeria [19]. They were identified at the herbarium unit of the Biological Sciences Department, Ahmadu Bello University, Zaria Nigeria.

2.2. Experimental Protocols

Twenty wistar albino rats of both sexes weighing 140–180 g were purchased from the Faculty of Pharmaceutical Sciences, Ahmadu Bello University, Zaria-Nigeria. They were housed in polypropylene cages in a room where a congenital temperature was 27 °C ± 1 °C and 12 h light and dark cycles were maintained. The animals were allowed to acclimatize to the environment for fourteen days. During this period they were supplied with a commercial growers mash (Grand cereals limited, Jos, Nigeria) available in pellet form and water *ad libitum*.

2.3. Ethical Consideration

The study was approved on 18th September, 2014 by the Institutional animal care and use committee (Protocol number; AREC/EA14/273). All protocols were in accordance with the ethical committee guidelines that are in compliance with the National and International Laws and Guidelines for Care and Use of Laboratory Animals in Biomedical Research [20,21].

2.4. Period of Experimentation

The research was conducted between November 2014 and August 2015.

2.5. Preparation and Extractions of Plant Parts

The banana peels were air-dried in the laboratory for a period of two weeks and then made into powder by grinding and sieved with a mesh size of 0.05 mm. The banana peels aqueous extracts were prepared by soaking 300 g of the powder in 1500 mL (1:5) distilled water in a 2 L conical flask [22]. It was stirred and allowed to stand for 48 h. The extracts were thereafter filtered using filter paper. The filtrates were concentrated to dryness on a water bath set at 45 °C.

2.6. Acute Toxicity (LD_{50}) Test

The mean lethal dose of aqueous peel extracts of *Oranta, Ominni* and *Saro* of *M. acuminata* was determined in albino rats using the method described by Lorke [23]. The LD_{50} was conducted in a pilot study using 9 Wistar rats. The rats were randomly divided into 3 groups of 3 rats each and 10, 100, and 1000 mg/kg b.w., respectively, was administered orally. The animals were monitored for behavioral changes and mortality for 24 h. When no death was observed in any of the groups, 5 other groups were given 1250, 1500, 2000, 2500 and 5000 mg/kg b.w. of the extract and monitored for 24 h for changes in behavior and mortality. The LD_{50} is generally calculated as the geographical mean of the least lethal dose that killed a rat and the highest dose that did not kill a rat. Usually, the extract dose administered to the animal is either calculated as 1/10th of the observed acute toxicity test or extrapolated from the human dose. In this study, the reference body surface area of rat (0.02 m^2) [24] was multiplied by the maximum dose (5000 mg/kg b.w.) tested during the acute toxicity study [25]; that is, $0.02 \times 5000 = 100$.

2.7. Animal Grouping and Treatment

A total of 20 rats were used. The rats were divided into 4 groups of 5 rats each as follows:

Group I: Normal control received feed and distilled water only for 28 days.

Group II: Normal rats treated with *Saro* 100 mg/kg bw/day aqueous extract orally for 28 days.
Group III: Normal rats treated with *Ominni* 100 mg/kg bw/day aqueous extract orally for 28 days.
Group IV: Normal rats treated with *Oranta* 100 mg/kg bw/day aqueous extract orally for 28 days.

2.8. Blood Sample Collection

At the end of the experimental period, the rats were sacrificed by anesthesia using chloroform before sample collection through cardiac puncture. Blood was collected into EDTA bottles and centrifuged at 3500 rpm for 10 min and the clear sera aspirated off for biochemical evaluation.

2.9. Biochemical Analysis

Alanine aminotransferase (ALT) and aspartate aminotransferase (AST) were determined by monitoring the concentration of pyruvate hydrazone formed with 2,4, dinitrophenyl hydrazine and oxaloacetate hydrazone formed with 2,4-dinitrophenyl hydrazine respectively using Randox Diagnostic kits (Randox laboratories Ltd., Antrim, UK) [26]. Serum Creatinine and urea were assayed using standard procedures as described by Varley and Alan [27].

2.10. Statistical Analysis

Data obtained were expressed as mean ± SD. The data were analyzed using analysis of variance (ANOVA). The difference between the various extracts and animal groups were compared using the Duncan Multiple Range Test. The values of $p < 0.05$ were considered as statistically significant.

3. Results and Discussion

In the acute toxicity test study, no death was recorded even at a dose of 5000 mg/kg b.w. This signifies that the LD_{50} is greater than 5000 mg/kg b.w., hence there was nothing to present as results under this section. This observation was in agreement with the reports of Ezekwesili et al. [28]. According to the Hodge and Sterner [29] toxicity scale, *Musa acuminata* is said to be in the non-toxic herbal drug category [30]. The changes in serum liver marker enzymes and proteins of Wistar rats administered with extracts of *Musa acuminata* are shown in Tables 1 and 2, respectively. The results from this study show that there were no significant ($p > 0.05$) changes in the levels of aspartate amino transferase, alanine aminotransferase, alkaline phosphatase, total protein and albumin of all the extract-treated groups when compared to the normal control group. As shown in Table 3, there was a significant ($p < 0.05$) increase in the creatinine level of the group treated with the extract of *Saro* (1.53 ± 0.23) when compared with *Oranta* (0.74 ± 0.22), *Ominni* (0.92 ± 0.39) and normal control (0.72 ± 0.15) groups. Similarly, there was a significant ($p < 0.05$) increase in the level of serum urea of *Saro* (41.56 ± 4.68) when compared to the normal control (26.05 ± 0.73), *Ominni* (28.44 ± 2.43) and *Oranta* (26.10 ± 2.94) groups.

Table 1. Effect of *Musa acuminata* peels on some Serum Liver Marker Enzymes concentration in rats.

Groups (n = 5)	Serum ALK-P (U/L)	Serum ALT (U/L)	Serum AST (U/L)
NC	64.40 ± 15.93 ^{a}	43.53 ± 6.11 ^{a}	21.65 ± 5.77 ^{a}
N + OMN_{100}	36.80 ± 14.74 ^{a}	52.67 ± 8.32 ^{a}	25.01 ± 8.66 ^{a}
N + ORT_{100}	61.07 ± 10.16 ^{a}	41.33 ± 2.31 ^{a}	23.34 ± 7.64 ^{a}
N + SRO_{100}	46.03 ± 16.00 ^{a}	45.46 ± 9.24 ^{a}	26.67 ± 2.89 ^{a}

Values are means of five determination ± SD; ^{a} Values with different superscripts down the column are significantly different ($p < 0.05$); NC: Normal rats Control, N + SRO_{100}: Normal rats + Saro Extract (100 mg/kg), N + ORT_{100}: Normal rats + Oranta Extract (100 mg/kg), N + OMN_{100}: Normal rats + Ominni Extract (100 mg/kg), ALK-P: Alkaline Phosphatase, AST: Aspartate aminotransferase, ALT: Alanine aminotransferase.

Table 2. Effect of aqueous extracts of *Musa acuminata* peels on serum total protein and albumin concentration in rats.

Groups (n = 5)	Total Protein (g/L)	Albumin (g/L)
NC	56.95 ± 6.84^{a}	31.16 ± 6.31^{a}
N + OMN_{100}	64.46 ± 10.75^{a}	27.57 ± 2.07^{a}
N + ORT_{100}	65.23 ± 9.54^{a}	26.77 ± 3.30^{a}
N + SRO_{100}	60.25 ± 7.18^{a}	23.97 ± 3.74^{a}

Values are means of five determination ± SD. [a] Values with different superscripts down the column are significantly different ($p < 0.05$) NC: Normal rats Control, N + SRO_{100}: Normal rats + *Saro* Extract (100 mg/kg), N + ORT_{100}: Normal rats + *Oranta* Extract (100 mg/kg), N + OMN_{100}: Normal rats + *Ominni* Extract (100 mg/kg).

Table 3. Effect of aqueous extracts of *Musa acuminata* peels on serum creatinine and urea concentration in rats.

Groups (n = 5)	Creatinine (mg/dL)	Urea (mg/dL)
NC	0.72 ± 0.15^{a}	26.05 ± 0.73^{a}
N + OMN_{100}	0.92 ± 0.39^{a}	28.44 ± 2.43^{a}
N + ORT_{100}	0.74 ± 0.22^{a}	26.10 ± 2.94^{a}
N + SRO_{100}	1.53 ± 0.23^{b}	41.56 ± 4.68^{b}

Values are means ± SD of n = 5 determinations. [a] Values with different superscripts down the column are significantly different ($p < 0.05$), NC: Normal rats Control, N + SRO_{100}: Normal rats + *Saro* Extract (100 mg/kg), N + ORT_{100}: Normal rats + *Oranta* Extract (100 mg/kg), N + OMN_{100}: Normal rats + *Ominni* Extract (100 mg/kg).

The liver is the major organ of xenobiotic metabolism and detoxification, which makes it vulnerable to hepatotoxicity [31]. AST and ALT are key enzymes involved in the breakdown of amino acids into α-keto acid, which are routed for complete metabolism through the Krebs cycle and electron transport chain. They are regarded as precise biomarkers for liver damage. Also, changes in membrane-bound alkaline phosphatase (ALP) affects membrane permeability and produces derangement in the transport of metabolites [32]. Any damage on the liver results in the release of these marker enzymes into the system above a certain threshold [3]. From the results of our study as indicated in Table 1, it was observed that there were no significant changes ($p < 0.05$) in the levels of serum ALT, AST and ALP of all the extract treated groups when compared to normal control group. These observed insignificant ($p > 0.05$) changes are in accordance with good functioning of the liver. This implies that the peel extracts are not hepatotoxic. Concentrations of albumin and total protein in the serum can be used to assess the health status of the liver and can also be used to ascertain different type of liver damage [33–35]. The liver is the sole site for the synthesis of albumin, which makes up approximately 60% of serum protein concentration [36]. The present study revealed (Table 2) that there were no significant ($p > 0.05$) changes in total protein and albumin levels of the extract treated groups as compared to the normal control rats. The data obtained with respect to liver function indices indicate no cellular toxicity of the extracts on the liver of the experimental rats. However, as presented in Table 3, there was an increase in serum creatinine concentration (1.53 ± 0.23 mg/dL), reflecting a failed capacity of the kidney to effectively excrete creatinine. By inference, it implies that the ability of the two kidneys to effectively excrete creatinine, might have been exceeded. Serum creatinine and urea are common biomarkers for prediction of renal dysfunction, due to the fact that they are elevated considerably when there is a dysfunction of the kidney [33]. The level of serum creatinine usually doesn't rise until at least half of the nephrons of kidney are destroyed or damaged [37]. For differential diagnosis, simultaneous determination of serum creatinine along with urea is a standard practice; hence, serum urea was also estimated. Though urea is inferior to other markers, such as creatinine, blood urea is grossly influenced by other factors, such as diet and nutrition [38]. The marked significant increase in urea (41.56 ± 4.68) of *Saro* means that its intake may pose an undesirable effect on the kidney. Since the elevated levels of urea and creatinine are markers of kidney function [38,39], it then indicates that the extract of *Saro* peel cultivar may impair renal function at the comparative human dose levels.

4. Conclusions and Recommendation

The results from this study revealed that rats treated with the aqueous extracts of the three cultivars of *Musa acuminata* pose no threat to the liver. Conversely, aqueous extracts of *Saro* cultivars showed increase in the biomarkers of the kidney. Thus, intake of peel extracts of *M. acuminata,* particularly the *Saro* cultivar, as a drug might lead to potential kidney problems in the management and/or treatment of hypertension and other cardiovascular related diseases. At present, the exact mechanism of action of *M. acuminata* is not fully known. On this note, further investigations in this direction are needed for possible isolation and structural elucidation of the components of *M. acuminata.*

Acknowledgments: This research did not receive any specific grant from funding agencies in the public, commercial, or not-for-profit sectors. The authors express their warm appreciation to the management of SIRONigeria Global Limited, Abuja, for the English language proof editing and typesetting of the manuscript.

Author Contributions: S.I.R.O. and C.E. conceived and designed the experiments; C.E. performed the experiments; O.O. participated in the literature search. S.I.R.O. critically revised and review the manuscript for important intellectual content. All the enlisted authors contributed substantially to the success of the work reported and approve the final version for publication.

References

1. Sarkiyayi, S.; Aileru, A.E. Effect of methanol leaf extract of anogeissusleio carpus on gentamicin induced biochemical derangement in rats. *Direct Res. J. Health Pharmacol.* **2016**, *4*, 1–7.
2. Megaraj, V.; Ding, X.; Fang, C.; Kovalchuk, N.; Zhu, Y.; Zhang, Q.Y. Role of hepatic and intestinal p450 enzymes in the metabolic activation of the colon carcinogen azoxymethane in mice. *Chem. Res. Toxicol.* **2014**, *27*, 656–662. [CrossRef] [PubMed]
3. Rama, V.G.; Reddy, V.R.; Kumar, V.; Reddy, M.K. Hepatoprotectivity activity of medicinal plant extracts on Albino rats. *World J. Pharm. Sci.* **2016**, *5*, 1275–1284.
4. Ramesh, R.; Dhanaraj, T.S. Hepatoprotective effect of ethyl acetate extract of terminaliaarjuna root on hcb induced liver carcinogenes is in female albino wistar rats. *Int. J. Appl. Biol. Pharm. Technol.* **2016**, *7*, 190–199.
5. Edenta, C.; James, D.B.; Owolabi, O.A.; Okoduwa, S.I.R. Hypolipidemic effects of aqueous extract of three Cultivars of Musa sapientumfruit peel on poloxamer-407 induced hyperlipidemicwistar rats. *Int. J. Pharm. Sci. Res.* **2014**, *5*, 1046–1051.
6. Imam, M.Z.; Akter, S. *Musa paradisiaca* L. and *Musa sapientum* L. A Phytochemical and Pharmacological Review. *J. Appl. Pharm. Sci.* **2011**, *1*, 14–20.
7. Onasanwo, S.A.; Emikpe, B.O.; Ajah, A.A.; Elufioye, T.O. Anti-ulcer and ulcer healing potentials of Musa sapientum peel extract in the laboratory rodents. *Pharm. Res.* **2013**, *5*, 173–178. [CrossRef] [PubMed]
8. Food and Agriculture Organization (FAO). *FAOSTAT*; Food and Agriculture Organization: Geneva, Switzerland, 2013.
9. D'Hont, A.; Denoeud, F.; Aury, J.M. The banana (*Musa acuminata*) genome and the evolution of monocotyledonous plants. *Nature* **2012**, *488*, 213–217. [CrossRef] [PubMed]
10. Alkarkhi, A.F.M.; Ramli, S.; Yeoh, S.Y.; Easa, A.M. Physiochemical properties of banana peel flour as influenced by variety and stage of ripeness: Multivariate statistical analysis. *Asian J. Food Agro-Ind.* **2010**, *3*, 349–362.
11. Adedayo, B.C.; Oboh, G.; Oyeleye, S.I.; Olasehinde, T.A. Antioxidant and antihyperglycemic properties of three banana cultivars (*Musa* spp.). *Scientifica* **2016**. [CrossRef] [PubMed]
12. El-Khishin, D.A.; Belatus, E.L.; El-Hamid, A.A. Radwan, K.H. Molecular characterization of banana cultivars (*Musa* spp.) from Egypt using AFLP. *Res. J. Agric. Biol. Sci.* **2009**, *5*, 271–279.
13. Emaga, T.H.; Ronkart, S.N.; Robert, C.; Wathelet, B.; Paquot, M. Characterisation of pectins extracted from banana peels (Musa AAA) under different conditions using an experimental design. *Food Chem.* **2008**, *108*, 463–471. [CrossRef] [PubMed]
14. Kumar, K.P.S.; Bhowmik, D.; Duraivel, S.; Umadevi, M. Traditional and Medicinal Uses of Banana. *J. Pharm. Phytochem.* **2012**, *1*, 51–63.
15. Atzingen, D.A.; Gragnani, A.; Veiga, D.F.; Abla, L.E.; Mendonça, A.R.; Paula, C.A.; Juliano, Y.; Correa, J.C.; Faria, M.R.; Ferreira, L.M. Gel from unripe Musa sapientum peel to repair surgical wounds in rats. *Acta Cir. Bras.* **2011**, *26*, 379–382. [CrossRef] [PubMed]

16. Pereira, A.; Maraschin, M. Banana (*Musa* spp.) from peel to pulp: Ethnopharmacology, source of bioactive compounds and its relevance for human health. *J. Ethnopharmacol.* **2015**, *160*, 149–163. [CrossRef] [PubMed]
17. Abe, R.; Ohtani, K. An ethnobotanical study of medicinal plants and traditional therapies on Batan Island, the Philippines. *J. Ethnopharmacol.* **2013**, *145*, 554–565. [CrossRef] [PubMed]
18. Selema, M.D.; Farago, M.E. Trace element concentrations in the fruit peels and trunks of Musa paradisiaca. *Phytochemistry* **1996**, *42*, 1523–1525. [CrossRef]
19. Maduekwe, A.A.L.; Garba, B. Characteristics of the monthly averaged hourly diffuse irradiance at Lagos and Zaria, Nigeria. *Renew. Energy* **1999**, *17*, 213–225. [CrossRef]
20. National Research Council (NRC). *Guide for the Care and Use of Laboratory Animals*; National Academies Press: Washington, DC, USA, 2010.
21. Clark, J.D.; Gebhart, G.F.; Gonder, J.C.; Kneeling, M.E.; Kohn, D.F. The 1996 guide for care and use of laboratory animal animals. *ILAR J.* **1997**, *38*, 41–48. [CrossRef] [PubMed]
22. Okoduwa, S.I.R.; Umar, I.A.; James, D.B.; Habila, J.D. Evaluation of extraction protocols for anti-diabetic phytochemical substances from medicinal plants. *World J. Diabetes* **2016**, *7*, 605–614. [CrossRef] [PubMed]
23. Lorke, D. A new approach to practical acute toxicity testing. *Arch. Toxicol.* **1983**, *54*, 275–287. [CrossRef] [PubMed]
24. Nair, A.B.; Jacob, S. A simple practice guide for dose conversion between animals and human. *J. Basic Clin. Pharm.* **2016**, *7*, 27. [CrossRef] [PubMed]
25. Spielmann, H.; Genschow, E.; Liebsch, M.; Halle, W. Determination of the staring dose for acute oral toxicity (LD50) testing in the up and down procedure (UDP) from cytotoxicity data. *Altern. Lab. Anim.* **1999**, *27*, 957–966. [PubMed]
26. Reitman, S.; Frankel, S. A colorimetric method for the determination of serum glutamicoxaloacetic and glutamine pyruvic transaminases. *Am. J. Clin. Pathol.* **1957**, *28*, 56–63. [CrossRef] [PubMed]
27. Varley, H.; Alan, H.G. Tests in renal disease. In *Practical Clinical Biochemistry*; William Heinemann Medical Book Ltd.: London, UK, 1984; p. 1123.
28. Ezekwesili, C.N.; Ghasi, S.; Adindu, C.S.; Mefoh, N.C. Evaluation of the anti-ulcer property of aqueous extract of unripe Musa paradisiaca Linn peel in wistar rats. *Afr. J. Pharm. Pharmacol.* **2014**, *8*, 1006–1011.
29. Hodge, A.; Sterner, B. *Toxicity Classes*; Canadian Centre for Occupational Health Safety: Hamilton, ON, Canda, 2005. Available online: http://www.ccohs.ca/oshanswers/chemicals/id50.htm (accessed on 16 May 2016).
30. Ahmed, M. Acute Toxicity (Lethal Dose 50 Calculation) of Herbal Drug Somina in Rats and Mice. *Pharmacol. Pharm.* **2015**, *6*, 185–189. [CrossRef]
31. Ullah, I.; Khan, J.A.; Adhikari, A.; Shahid, M. Hepatoprotective effect of Monothecabuxifolia fruit against antitubercular drugs-induced hepatotoxicity in rats. *Bangladesh J. Pharmacol.* **2016**, *11*, 248–256. [CrossRef]
32. Okoduwa, S.I.R.; Umar, I.A.; James, D.B. Antidiabetic potential of occimum gratissimum leaf fraction in fortified diet fed streptozotocin-treated diabetic rats. *Medicines* **2017**, *4*, 73. [CrossRef] [PubMed]
33. Tierney, L.M.; Mcphee, S.J.; Papadakis, M.A. Current Medical Diagnosis and Treatment, International edition. In *New York: Lange Medical Books*; McGraw-Hill: New York, NY, USA, 2002; pp. 1203–1215.
34. Yakubu, M.T.; Bilbis, L.S.; Lawal, M.; Akanji, M.A. Evaluation of selected parameters of rat liver and kidney function following repeated administration of Yohimbine. *Biokemistri* **2003**, *15*, 50–56.
35. Nwaogu, L.A. Toxico-pathological evaluation of Citrulluscolocynthis seed and Pulp aqueous extracts on albino rats. *World J. Biol. Med. Sci.* **2016**, *3*, 76–85.
36. Khan, N.; Ahmed, M.; Khan, R.A.; Khan, S.; Gul, S. Evaluating the effect of Acacia modestaleaves extract on blood glucose, serum Lipids, liver and kidney functions in diabetic and non-diabetic rats. *Biomed. Nurs.* **2016**, *2*, 1.
37. Chukwuedozie, N.F. Evaluation of Time-Dependent Effects of a Leaf Extract of Spermacoceocymoideson Kidney Function. *J. Med. Biol. Sci. Res.* **2016**, *2*, 68–74.
38. Odoula, T.; Adeniyi, F.A.; Bello, I.S.; Subair, H.G. Toxicity studies on an unripe Caripa papaya aqueous extract; Biochemical and hematological effects in wistar albino rats. *J. Med. Plant Res.* **2007**, *1*, 1–4.
39. Grant, G.H. *Amino Acids and Proteins; Fundamentals of Clinical Chemistry*, 3rd ed.; Tietz, N.W., Ed.; WB Saunders Company: Philadelphia, PA, USA, 1987; pp. 328–329.

3

The Protective Role of Sulfated Polysaccharides from Green Seaweed *Udotea flabellum* in Cells Exposed to Oxidative Damage

Fernando Bastos Presa [1,2,†], Maxsuell Lucas Mendes Marques [1,2,†], Rony Lucas Silva Viana [1], Leonardo Thiago Duarte Barreto Nobre [1], Leandro Silva Costa [3] and Hugo Alexandre Oliveira Rocha [1,2,*]

1 Departamento de Bioquímica, Universidade Federal do Rio Grande do Norte, Natal 59078-970, Rio Grande do Norte, Brazil; fernandobpresa@gmail.com (F.B.P.); maxsuell_lucas@hotmail.com (M.L.M.M.); rony_lucas@hotmail.com (R.L.S.V.); leo.dnobre@gmail.com (L.T.D.B.N.)

2 Programa de Pós-graduação em Ciências da Saúde, Universidade Federal do Rio Grande do Norte, Natal 59078-970, Rio Grande do Norte, Brazil

3 Instituto Federal de Educação, Ciência, e Tecnologia do Rio Grande do Norte (IFRN), Ceara-Mirim 59900-000, Rio Grande do Norte, Brazil; leandro-silva-costa@hotmail.com

* Correspondence: hugo@cb.ufrn.br

† These authors contributed equally.

Abstract: Seaweed is a rich source of bioactive sulfated polysaccharides. We obtained six sulfated polysaccharide-rich fractions (UF-0.3, UF-0.5, UF-0.6, UF-0.7, UF-1.0, and UF-2.0) from the green seaweed *Udotea flabellum* (UF) by proteolytic digestion followed by sequential acetone precipitation. Biochemical analysis of these fractions showed that they were enriched with sulfated galactans. The viability and proliferative capacity of 3T3 fibroblasts exposed to $FeSO_4$ (2 μM), $CuSO_4$ (1 μM) or ascorbate (2 mM) was not affected. However, these cells were exposed to oxidative stress in the presence of $FeSO_4$ or $CuSO_4$ and ascorbate, which caused the activation of caspase-3 and caspase-9, resulting in apoptosis of the cells. We also observed increased lipid peroxidation, evaluated by the detection of malondialdehyde and decreased glutathione and superoxide dismutase levels. Treating the cells with the ultrafiltrate fractions (UF) fractions protected the cells from the oxidative damage caused by the two salts and ascorbate. The most effective protection against the oxidative damage caused by iron was provided by UF-0.7 (1.0 mg/mL); on treatment with UF-0.7, cell viability was 55%. In the case of copper, cell viability on treatment with UF-0.7 was ~80%, but the most effective fraction in this model was UF-2.0, with cell viability of more than 90%. The fractions, mainly UF-0.7 and UF-2.0, showed low iron chelating activity, but high copper chelating activity and total antioxidant capacity (TAC). These results suggested that some of their protective mechanisms stem from these properties.

Keywords: sulfated galactan; 3T3 fibroblasts; green seaweed

---

1. Introduction

Copper and iron are two of the most abundant metals in the human body. They play several important roles in cellular metabolism. Copper is an essential micronutrient in human nutrition; it is a component of metalloenzymes and acts as an electron donor or acceptor, while iron forms complexes with proteins, such as flavin-iron enzymes, transferrin, ferritin, myoglobin or hemoglobin (responsible for oxygen transport), and with enzymes involved in electron transfer and oxidation-reduction reactions [1]. However, high levels of these transition metal ions in the form Cu^{2+} and Fe^{2+} are responsible for the production of reactive oxygen species (ROS), which leads to oxidative stress in cells, causing cellular damage and diseases. High levels of copper in the body, either by ingestion or genetic predisposition (Wilson's disease and Menkes syndrome), may contribute to mitochondrial dysfunction, subsequently leading to the production of ROS and induction of apoptosis. Consequently, several organs may suffer from its toxic effects [2]. An excess of iron in the body results in disorders, such as cirrhosis, liver cancer, diabetes, arrhythmia, and osteoporosis [3]. The use of chelating agents is always recommended in case of excess of physiological copper or iron [4]. However, these agents have several side effects [5]; thus, there is a continued search for new chelating agents.

Campo and colleagues [6] demonstrated that glycosaminoglycans, a group of sulfated polysaccharides (SPs), have antioxidant activity and can chelate both Cu^{++} and Fe^{++}, indicating that these compounds may serve as prospective drugs to combat the damaging effects of copper and iron. However, glycosaminoglycans are found in small amounts in all their sources, which could make their commercial use difficult. Other SPs are found in all seaweeds, and in some species of animals, plants, bacteria, fungi, and other microorganisms [7]. However, only seaweeds can synthetize SPs in large quantities. In addition, several SPs from seaweeds showed iron chelation activity, which makes seaweeds potential sources of chelating SPs.

Ulvans, green seaweed-origin SPs from the genus *Ulva*, showed antioxidant activity in several in vitro models [8]. In the present study, we draw attention to the SPs from *Ulva pertusa*, as they are known to form chelates with iron [9]. We have previously demonstrated that SPs from tropical green seaweeds, namely *Caulerpa cupressoides* [10], *Caulerpa prolifera* and *Caulerpa sertularioides* [11], have iron chelation activity.

Green seaweeds synthesize a range of sulfated homo- [12] and heteropolysaccharides [13]. These SPs have distinct chemistries and functions without parallelism in other organisms. This uniqueness results in the low degree of redundancy in the structure and mechanism of action of SPs, which has in turn resulted in renewed interest in the recognition of green seaweeds as novel sources of SPs [14]. However, there are fewer studies on SPs of green algae compared to those on other types, of seaweed.

Recently, we found that an extract enriched in SPs from another tropical seaweed, *Udotea flabellum* showed copper chelating activity (unpublished data). This seaweed is found easily on the Brazilian coast, and antioxidative properties of polysaccharides from its extracts have not been evaluated to date. Therefore, the aim of this study was to obtain SP-rich fractions from *U. flabellum* and evaluate their potential as protective agents in two models of oxidative stress caused by the presence of copper or iron.

2. Results

2.1. Chemical Analyses

We used a low-cost, widely reproducible method, which combined proteolysis and sequential acetone precipitation, to obtain six sulfated polysaccharide-rich fractions (named UF-0.3, UF-0.5, UF-0.6, UF-0.7, UF-1.0, and UF-2.0) from the green seaweed *U. flabellum*. The results of the chemical analysis of the fractions and their polysaccharide yields are summarized in Table 1. The yield ranged from 4.2% (UF-0.3) to 36.9% (UF-0.5); UF-0.3 and UF-1.0 were contaminated with proteins. The sulfate percentage indicated that it was present in all fractions.

Table 1. Chemical composition of polysaccharides extracted from the *U. flabellum*; Gal: galactose; Xyl: xylose; Man: mannose; Gluc: glucose; -Traces; n.d—not detected.

Sulfated Polysaccharides	Yield [a] (%)	Sulfate (%)	Protein (%)	Molar Ratio			
				Gal	Glu	Man	Xyl
UF-0.3	4.20	7.3 ± 0.8	4.9 ± 0.8	1.0	1.1	n.d	n.d
UF-0.5	36.9	18.7 ± 0.8	-	1.0	0.5	-	-
UF-0.6	9.9	10.7 ± 1.2	n.d	1.0	0.4	0.2	-
UF-0.7	17.7	17.0 ± 1.8	-	1.0	0.4	0.2	-
UF-1.0	11.5	9.8 ± 0.7	5.6 ± 0.8	1.0	0.7	0.7	0.3
UF-2.0	19.7	21.5 ± 1.3	n.d	1.0	1.0	1.0	n.d

[a] All polysaccharides obtained by acetone precipitation were dried and weighed and total mass of each sample corresponded to 100%.

In order to confirm whether the sulfate was covalently linked to polysaccharides, we subjected the fractions to agarose gel electrophoresis. After the gel was stained with toluidine blue (Figure 1) we found that all fractions contained electrophoretically mobile purple colored bands, characteristic to sulfated polysaccharides. We observed slight differences in the mobility of the bands of each fraction, and multiple bands were observed for some fractions (UF-0.3 and UF-1.0).

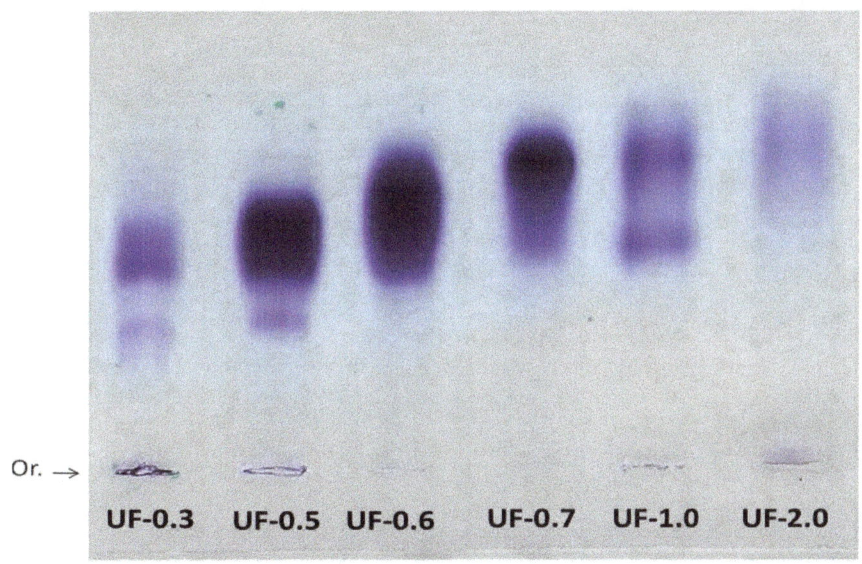

Figure 1. Electrophoresis in 0.05 M diaminopropane acetate buffer, pH 9.0, of fractions obtained by acetone precipitation. About 5 μL (50 μg) of each polysaccharide was applied in agarose gel prepared in diaminopropane acetate buffer and subjected to electrophoresis, as described in methods. Or.—origin.

Table 1 also shows that galactose and glucose are present in all fractions, but in different proportions. Galactose was found to be the predominant sugar in all fractions; therefore, it was chosen as a reference to determine the proportion of other sugars. Glucose was found in large proportions in the fractions UF-0.3, UF-1.0, and UF-2.0. Mannose was not detected in UF-0.3, and its percentage increased with respect to other sugars in subsequent fractions reaching the maximum in UF-2.0. Xylose was absent in fractions UF-0.3 and UF-2.0.

2.2. *Effect of Sulfated Polisaccharides on Cell Viability and Cell Proliferation*

Initially, we evaluated whether sulfated polysaccharides were toxic to 3T3 fibroblast cells. As seen in Figure 2A, the polysaccharides, at the proportions determined previously, failed to have any effect on the ability of fibroblasts to reduce 3-(4,5-dimethylthiazol-2-yl)-2,5-diphenyltetrazolium bromide

(MTT). In contrast, treatment with cisplatin, which was used as a positive control, caused 3T3 cells to reduce only 27% of the MTT molecules.

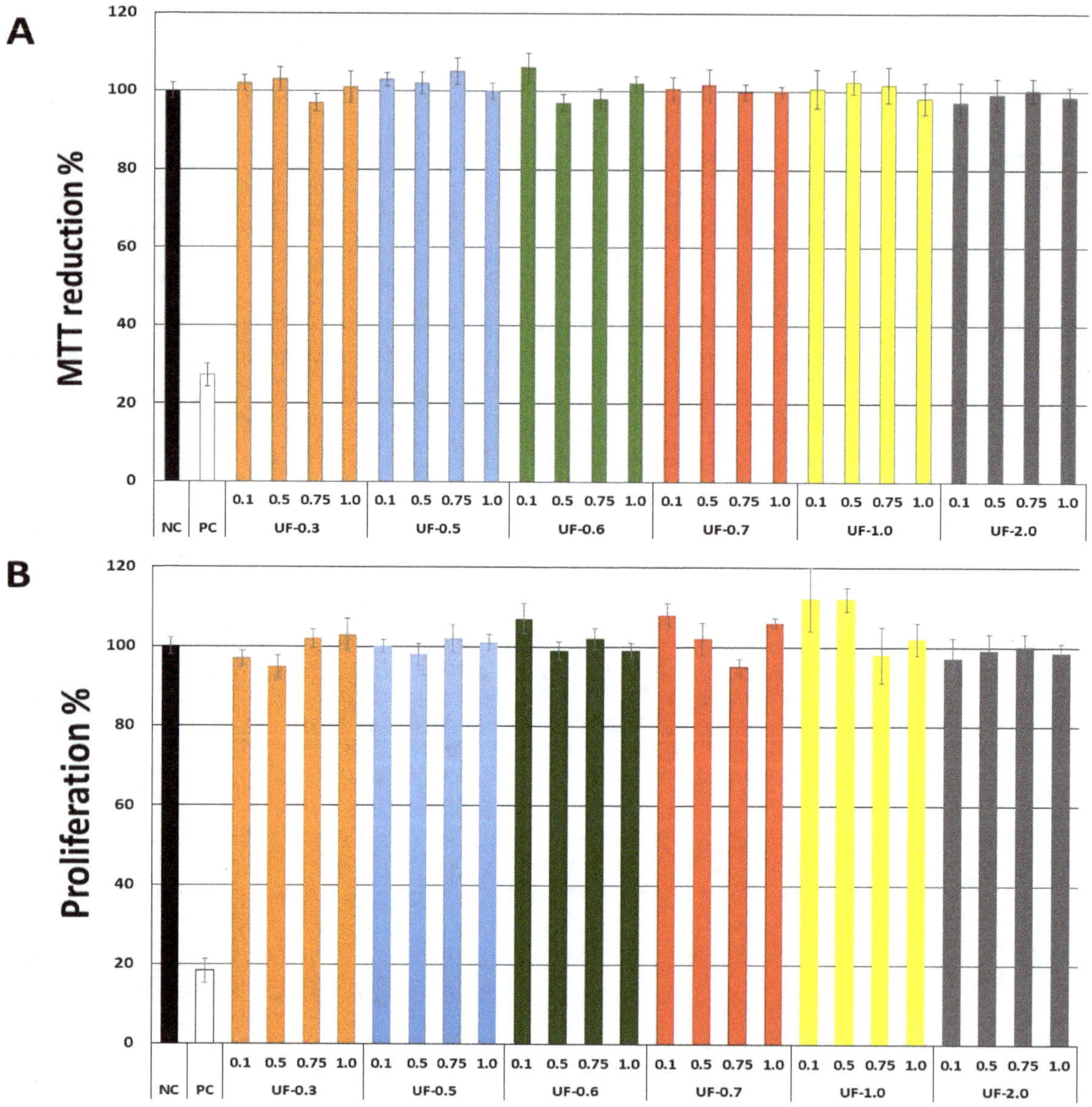

Figure 2. Effect of different concentrations (mg/mL) of sulfated polysaccharides from *U. flabellum* on the ability of fibroblast (3T3) cells to reduce 3-(4,5-dimethylthiazol-2-yl)-2,5-diphenyltetrazolium bromide (MTT) (**A**) and incorporate 5-bromo-2-deoxyuridine (BrdU) BrdU (**B**). NC—negative control composed only of culture medium with fetal bovine serum. PC—positive control-culture medium with fetal bovine serum and cisplatin (2 μg/mL).

Figure 2B shows that the sulfated polysaccharides also did not affect the proliferation of 3T3 cells, as the incorporation of 5-bromo-2-deoxyuridine (BrdU) by the cells incubated in the presence of fractions was similar with the cells of the negative control group (cells exposed only to medium and fetal bovine serum).

2.3. *Evaluation of SP Chelation Activity*

As UF-0.3 and UF-1.0 showed protein contamination, we did not use these fractions in subsequent experiments.

As seen in Figure 3, all samples had low iron chelating activity (<20%) compared to that of ethylenediaminetetraacetic acid (EDTA), used as the positive control. In contrast, the polysaccharides showed a dose-dependent effect when copper was used. The most significant chelation (~90%) was observed for UF-2.0.

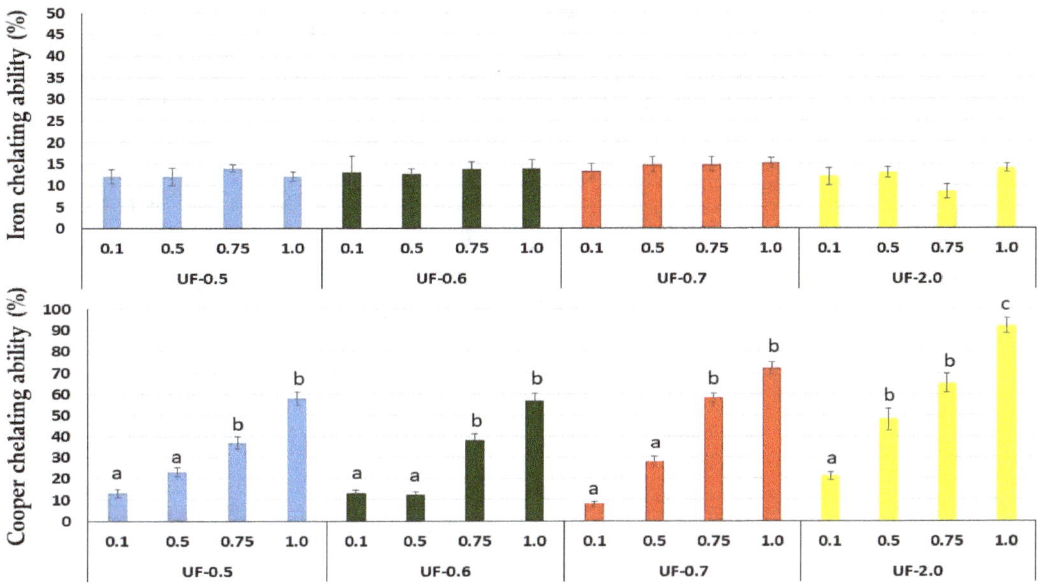

Figure 3. Copper- and iron-chelating ability of sulfated polysaccharides from *U. flabellum.* Data are presented as means ± standard deviation. Different lowercase letters indicate a significant difference ($p < 0.05$) between the ability of polysaccharides to chelate copper or iron. Ethylenediaminetetraacetic acid (EDTA) was used as the positive control, which corresponded to 100% chelating ability (maximum chelating ability was 0.025 and 0.02 mg/mL in the copper and iron analyses, respectively).

2.4. *Effect of Sulfated Polysaccharides on MTT Reduction in 3T3 Fibroblast Cells*

As Figure 4 shows, the sulfated polysaccharides protected the cells from the action of $FeSO_4$ and $CuSO_4$ -. On using $FeSO_4$, UF-0.7 was the only fraction that caused the 3T3 cells to reduce more than 50% of the MTT molecules that were present in the culture medium. In contrast, when we used $CuSO_4$, the cells that were subjected to the higher concentrations of samples were able to reduce more than 50% of the MTT molecules. Notably, fractions UF-0.7 and UF-2.0, (1.0 mg/mL) enabled cells to reduce ~81% and ~95% of the MTT molecules, respectively.

We also exposed the 3T3 cells to $FeSO_4$ (2 μM), $CuSO_4$ (1 μM) or ascorbate (2 mM) and we observed that the ability of 3T3 cells to reduce MTT was not affected in any of the conditions evaluated.

2.5. *Effect of Sulfated Polysaccharides on 3T3 Fibroblast Caspase-3 and Caspase-9*

Several studies show that $FeSO_4$ and $CuSO_4$ induce cell death along with ascorbate by promoting the activation of caspases. Therefore, we evaluated the activity of capase-3 and caspase-9 from the 3T3 fibroblasts that were exposed to $FeSO_4$ and $CuSO_4$, in the absence and presence of sulfated polysaccharides (1 mg/mL). Figure 5 shows that the activity of caspase-3 and caspase-9 is very high after the cells have been exposed to oxidizing conditions positive control (PC), metal plus ascorbate). Moreover, the presence of polysaccharides decreased the activity of both caspases in various conditions. However, polysaccharides were less effective when the cells were exposed to $FeSO_4$ than when exposed to $CuSO_4$.

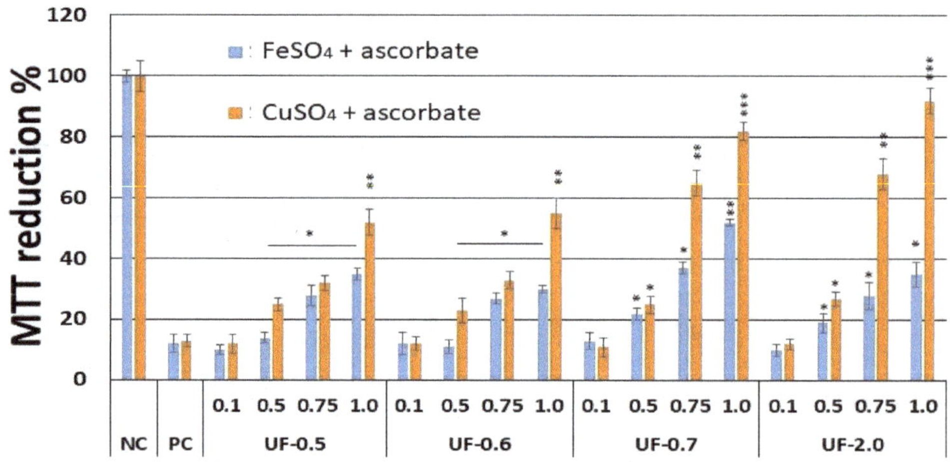

Figure 4. Effect of different amounts (mg/mL) of sulfated polysaccharides from *U. flabellum* on the ability of fibroblast (3T3) cells to reduce MTT in the two models of oxidative stress. NC—negative control composed only of culture medium with fetal bovine serum. PC—positive control-culture medium with fetal bovine serum, $FeSO_4$ or $CuSO_4$, and ascorbate. *** $p < 0.001$; ** $p < 0.01$; * $p < 0.05$ vs. PC.

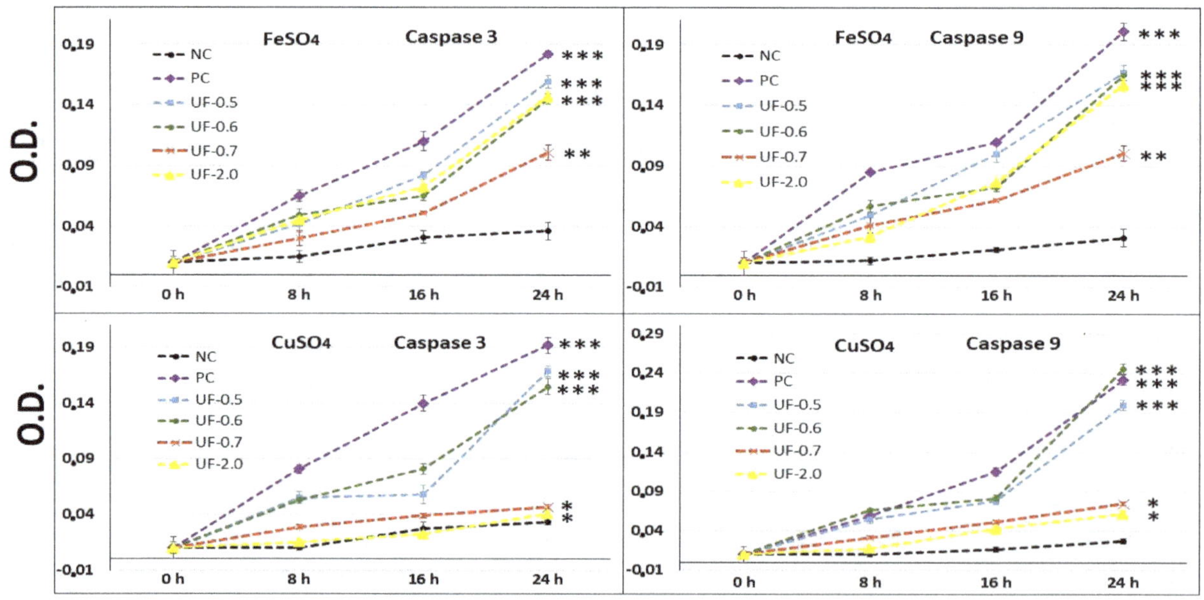

Figure 5. Effect of different amounts (mg/mL) of sulfated polysaccharides from *U. flabellum* on caspase-3 and caspase-9 activity in 3T3 cells exposed to two models of oxidative stress. O.D.—optical density. NC—negative control composed only of culture medium with fetal bovine serum. PC—positive control-culture medium with fetal bovine serum $FeSO_4$ or $CuSO_4$ and ascorbate. *** $p < 0.001$; ** $p < 0.01$; * $p < 0.05$ vs. NC.

When the effect of each fraction was studied individually, the activity of the caspases in fractions UF-0.5, UF-0.6, and UF-2.0 in the presence of $FeSO_4$ was about 25% lower than that observed with the PC group. On the other hand, the activity of both caspases corresponded to about 50% to that observed in the PC group.

2.6. Lipid Peroxidation Analysis

Estimation of malondialdehyde levels was performed to determine the degree of free radical production in 3T3 cells (Table 2). The concentration of malondialdehyde found in the cells of the control group was approximately 250 mmol/10^6 cells, and this was considered to be the physiological concentration. These levels were about ten times higher in the presence of metals and ascorbate. This indicates that the presence of these compounds promoted oxidative damage.

Table 2. Evaluation of the protective effect of the polysaccharides on the 3T3 cells exposed to the two models of oxidative damage.

Effect of Sulfated Polysaccharides (1 mg/mL) on Total Glutathione (GSH) (mmol/10^6 Cell) Levels of 3T3 Cells Exposed to Oxidative Damage				
		$FeSO_4$		$CuSO_4$
NC	6.78 ± 2.21		7.01 ± 2.11	
PC		2.37 ± 0.60 [a]		2.47 ± 0.43 [a]
UF-0.5		3.63 ± 0.61 [b]		4.71 ± 1.01 [c]
UF-0.6		4.18 ± 0.98 [c]		4.52 ± 0.93 [c]
UF-0.7		4.75 ± 0.78 [c]		4.89 ± 1.12 [c]
UF-2.0		4.76 ± 1.08 [c]		5.77 ± 1.08 [c]
Effect of Sulfated Polysaccharides (1 mg/mL) on Malondialdehyde (MDA) (mmol/10^6 cell) Levels of 3T3 Cells Exposed to Oxidative Damage				
		$FeSO_4$		$CuSO_4$
NC	250.1 ± 21.1		217.2 ± 41.7	
PC		2123.8 ± 99.7 [a]		2312.1 ± 103.5 [a]
UF-0.5		1542.5 ± 123.1 [b]		1428.5 ± 111.2 [b]
UF-0.6		1488.1 ± 209.2 [b]		15,012 ± 93.9 [b]
UF-0.7		1107.0 ± 89.1 [c]		1001 ± 101.1 [c]
UF-2.0		1083.0 ± 56.3 [c]		987 ± 95.1 [c]
Effect of Sulfated Polysaccharides (1 mg/mL) on Total Superoxide Dismutase (SOD) Levels (U/mg Protein) of 3T3 Cells Exposed to Oxidative Damage				
		$FeSO_4$		$CuSO_4$
NC	33.5 ± 1.1		31.2 ± 0.9 [a]	
PC		8.2 ± 2.1 [a]		10.2 ± 1.1 [a]
UF-0.5		11.8 ± 2.1 [b]		13.9 ± 1.5 [b]
UF-0.6		10.9 ± 1.0 [b]		14.7 ± 1.2 [b]
UF-0.7		14.2 ± 0.4 [b]		20.8 ± 1.5 [c]
UF-2.0		15.8 ± 0.7 [b]		20.9 ± 0.8 [c]

PC—positive control-culture medium with fetal bovine serum $FeSO_4$ or $CuSO_4$ and ascorbate. [a] $p < 0.001$ vs. NC; [b] $p < 0.05$; [c] $p < 0.001$ vs. PC.

When the cells were exposed to $FeSO_4$ or $CuSO_4$ and ascorbate along with the polysaccharides the levels of malondialdehyde were significantly lower than those observed in the PC group. The most efficient samples to reduce malondialdehyde levels were UF-0.7 and UF-2.0.

2.7. Assessment of the Cell Antioxidant Status

The concentration of glutathione (GSH) and Superoxide dismutase (SOD) were assayed in order to evaluate antioxidant balance after free radical production (Table 2). The levels of GSH (6.78 ± 2.21 mmol/10^6 cell) and SOD (33.5 ± 1.1 mmol/10^6 cell) found in the control cells were considered physiological. A significant reduction in levels of both antioxidants was observed in several experimental conditions, and this effect was more pronounced in the PC group.

When cells were treated with copper, ascorbate, and polysaccharides, we found no significant difference in GSH levels between the treated groups and the negative group (NC) group. When cells were exposed to iron, similar results were obtained with UF-0.7 and UF-2.0. This shows that these two fractions prevented a decrease in the levels of GSH even when the cells were subjected to oxidative damage.

The protective effect of polysaccharides was less pronounced in the case of SOD. However, treatment with both UF-0.7 and UF-2.0, in the presence of iron or copper, showed decreased levels of this enzyme

2.8. In Vitro Evaluation of Antioxidant Capacity of Polysaccharides

The total antioxidant capacity (TAC) test aims to evaluate the ability of a compound to donate electrons to another molecule, which stabilizes it. UF-2.0 presented significantly lower TAC than the other samples. The other samples presented significantly similar TAC as shown in Figure 6.

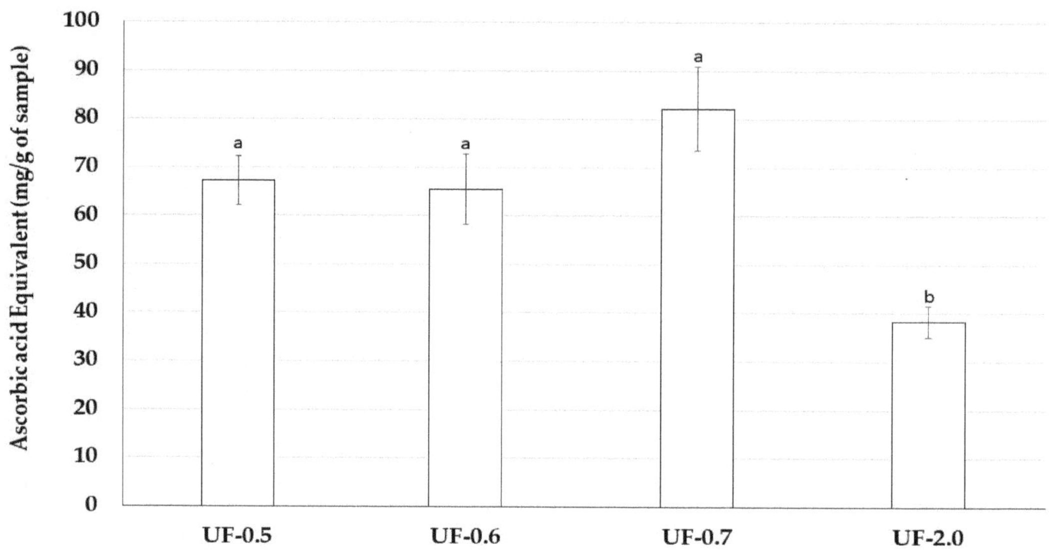

Figure 6. Total antioxidant capacity of sulfated polysaccharides-rich fractions from *U. flabellum*. Data are presented as means ± standard deviation. [a, b] Different lowercase letters indicate a significant difference ($p < 0.05$) between the total antioxidant capacities of samples.

The polysaccharides at all concentrations tested (from 0.1 to 1.0 mg/mL) did not exhibit any hydroxyl radical scavenging activity. In addition, only UF-2.0 exhibited superoxide radical scavenging activity, but this activity was 15%, and it was only detected at the highest concentration (1.0 mg/mL).

The last antioxidant evaluation test we performed was to determine the reducing power of the samples. UF-0.5 and UF-2.0 showed activity (~35%), but we only detected this activity at the highest concentration (1.0 mg/mL).

3. Discussion

The data presented in Table 1 indicate that all fractions contained polysaccharides and sulfate. The confirmation that sulfate ions were covalently bound to the polysaccharides was achieved by using agarose gel electrophoresis, as the free sulfate ions and small sulfated molecules would not be retained in the gel mesh [15]. Based on these data, we obtained six sulfated polysaccharide-rich fractions from *U. flabellum*.

We obtained the fractions using differential precipitation with acetone, which was due to different interaction forces between polysaccharide molecules with water. Therefore, the addition of increasing volumes of acetone to the samples is necessary during precipitation. The polysaccharides, which are most weakly bound, precipitate with lower concentrations of acetone and those, which are more strongly bound, requiring higher concentrations of acetone for precipitation.

Agarose gel electrophoresis allowed the visualization and verification of the existence of sulfated polysaccharides in all fractions. The purple color obtained is typical of SPs due to the interaction of the toluidine blue dye with the sulfated group present in the polysaccharides [15].

Generally, in agarose gel electrophoresis systems, the mobility of the polysaccharides depends on their charges; for example, the more negative ones have greater mobility than the negative ones. However, as suggested by Dietrich and Dietrich [15], the use of 1,3-diaminopropane was important for the visualization of different polysaccharide molecules in the fractions. In the pH of the test (9.0) the sulfated polysaccharides assume a conformation in which some sulfate groups are exposed and others not. These exposed sulfates react with the diamine and their negative charges are quenched. This will induce a change in the conformation of the polysaccharide, and new sulfate groups are exposed and, accordingly, will react with the diamine. This process continues until equilibrium is reached, and the conformation of the polysaccharide no longer changes. However, the polysaccharide, in this conformational equilibrium condition, will still have sulfate groups that did not react with the diamine, and it will be these groups that will permit the mobility of the polysaccharide in the agarose during the electrophoresis. In short, polysaccharide molecules that have the same structure will have the same interaction with the diamine, and consequently have the same electrophoretic motility; whereas, structurally different polysaccharides have different electrophoretic mobilities [15]. In Figure 2, the presence of multiple bands with different mobilities in some fractions indicated that there are at least two polysaccharides in these Udotea fractions.

The results discussed so far (acetone precipitation, electrophoresis, and monosaccharide composition) show that *U. flabellum* synthesizes more than one type of sulfated polysaccharide. This agrees with reports that describe green seaweeds synthesizing more than one type of SP [13].

The analysis of the monosaccharide composition showed that all the fractions are heterogeneous, and that their main constituent is galactose. The predominance of one or more monomers over others as observed in the fractions of the *U. flabellum* was not surprising, as there are previous reports with data from other seaweeds, supporting a similar predominance [16,17]. Moreover, galactose has been described as the main component of SPs in other seaweeds, such as *Caulerpa cupressoides* [10] and *Codium isthmocladum* [12].

Our first objective was to rule out the toxicity of *Udotea* SPs to fibroblast 3T3 cells. As seen in Figure 2, *Udotea* SPs were not cytotoxic, and did not influence the proliferation of fibroblasts. Therefore, we hypothesized these SPs to be putative protective agents under conditions of oxidative stress. Two samples (UF-0.3 and UF-1.0) were not used due to protein contamination.

Production of reactive oxygen species leads to oxidative stress in cells, and, consequently, are harmful to organisms. In many oxidative stress models, one of the first reactive species of oxygen that is formed in great quantity is the superoxide anion. It is considered a reactive primary species, as it can generate reactive derivatives by direct interactions with other molecules or by processes catalyzed by metals or enzymes. In addition, under conditions of stress, superoxide anions can interact with proteins with iron as a cofactor and release iron groups from them [18]. Superoxide anion is a substrate for SOD that transforms it into hydrogen peroxide. These two species have a short-lived action. However, they can react with iron or copper through the Fenton and Haber-Weiss reactions, which leads to formation of the hydroxyl radical (OH•), which is a much more damaging ROS [19].

Several studies have demonstrated that the presence of iron or copper sulfate under culture conditions promotes oxidative stress. In addition, the presence of ascorbate also contributes to enhance the production of the detrimental OH• [6,20]. Therefore, we chose the model of cellular damage in the presence of these two salts and ascorbate to evaluate the protective action of Udotea SPs.

Because the oxidation of a substrate is caused by a reactive species in a chain reaction that includes three steps (initiation, propagation, and termination), the action of the antioxidants is evaluated through several mechanisms. Chelating agents act in both the initiation and propagation steps. Thus, they are antioxidant compounds because they prevent the formation of radicals and thus indirectly reduce the risk posed by radicals [9].

That is why we evaluated the chelating capacity of *Udotea* SPs. All SPs showed high copper chelating activity, with emphasis on UF-0.7 and UF-2.0 at 1 mg/mL, which presented activities superior to 80% and 90%, respectively. SPs from the brown seaweed *Undaria pinnatifida* also showed high copper chelating activity, but this activity was obtained only with high concentration (2.5 mg/mL) [21]. SPs from *Dictyopteris justii* (brown seaweed) also showed iron chelating activity, and one of these polysaccharides had a maximum activity of ~80% (1 mg/mL) [22]. We have not identified other reports that have evaluated the copper chelating activity of SPs from seaweeds. Many reports show a positive correlation between the activity of SPs and their sulfate content. We did not identify this correlation with *Udotea* SPs. Indeed, the copper chelating activity of polysaccharides appears to be more related to the conformation of the polysaccharide than to the presence of negatively charged groups, since neutral polysaccharides showed this activity. For example, yeast-neutral polysaccharides showed 80% activity when evaluated at concentrations similar to those used in the present study [23].

This copper chelating activity of *Udotea* SPS was reflected in cell-based assays. We found that UF-0.7 and UF-2.0, which were the most potent chelators, were also the ones that most protected the cells from damage caused by oxidative stress. Moreover, as shown in Figure 3, this activity was dose dependent. UF-1.0 contained the most potent SPs, which was demonstrated when SPs were used at similar concentrations (Figures 4 and 5, and Table 2).

Campo and colleagues [6] showed that the glycosaminoglycans, hyaluronic acid and chondroitin-4-sulfate, protect fibroblastic cells against the damage caused by the presence of $CuSO_4$ and ascorbate. However, when we performed the cytotoxicity assay (Figure 4.), the rate of reduction of MTT was 80%, and this was only achieved at a concentration of 2.0 mg/mL, which is twice the concentration used with UF-2.0. In addition, with UF-2.0, we achieved an MTT reduction rate of over 90%.

Our results showed that when 3T3 cells were exposed to $CuSO_4$, the levels of caspase-3 (executioner) and caspase-9 (initiator) in the cells were very high, corroborating with the MTT test data (Figure 5). This implies that the cells under conditions of oxidative damage tend to die by apoptosis. Caspases are a group of proteases important for cellular apoptosis to occur. There are initiator caspases and executioner caspases, which are activated by the initiator caspases. The activation of caspases under conditions of oxidative stress and their involvement in the process of cell death induced by it have been reported since a long time [24]. The activity levels of these caspases in the groups of cells treated with UF-0.7 and UF-2.0 were similar to those observed in the NC group. This data demonstrated that fractions UF-0.7 and UF-2.0 could act as chelating agents, thus decreasing the oxidative stress, activation of caspases, and the number of dead cells (as seen indirectly via the MTT test).

To confirm that the oxidative stress in the cells was reduced by the presence of sulfated polysaccharides, we evaluated the levels of three markers of oxidative stress SOD, GSH, and malondialdehyde.

Free radical-mediated cell damage can generally cause lipid peroxidation, and malondialdehyde levels are a good marker of this event, the higher the amount of this molecule, the greater the lipid peroxidation [6]. The presence of sulfated polysaccharides prevented the levels of malondialdehyde from getting so high. In fractions UF-0.7 and UF-2.0, these levels were only 5 times higher than those observed in the PC.

The concentration of SOD and GSH decreases considerably when cells are exposed to oxidative damage. This is because SOD and GSH are consumed by the reactive species that are formed [25].

This explains the decrease in the levels of SOD and GSH when 3T3 cells are exposed to oxidative damage. In both cases, we observed that the sulfated polysaccharides, mainly UF-0.7 and UF-2.0, protected the cells against the oxidative damage.

The mechanism by which SPs from *Udotea* reduce cellular damage against free radical overproduction is similar to that of hyaluronic acid and chondroitin-4-sulfate, typical SPs that can behave as chelating agents [6,26]. We had hypothesized that the protective action of polysaccharides from this seaweed against oxidative damage occurs mainly because of its copper chelating properties.

Udotea SPs presented low iron chelating activity. However, their presence protected 3T3 cells against oxidative damage caused by exposure to $FeSO_4$. This was observed in all the tests performed. In addition, the data showed that, unlike in the $CuSO_4$ assays, the most effective polysaccharide was UF-0.7. These data indicated that oxidative stress caused by iron was attenuated by the polysaccharides via other mechanisms besides chelation to wield their antioxidant action, consequently, protecting the cell against oxidative damage.

Therefore, we assessed antioxidant properties of *Udotea* SPs using five antioxidant tests. *Udotea* SPs were effective only in the TAC. In this test, we verified that the activity of UF-2.0 was lower than that of the other SPs. In contrast, UF-0.7 was the most potent antioxidant among all SPs. In the TAC assay, the sample is evaluated as an electron donor; the higher the value obtained in the TAC, the greater its ability to donate electrons and, consequently, to neutralize the ROS.

TAC data may partly explain why *Udotea* SPs, although not strong iron chelators, are able to protect cells from the oxidative stress caused by the presence of iron. We are interested in identifying other mechanisms that allow the *Udotea* SPs to act as protectors of cells exposed to oxidative stress caused by iron.

4. Materials and Methods

4.1. Materials

Iron (II) sulfate, potassium ferricianyde, sulfuric acid and acetonitrile were obtained from Merck (Darmstadt, Germany). Nitro Blue Tetrazolium (NBT), monosaccharides, methionine and ammonium molybdate were purchased from Sigma-Aldrich Co. (St. Louis, MO, USA). Cell culture medium components (Dulbecco's Modified Eagle Medium-DMEM), trypsin and newborn calf serum (FCS) were obtained from Cultilab (Campinas, Brazil). L-glutamine, sodium bicarbonate, sodium pyruvate and phosphate buffered saline (PBS) were purchased from Invitrogen Corporation (Burlington, ON, USA). All other solvents and chemicals were of analytical grade.

Eukaryotic cells—Mouse embryonic fibroblast cells (NIH/3T3 ATCC® CRL-1658™-3T3, Manassas, VA, USA) were grown in Dulbecco's modified Eagle's medium (DMEM) with 10% of fetal bovine serum (FBS), 10 mg/mL streptomycin, and 10,000 IU penicillin.

4.2. Extraction of Sulfated Polysaccharide-Rich Fractions

The seaweed *Udotea flabellum* was collected at Búzios Beach, Nísia Floresta-RN, Brazil. The alga was stored in our laboratory and dried at 50 °C under ventilation in an oven, ground in a blender and incubated with ethanol to eliminate lipids and pigments. About 90 g of powdered alga was suspended with five volumes of 0.25 M NaCl and the pH was adjusted to 8.0 with NaOH. Next, 900 mg of Prolav 750 (Prozyn Biosolutions, São Paulo, SP, Brazil), a mixture of alkaline proteases, was added for proteolytic digestion. After incubation for 24 h at 60 °C under agitation and periodical pH adjustments, the mixture was filtered through cheesecloth. The filtrate was fractionated by precipitation with acetone as follows: 0.3 volumes of ice-cold acetone was added to the solution under gentle agitation and maintained at 4 °C for 24 h. The precipitate formed was collected by centrifugation (10,000× *g*, 20 min), vacuum dried, resuspended in distilled water, and analyzed. The operation was repeated by adding 0.5, 0.6, 0.7, 1.0, and 2.0 volumes of acetone to the supernatant.

4.3. Chemical Analysis and Monosaccharide Composition

Sulfate content was determined according to the gelatin-barium method [27], using sodium sulfate (1 mg/mL) as standard and after acid hydrolysis of the polysaccharides (4 M HCl, 100 °C, 6 h). Protein content was measured using Spector's method [28]. The polysaccharides were hydrolyzed with 0.5, 1, 2, and 4 M, respectively, for various lengths of time, (0.5, 1, 2 and 4 h), at 100 °C. Reducing sugars were determined using the Somogyi-Nelson method [29]. After acid hydrolysis, sugar composition was determined by a LaChrom Elite® HPLC system from VWR-Hitachi (Hitachi, Ltd., Tokyo, Japan) with a refractive index detector (RI detector model L-2490). A LichroCART® 250-4 column (250 mm × 40 mm) packed with Lichrospher® 100 NH2 (5 µm) was coupled to the system. The sample mass used was 0.2 mg and analysis time was 25 min. The following sugars were analyzed as references: arabinose, fructose, fucose, galactose, glucose, glucosamine, glucuronic acid, mannose, and xylose.

4.4. 3-(4,5-dimethylthiazol-2-yl)-2,5-diphenyltetrazolium Bromide Test

For the tests, 0.5×10^4 cells were grown in 96-well plates with DMEM medium containing the samples in concentrations of 0.1, 0.5, 0.75 and 1 mg/mL for 24 h (each concentration in triplicate). The cell capacity to reduce MTT was determined by the colorimetric test of MTT as described earlier [30].

4.5. 5-bromo-2-deoxyuridine Incorporation

The cells (5×10^3 cells/well) were seeded into 96-well plates with 300 μL of fresh medium and incubated for 12 h at 37 °C and 5.0% CO_2. The medium was removed, the samples in DMEM medium was added to a final concentration between 0.1 and 1.0 mg/mL, and plates were incubated for 24 h, at 37 °C and 5.0% CO_2. After incubation, unbound samples were removed by washing the cells twice with 200 μL PBS and BrdU incorporation was determined according to manufacturer's instruction (BrdU cell proliferation assay kit-Cell Signaling, Danvers, MA, USA).

4.6. Induced Oxidative Stress Assay

3T3 cells (1×10^6 cells/mL) were placed in 6-well plates in de presence of 1 mL of DMEM supplemented with 10% FCS. After 24 h, the plates were washed and 1 mL of DMEM supplemented with 10% FCS and sulfated polysaccharides (0.1; 0.5; 0.75 or 1.0 mg/mL), $CuSO_4$ (1 μM, final concentration) or $FeSO_4$ (2 μM, final concentration) were added. 15 min after, 10 μL of 200 mM ascorbate acid (2 mM final concentration) was added. The plates were kept in culture condition (37 °C; 5% CO_2; dark) for 90 min; thus, the medium was replaced by 1 mL of the same fresh medium. After 24 h, the cells were submitted to MTT test as described above.

4.7. Caspase-3 and -9 Activity Assays

3T3 cells (1×10^6 cells/mL) were placed in 6-well plates in de presence of 1 mL of DMEM supplemented with 10% FCS. After 24 h, the plates were washed and 1 mL of DMEM supplemented with 10% FCS, $FeSO_4$, $CuSO_4$, ascorbate and/or sulfated polysaccharides (1 mg/mL) was added. After 90 min, the medium was replaced by fresh medium. 8, 16 and 24 h the plates were washed with ice-cold PBS and scraped into 200 mL lysis buffer (50 mM Tris-HCl (pH 7.4), 1% Tween 20, 0.25% sodium deoxycholate, 150 mM NaCl, 1 mM EDTA, 1 mM Na3VO4, 1 mM NaF], and protease inhibitors (1 mg/mL aprotinin, 10 mg/mL leupeptin and 1 mM 4-(2-aminoethyl) benzenesulfonyl fluoride) for 2 h in ice. The same conditions were used for untreated cells in the 0, 8, 16 and 24 h. Protein extracts were cleared by centrifugation and protein concentrations were determined using Bradford reagent [28] with bovine serum albumin as standard. In vitro caspase-3 and -9 protease activity was measured using a caspase activation kit according to the manufacturer's protocol (Invitrogen, São Paulo, Brazil). For this, 50 μL of cell lysate was mixed with 50 μL of 2x reaction buffer (containing 10 μL of 1 M dithiothreitol and 5 μL of 4 mM synthetic tetrapeptide Asp-Glue-Val (for caspase 3) or Leu-Glu-His-Asp (for caspase 9) conjugated top-nitroanilide (pNA)) in a 96-well plate, after which the mixture was incubated for 2 h at 37 °C in the dark. Active caspase cleaves the peptide and releases the chromophore pNA that can be detected spectrophotometrically at a wavelength of 405 nm. Theoretically, the apoptotic cell lysates containing active tested caspases should yield a considerable emission compared with the non-apoptotic cell lysates. Data presented are representative of those obtained in at least three independent experiments done in duplicates.

4.8. Superoxide Dismutase Evaluation

The SOD activity was measured using commercially available kit (SOD activity Enzo Life Sciences, Farmingdale, NY, USA). The principle of the method is based on the ability of SOD to neutralize superoxide ions created by the xanthine/xanthine oxidase system and subsequently inhibits the reduction of WST-1 (water soluble tetrazolium salt) to WST-1 formazan. Briefly, 3T3 fibroblasts (5×10^6 in six-well plate), obtained 24 h after oxidative stress induction, were washed with ice-cold

1× PBS, and lysed as described in kit protocol. The supernatant of each sample was collected, and the total SOD activity was assayed spectrophotometrically at 450 nm. SOD concentration, expressed in units per milligram of protein, was determined using the SOD standard curve.

4.9. Glutathione Evaluation

To assess the total level of glutathione, the 3T3 cells (5×10^6 in six-well plate), obtained 24 h after oxidative stress induction, were washed with ice-cold 1× PBS, removed, resuspended in PBS and centrifuged (3000× *g* at 4 °C) twice for 5 min. After this process, the suspension obtained was then diluted in 50% trichloroacetic acid (Vetec, São Paulo, SP, Brazil) and centrifuged during 15 min (3000× *g* at 4 °C). After, the cell supernatant was diluted with the same volume 0.4 M Tris buffer contained 0.01 M dithiobisnitrobenzoic (Sigma-Aldrich, São Paulo, SP, Brazil). The material was read at 412 nm. The results were expressed as nmol/10^6 cells.

4.10. Malonaldehyde Levels

To assess lipid peroxidation, malonaldehyde (MDA) production was measured with thiobarbituric acid reaction. Briefly, the cells under the same conditions as described above were triturated in 20 mM Tris-HCl buffer and centrifuged during 15 min (3000× *g* at 4 °C). The chromogenic reagent (10.3 mM 1-methyl-2-phenylindole in acetonitrile, 3:1 *v/v*), and a 37% solution of HCl were dropped to each supernatant sample (150 mL). The samples were kept at 45 °C for 40 min, and then were centrifuged (15 min; 3000× *g*; 4 °C). The absorbance was measured at 586 nm, and the results were expressed as nmol/10^6 cells.

4.11. Antioxidant Activity

Four assays were performed to analyze the antioxidant activity of the sulfated polysaccharides obtained: total antioxidant capacity, hydroxyl radical scavenging, superoxide radical scavenging, and ferric chelating, as previously described [11,23].

4.11.1. Determination of Total Antioxidant Capacity

This assay is based on the reduction of Mo (VI) to Mo (V) by sulfated polysaccharides and subsequent formation of a green phosphate/Mo(V) complex at acid pH. Tubes containing sulfated polysaccharides and reagent solution (0.6 M sulfuric acid, 28 mM sodium phosphate and 4 mM ammonium molybdate) were incubated at 95 °C for 90 min. After the mixture had cooled to room temperature, the absorbance of each solution was measured at 695 nm against a blank. Total antioxidant capacity was expressed as ascorbic acid equivalent.

4.11.2. Hydroxyl Radical Scavenging Activity Assay

The scavenging activity of seaweed polysaccharides against the hydroxyl radical was investigated using Fenton's reaction ($Fe^{2+} + H_2O_2 \rightarrow Fe^{3+} + OH^- + OH$). These results were expressed as inhibition rate. Hydroxyl radicals were generated using 3 mL sodium phosphate buffer (150 mM, pH 7.4), which contained 10 mM $FeSO_4.7H_2O$, 10 mM EDTA, 2 mM sodium salicylate, 30% H_2O_2 (200 mL) and varying polysaccharide concentrations. In the control, sodium phosphate buffer replaced H_2O_2. The solutions were incubated at 37 °C for 1 h, and the presence of the hydroxyl radical was detected by monitoring absorbance at 510 nm. Gallic acid was used as positive control.

4.11.3. Superoxide Radical Scavenging Activity Assay

This assay was based on the capacity of sulfated polysaccharides to inhibit the photochemical reduction of NBT in the riboflavin–light–NBT system. Each 3 mL of reaction mixture contained 50 mM phosphate buffer (pH 7.8), 13 mM methionine, 2 mM riboflavin, 100 mM EDTA, NBT (75 mM) and 1 mL sample solution. After the production of blue formazan, the increase in absorbance at 560 nm after 10 min illumination from a fluorescent lamp was determined. The entire reaction assembly was enclosed in a box lined with aluminum foil. Identical tubes with the reaction mixture were kept in the dark and served as blanks. Gallic acid was used as positive control.

4.11.4. Ferric Chelating

The ferrous ion chelating ability of samples was investigated using the following methodology: sulfated polysaccharides at different concentrations were applied with the reaction mixture, which contained $FeCl_2$ (0.05 mL, 2 mM) and ferrozine (0.2 mL, 5 mM). The mixture was shaken and incubated for 10 min at room temperature and absorbance of the mixture was measured at 562 nm against a blank. EDTA was used as positive control.

4.11.5. Cupric Chelating

Pyrocatechol violet, the reagent used in this assay, has the ability to associate with certain cations such as aluminum, copper, bismuth, and thorium. In the presence of chelating agents this combination is not formed, resulting in decreased staining. This reduction thus allows the estimation of the chelating activity of the copper ion from the fraction from *U. flabellum*. The test is performed in 96-well microplates with a reaction mixture containing different concentrations of samples (0.1–20 mg/mL), pyrocatechol violet (4 mM), and copper II sulfate pentahydrate (50 mg/mL). All wells were homogenized with the aid of a micropipette and the solution absorbance was measured at 632 nm. The ability of the samples in chelating the copper ion was calculated using the following equation:

$$(\text{Absorbance of blank}) - (\text{Absorbance of the sample})/(\text{Absorbance of the blank}) \times 100$$

4.12. Electrophoresis in Agarose Gel

Agarose gel electrophoresis of the acidic polysaccharides was performed in 0.6% agarose gel (7.5 cm × 10 cm × 0.2 cm thick) prepared in 0.05 M 1.3-diaminopropane acetate buffer pH 9.0, as previously described [15]. Aliquots of the polysaccharides (about 50 μg) were applied to the gel and subjected to electrophoresis. The gel was fixed with 0.1% cetyltrimethylammonium bromide solution for 2 h, dried, and stained for 15 min with 0.1% toluidine blue in 1% acetic acid in 50% ethanol. The gel was then destained with the same solution without the dye.

4.13. Statistical Analysis

All data were expressed as mean ± standard deviation of three observation ($n = 3$). Statistical analysis was done by one-way analysis of variance (ANOVA) followed by the Turkey-Kramer test. All tests were conducted on the SigmaPlot® (Systat software, San Jose, CA, USA). In all cases, statistical significance was set at $p < 0.05$.

5. Conclusions

We obtained six antioxidant sulfated polysaccharide-rich fractions from the green alga *U. flabellum*. These fractions mainly comprised heterogalactans, and were designated UF-0.3, UF-0.5, UF-0.6, UF-0.7, UF-1.0, and UF-2.0. None of the fractions exhibited cytotoxicity or inhibited 3T3 fibroblast proliferation. The four fractions that were assessed protected the cells from oxidative damage. UF-2.0 was the most effective in reducing oxidative stress when the cells were exposed to CuSO4; this can be attributed to the copper chelating ability of the fraction. The most effective fraction in mitigating oxidative stress in the presence of FeSO4 was UF-0.7. However, this effectiveness cannot be attributed solely to the ability of the fractions to chelate iron.

Our aims for future studies include identification of other mechanisms involved in mitigation of oxidative stress caused by compounds of iron and the role of sulfated polysaccharides in such mitigation. In addition, as UF-0.7 showed notable protective activity both in the presence of copper and iron, we intend to assess its effect in vivo to identify its role as a putative drug to be used for the treatment of diseases associated with elevated levels of copper and/or iron.

Acknowledgments: The authors wish to thank Conselho Nacional de Desenvolvimento Científico e Tecnológico-CNPq (National Council for Scientific and Technological Advancement, in loose translation), Coordenação de Aperfeiçoamento Pessoal de Nível Superior-CAPES (Higher Level Personal Development Coordination, in loose translation), Programa Nacional de Cooperação Acadêmica (PROCAD), Ciências do Mar/CAPES, and Ministério de Ciência, Tecnologia, Inovação e Comércio (MCTIC) (the Science and Technology Ministry in Brazil, in loose translation) for the financial support. Hugo Rocha is an honored researcher of the CNPq. The authors would like to thank the Department of Biochemistry at Universidade Federal do Rio Grande do Norte for letting us use the cell culture room. This research was presented at Programa de Pós-Graduação em Ciências da Saúde at Universidade Federal do Rio Grande do Norte, as part of the M.Sc. thesis of Fernando Presa.

Author Contributions: Fernando Bastos Presa prepared the samples. Fernando Bastos Presa and Maxsuell Lucas Mendes Marques performed the chemical analysis. Fernando Bastos Presa, Leonardo Thiago Duarte Barreto Nobre, Rony Lucas Silva Viana, Leandro Silva Costa and Maxsuell Lucas Mendes Marques performed tests with the 3T3-cells. Fernando Bastos Presa performed the antioxidant tests. Fernando Bastos Presa and Maxsuell Lucas Mendes Marques analyzed the data. Fernando Bastos Presa, Maxsuell Lucas Mendes Marques and Hugo Alexandre Oliveira Rocha wrote the paper. Leandro Silva Costa and Hugo Alexandre Oliveira Rocha funded and revised the paper.

References

1. Kremastinos, D.T.; Farmakis, D. Iron overload cardiomyopathy in clinical practice. *Contemp. Rev. Cardiovasc. Med.* **2011**, *124*, 2253–2263. [CrossRef]
2. Dong, Q.; Wu, Z. Advance in the pathogenesis and treatment of Wilson disease. *Transl. Neurodegener.* **2012**, *1*, 1–8. [CrossRef]
3. Dixon, S.J.; Stockwell, B.R. The role of iron and reactive oxygen species in cell death. *Nat. Chem. Biol.* **2014**, *10*, 9–17. [CrossRef]
4. Brewer, G.J. Novel therapeutic approaches to the treatment of Wilson's disease. *Expert Opin. Pharmacother.* **2006**, *7*, 317–324. [CrossRef]
5. Hansen, J.B.; Moen, I.W.; Mandrup-Poulsen, T. Iron: The hard player in diabetes pathophysiology. *Acta Physiol.* **2014**, *210*, 717–732. [CrossRef]
6. Campo, G.M.; D'Ascola, A.; Avenoso, A.; Campo, S.; Ferlazzo, A.M.; Micali, C.; Zanghí, L.; Calatroni, A. Glycosaminoglycans reduce oxidative damage induced by copper (Cu^{+2}), iron (Fe^{+2}) and hydrogen peroxide (H_2O_2) in human fibroblast cultures. *Glycoconj. J.* **2004**, *2*, 133–141. [CrossRef]
7. Negreiros, M.M.F.; Almeida-Lima, J.; Rocha, H.A.O. Sulfated Polysaccharides from Unusual Natural Sources. In *Sulfated Polysaccharides*, 1st ed.; Gama, M., Nader, H.B., Rocha, H.A.O., Eds.; Nova Science Publishers: New York, NY, USA, 2015; Volume 1, pp. 217–234, ISBN 978-1-63482-975-5.
8. Shao, P.; Chen, X.X.; Sun, P.L. In vitro antioxidant and antitumor activities of different sulfated polysaccharides isolated from three algae. *Int. J. Biol. Macromol.* **2013**, *62*, 155–161. [CrossRef]
9. Qi, H.; Zhang, Q.; Zhao, T.; Chen, R.; Zhang, H.; Niu, X.; LI, Z. Antioxidant activity of different sulfate content derivatives of polysaccharide extracted from *Ulva pertusa* (Chlorophyta) in vitro. *Int. J. Biol. Macromol.* **2005**, *4*, 15–37. [CrossRef]
10. Costa, M.S.S.P.; Costa, L.S.; Cordeiro, S.L.; Almeida-Lima, J.; Santos, N.D.; Magalhães, K.D.; Sabry, D.A.; Albuquerque, I.R.L.; Pereira, M.R.; Leite, E.L.; et al. Evalutaing the possible anticoagulant and antioxidant effects of sulfated polysaccharides from the tropical green alga *Caulerpa cupressoides* var. Flabellata. *J. Appl. Phycol.* **2012**, *24*, 1159–1167. [CrossRef]
11. Costa, L.S.; Fidelis, G.P.; Cordeiro, S.L.; Oliveira, R.M.; Sabry, D.A.; Câmara, R.B.; Nobre, L.T.; Costa, M.S.; Almeida-Lima, J.; Farias, E.H.; et al. Biological activities of sulfated polysaccharides from tropical seaweeds. *Biomed. Pharmacother.* **2010**, *64*, 21–28. [CrossRef]
12. Farias, E.H.; Pomin, V.H.; Valente, A.P.; Nader, H.B.; Rocha, H.A.; Mourão, P.A. A preponderantly 4-sulfated, 3-linked galactan from the green alga *Codium isthmocladum*. *Glycobiology* **2008**, *3*, 250–259. [CrossRef]
13. Arata, P.X.; Quintana, I.; Raffo, M.P.; Ciancia, M. Novel sulfated xylogalactoarabinans from green seaweed *Cladophora falklandica*: Chemical structure and action on the fibrin network. *Carbohydr. Polym.* **2016**, *154*, 139–150. [CrossRef]

14. Alves, A. Sulfated Polysaccharides from Green Seaweed. In *Sulfated Polysaccharides*, 1st ed.; Gama, M., Nader, H.B., Rocha, H.A.O., Eds.; Nova Science Publishers: New York, NY, USA, 2015; Volume 1, pp. 135–153, ISBN 978-1-63482-975-5.
15. Dietrich, C.P.; Dietrich, S.M. Electrophoretic behaviour of acidic mucopolysaccharides in diamine buffers. *Anal. Biochem.* **1976**, *70*, 645–647. [CrossRef]
16. Hayakawa, Y.; Hayashi, T.; Lee, J.; Srisomporn, P.; Maeda, M.; Ozawa, T.; Sakuragawa, N. Inhibition of thrombin by sulfated polysaccharides isolated from green algae. *Biochim. Biophys. Acta* **2000**, *1543*, 86–94. [CrossRef]
17. Wenjun Mao, W.; Zang, X.; Li, Y.; Zhang, H. Sulfated polysaccharides from marine green algae *Ulva conglobata* and their anticoagulant activity. *J. Appl.* **2006**, *18*, 9–14. [CrossRef]
18. Valko, M.; Leibfritz, D.; Moncol, J.; Cronin, M.T.; Mazur, M.; Telser, J. Free radicals and antioxidants in normal physiological functions and human disease. *Int. J. Biochem. Cell Biol.* **2007**, *39*, 44–84. [CrossRef]
19. Jomova, K.; Vondrakova, D.; Lawson, M.; Valko, M. Metals, oxidative stress and neurodegenerative disorders. *Mol. Cell. Biochem.* **2010**, *345*, 91–104. [CrossRef]
20. Nappi, A.J.; Vass, E. Comparative studies of enhanced iron-mediated production of hydroxyl radical by glutathione, cysteine, ascorbic acid, and selected catechols. *Biochim. Biophys. Acta* **1997**, *1336*, 295–301. [CrossRef]
21. Mak, W.; Hamid, N.; Liu, T.; Lu, J.; White, W.L. Fucoidan from New Zealand *Undaria pinnatifida*: Monthly variations and determination of antioxidant activities. *Carbohydr. Polym.* **2013**, *95*, 606–614. [CrossRef]
22. Melo, K.R.; Câmara, R.B.; Queiroz, M.F.; Vidal, A.A.; Lima, C.R.; Melo-Silveira, R.F.; Almeida-Lima, J.; Rocha, H.A. Evaluation of sulfated polysaccharides from the brown seaweed *Dictyopteris justii* as antioxidant agents and as inhibitors of the formation of calcium oxalate crystals. *Molecules* **2013**, *25*, 14543–14563. [CrossRef]
23. Galinari, E.; Almeida-Lima, J.; Macedo, G.R.; Mantovani, H.C.; Rocha, H.A. Antioxidant, antiproliferative, and immunostimulatory effects of cellwall-d-mannan fractions from *Kluyveromyces marxianu*. *Int. J. Biol. Macromol.* **2018**, *109*, 837–846. [CrossRef]
24. Oral, B.; Guney, M.; Demirin, H.; Ozguner, M.; Giray, S.G.; Take, G.; Mungan, T.; Altuntas, I. Endometrial damage and apoptosis in rats induced by dichlorvos and ameliorating effect of antioxidant vitamins E and C. *Reprod. Toxicol.* **2006**, *22*, 783–790. [CrossRef]
25. Knigth, J.A. Review: Free radicals, antioxidants, and the immune System. *Ann. Clin. Lab. Sci.* **2000**, *30*, 145–158.
26. Campo, G.M.; Avenoso, A.; Campo, S.; D'Ascola, A.; Traina, P.; Samà, D.; Calatroni, A. NF-kB and caspases are involved in the hyaluronan and chondroitin-4-sulphate-exerted antioxidant effect in fibroblast cultures exposed to oxidative stress. *J. Appl. Toxicol.* **2008**, *28*, 509–517. [CrossRef]
27. Dodgson, K.S.; Price, R.G. A note on the determination of the ester sulphate content of sulphated polysaccharides. *Biochem. J.* **1962**, *84*, 106–110.
28. Spector, J. Refinement of the coomassie blue method of protein quantification. A simple and linear spectrophotometric assay of 0.5 to 50 μg of protein. *Anal. Biochem.* **1978**, *86*, 142–143. [CrossRef]
29. Somogyi, M. Notes on sugar determination. *J. Biol. Chem.* **1952**, *195*, 19–23.
30. Rocha-Amorim, M.O.; Gomes, D.L.; Dantas, L.A.; Viana, R.L.S.; Chiquetti, S.C.; Almeida-Lima, J.; Silva Costa, L.; Rocha, H.A.O. Fucan-coated silver nanoparticles synthesized by a green method induce human renal adenocarcinoma cell death. *Int. J. Biol. Macromol.* **2016**, *93*, 57–65. [CrossRef]

4

Medicinal Plants Used for Neuropsychiatric Disorders Treatment in the Hauts Bassins Region of Burkina Faso

Prosper T. Kinda [1], Patrice Zerbo [2], Samson Guenné [1], Moussa Compaoré [1], Alin Ciobica [3] and Martin Kiendrebeogo [1,*]

1 Laboratoire de Biochimie et Chimie Appliquées, Université Ouaga I-Pr Joseph KI-ZERBO, 03 PB 7021 Ouagadougou 03, Burkina Faso; pros.kinda@hotmail.fr (P.T.K.); guesams@gmail.com (S.G.); mcompaore_3@yahoo.fr (M.C.)

2 Laboratoire de Biologie et écologie végétale, Université Ouaga I-Pr Joseph KI-ZERBO, 03 BP 7021 Ouagadougou 03, Burkina Faso; patzerbo@yahoo.fr

3 "Alexandru Ioan Cuza" University of Iasi, Faculty of Biology, Department of Research, Carol I Avenue, No. 20A, Iasi 700505, Romania; alin.ciobica@uaic.ro

* Correspondence: martinkiendrebeogo@yahoo.co.uk

Academic Editor: James D. Adams

Abstract: Background: In Burkina Faso, phytotherapy is the main medical alternative used by populations to manage various diseases that affect the nervous system. The aim of the present study was to report medicinal plants with psychoactive properties used to treat neuropsychiatric disorders in the Hauts Bassins region, in the western zone of Burkina Faso. **Methods:** Through an ethnobotanical survey using structured questionnaire, 53 traditional healers (TH) were interviewed about neuropsychiatric disorders, medicinal plants and medical practices used to treat them. The survey was carried out over a period of three months. **Results:** The results report 66 plant species used to treat neuropsychiatric pathologies. Roots (36.2%) and leaves (29%) were the main plant parts used. Alone or associated, these parts were used to prepare drugs using mainly the decoction and the trituration methods. Remedies were administered via drink, fumigation and external applications. **Conclusions:** It appears from this study a real knowledge of neuropsychiatric disorders in the traditional medicine of Hauts Bassins area. The therapeutic remedies suggested in this work are a real interest in the fight against psychiatric and neurological diseases. In the future, identified plants could be used for searching antipsychotic or neuroprotective compounds.

Keywords: Neuropsychiatry; phytotherapy; traditional healers; Burkina Faso

1. Introduction

Nowadays, medicinal plant use in traditional therapy is increasing and diversifying. These plants were a precious patrimony for the humanity in general and particularly very important for developing countries people's healthcare and their subsistence [1]. They are invaluable resources for the great majority of rural populations in Africa, where more than 80% use them to ensure their primary healthcare [2]. According to the World Health Organization (WHO), neuropsychiatric disorders are a whole of "mental health problems", which are characterized by anomalies of the thought, emotions, behavior and relationship with others. These pathologies handicap the person concerned and assign people of its circle. Factors causing these disorders are essentially genetic, social, environmental and psychotropic drugs. Mental and neurological disorders represent 13% of the burden of total morbidity in the world [3]. Thirteen per cent to 49% of the world's populations develop neuropsychiatric disorders at some point in their life [4]. These pathologies affect all categories of person, race, sex and age [5]. Epilepsy is one of the most common neurological disorders. It affects more than 50 million persons in the world including 80% in developing countries [6]. High prevalence was observed in Africa where about 75% of patients do not receive adequate treatment [7]. The prejudices that surround neuropsychiatric diseases are causes of stigmatization of unwell persons who are often marginalized [3,8]. In Burkina Faso, 175‰ of the cases of disability are caused by neuropsychiatric disorders [6].

Many natural or synthetic psychoactive molecules such as neuroleptics, antidepressants, anxiolytics are used in modern medicine to treat these pathologies, particularly epilepsy, schizophrenia and the others psychotic disorders [8–10]. However, these modern treatments are expensive, complex and inaccessible for African populations in rural area [8,11]. Many of these psychoactive molecules have plant origins [12,13], which could justify plants use in the African traditional medicine to treat neuropsychiatric diseases [14,15]. In Burkina Faso, medicinal plants are widely used by peoples. Disapproved a long time after independences period for allopathic drugs [16], the government allowed in 1994 the traditional medicine practice. Since this time, it appeared a craze more and more growing for phytotherapy within the population, already predisposed to be directed there [17]. Moreover, many studies were undertaken to document plant species used in this therapy practice [18–22].

However, little research has approached the specific case of plants used to treat nervous system disorders in Burkina Faso. In the Hauts Bassins region, these pathologies were frequently denoted in psychiatric consultation [23,24]. Except Millogo's group works on "epilepsy and traditional medicine in Bobo-Dioulasso" [25], the traditional therapy of these pathologies is quoted only in other parallel studies. The present study aims to provide information about medicinal plants used to treat neuropsychiatric disorders in the Hauts Bassins region of Burkina Faso. It was necessary to report psychic and neurological disorders treated by traditional healers, medicinal plants and medical practices used for these treatments.

2. Materials and Methods

2.1. Study Area

The study was carried out in the Hauts Bassins region, located in western part of Burkina Faso (Figure 1). This area is known for its high phytogenetical and cultural diversity. Located at the West of Burkina Faso, between 9°21′N latitude and 2°27′W longitude, the Hauts Bassins region belongs to the phytogeographical sector of south-soudanien, characterized by average annual precipitations higher than 900 millimeters and average temperatures oscillating between 25 °C and 30 °C [26]. This sector is dominated by vegetable formations of savannas type timbered, arboreous or shrubby [27]. Several ethnics groups live in this area with a great diversity of cultural practices. The main spoken languages are Mooré (29.5%), Dioula (27.1%) and Bobo (18.8%) [28]. This region is characterized by a high number of traditional healers (TH) resulting from various ethnic groups. In addition to plant diversity and neuropsychiatric diseases frequency [24], the area was chosen because of the presence of various TH.

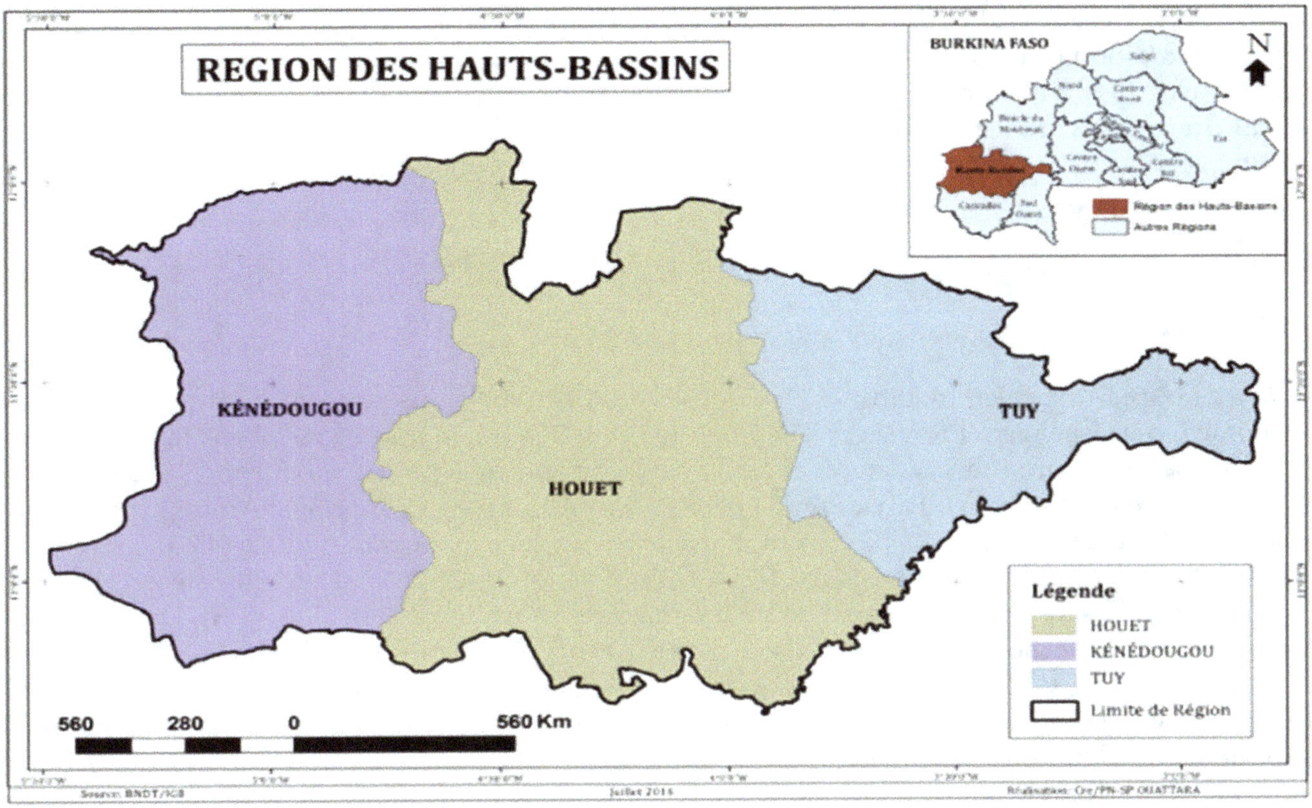

Figure 1. Study area localization (Hauts Bassins region of Burkina Faso).

2.2. Ethnobotanical Data Collection

The ethnobotanical survey was carried out during a three month period from October to December 2015. Data were collected using a structured interview with traditional healers (TH) who are organized in association. Through the association, a preliminary phone call was had with TH to inform them about objectives of the study. After that, an appointment were fixed with each one for individual interview. The approach was based on a dialogue using one of the three languages (Mooré, Dioula or French) to the TH choice. Pre-established questionnaires were used and a local person acting as a guide was necessary. Data were collected and transcribed on survey card-guides. It concerned medicinal plants used to treat the main psychiatric and neurological diseases such as epilepsy, mental disorders or madness, evils related to charm or witchcraft, hallucination or consciousness loss. These pathologies were reported to be more frequent in this area of Burkina Faso [24]. We gathered some of them because of their names in the local languages. Other collected information related to local names (in Mooré and/or Dioula) of plants, organs used of plants and medical practices such as drugs preparation and administration methods. Fifty-three TH including 35 men and 18 women, old from 31 to 82 years and having experience of plants use in traditional medicine were interviewed. Plants mentioned in the interview were collected in order to make the herbal constitution.

2.3. Data Analysis

Samples of plants collected were identified by botanists of the Ecology Department of University of Ouaga I-Pr Joseph Ki Zerbo (Burkina Faso). Then, voucher specimens were deposited in the herbarium of this University. The adopted nomenclature is that of "the tropical flora of Western Africa" [29], "medicinal plants and traditional medical practices in Burkina Faso" [30], "the catalogue of vascular plants of Burkina Faso" [31] and some enumerations of tropical Africa plants [32–34]. Plant parts used and medical practices were listed. Data were analyzed using SPSS software version 17.0 for window (SPSS Inc., Chicago, USA), and graphs were made on Excel of Office 2013.

3. Results

3.1. Plants Species Used

Sixty-six plant species including 51 woody and 15 herbaceous used to treat psychiatric and neurological diseases were identified. They belonged to 56 genera and 32 families (Table 1). Acacia and Ficus Genera were the most represented with 4 species each. The most represented families were Mimosaceae (8 species), Fabaceae (5 species) and Rubiaceae (5 species). Among these plants, the most used were showed on Table 2. A high use of Securidaca longepedunculata (45.3%), Calotropis procera (20.75%), Khaya senegalensis (20.75%), Allium sativum (20.75%), Daniellia oliveri (19%) and Annona senegalensis (17%) was observed by the majority of traditional healers (TH). Datura innoxia and Zanthoxlum zanthoxyloïdes were used by the oldest TH (more than 60 year old). Six species: S. longepedunculata, C. procera, K. senegalensis, A. senegalensis, Diospyros mespiliformis and Guiera Senegalensis were used to treat the main diseases targeted. Most of the plants were used alone and in association with other plants.

3.2. Plant Parts Used and Medical Practices

Various plant parts were used to prepare remedies (Figure 2a). Roots were mainly used (36.2%), followed by leaves (29%), mistletoes (9.3%) and stem barks (9%). Drugs preparation modes were the decoction (46.7%), the trituration (31%), the calcination (11.6%) and the aqueous maceration (10.7%) (Figure 2b). The drink (40.8%), the bath (33.8%), the fumigation (14.8%) and the massage (8.4%) are the main modes of administration (Figure 2c).

3.3. Neuropsychiatric Pathologies Treated

Diseases or regrouping diseases treated by traditional healers were registered in Table 3. From these results, hallucination or consciousness loss were most treated, followed by epilepsy, mental disorders and witchcraft or evils related to charm. In addition to these target pathologies, other cases such as insomnia and nerves diseases are also treated. Several plant species intervene in the treatment of each listed disorders. Thus, 37 plants were used to treat hallucination or consciousness loss, 32 to treat mental disorders, 31 to fight against epilepsy and 25 against diseases related to charm or witchcraft.

Table 1. Global information on plants used in various treatments.

Scientific Name (Genera and Specie)	Family	Local Name (Mooré)	Local Name (Dioula)	Parts Used	Mode of Preparation	Mode of Administration	Pathologies Treated
Abrus precatorius L.	Fabaceae	Noraog-nini	Noronha	Fr	Cal	Mas	MA-MD
Acacia ataxacantha DC.	Mimosaceae	Kanguin pèelga		Ro, Ba	Dec	Bat, Dri	EP
Acacia nilotica (L.) Willd. Ex Del.	Mimosaceae	Peg-nenga	Bangana	Ro	Dec	Bat, Dri	MA-MD
Acacia pennata (L.) Willd	Mimosaceae	Kanguinga		Ro	Dec	Bat, Dri	EP
Acacia sieberiana DC.	Mimosaceae	Gor-ponsego	Wenekassango	Le, Ro, Ba	Mac, Dec, Tri	Bat, Dri, Fum, Mas	MA-MD, HA-CL
Adansonia digitata L.	Bombacaceae	Tohèga	Sira-yiri	Le, Ro	Dec, Cal	Bat, Dri, Fum	MA-MD, HA-CL
Afzelia africana Smith ex Pers.	Caesalpiniaceae	Kankalga	Lingué, Lingué yiri	Le, Ro, Ba, Mi	Dec, Cal, Tri	Bat, Dri, Fum	MA-MD, HA-CL
Allium cepa L.	Liliaceae	Zéyon	Djaba	Bu	Tri	Fum	EP
Allium sativum L.	Liliaceae	Layi		Bu	Dec, Cal, Tri	Bat, Dri, Fum, Pur, Mas	MA-MD, HA-CL
Annona senegalensis Pers.	Annonaceae	Barkudga	Mandé sunsun, Barkandé	Wp, Le, Ro, Ba	Dec, Cal, Tri	Bat, Dri, Fum, Mas	EP, MA-MD, CH-WI, HA-CL
Anogeissus leiocarpus (DC) Guill. & Perr.	Combretaceae	Siiga		Ba	Mac	Bat, Dri	HA-CL
Balanites aegyptiaca L.	Balanitaceae	Kyeguelga	Zèguenè	Le, Ro	Dec	Bat, Dri	MA-MD, CH-WI
Boscia senegalensis (Pers) Lam. ex Poir.	Capparidaceae	Lambwetga	Bere	Le, Ro	Dec	Bat, Dri	EP
Boswellia dalzielii Hutch	Burseraceae	Gondregneogo, Kondregneogo		Ro, Ba	Mac, Dec, Tri	Bat, Dri, Fum	HA-CL
Calotropis procera (Ait) Ait. F.	Asclepiadaceae	Putrepuuga	Fogofogo	Wp, Le, Ro, Mi, La	Mac, Dec, Tri	Bat, Dri, Fum, Ing	EP, MA-MD, CH-WI, HA-CL
Ceiba pentandra (L.) Gaertn	Bombacaceae	Gounga	Bana-yiri	Ro	Cal	Dri	EP
Cissus quadrangularis L.	Vitaceae	Wob-Zanré	Oulouyoroko	St	Cal	Dri	EP
Citrus aurantifolia (Christm.) Swingle	Rutaceae	Lembur-tiiga	Laimbourou	Fr, Mi	Mac, Dec, Cal	Bat, Dri, Mas	MA-MD, CH-WI, HA-CL
Crateva adansonii DC.	Capparidaceae	Kalguem-tohèga		Le	Dec	Dri	CH-WI
Cymbopogon giganteus Chiov.	Poaceae	Kuwaré	Tiékala	Le, Ro	Dec	Bat, Dri	MA-MD, HA-CL
Cymbopogon proximus (Hochst ex A. Rich) Stapf	Poaceae	Soompiiga		Wp, Ro	Cal	Dri	CH-WI
Dalbergia melanoxylon Guill. & Perr.	Fabaceae	Guirdiandéga		Ro	Mac	Fum	MA-MD, HA-CL
Daniellia oliveri (Rolfe) Hutch et Dalz	Caesalpiniaceae	Aoga, Anwga	sana, sana yiri	Le, Ro, Ba, Mi	Mac, Dec, Cal, Tri	Bat, Dri, Fum	MA-MD, CH-WI, HA-CL
Datura innoxia Mill.	Solanaceae	Barassé, Zèèbla	Alomoukaïkaï	Le, Fr	Cal	Dri, Mas	MA-MD,CH-WI, HA-CL,IN,ND
Detarium microcarpum Guill. & Perr.	Caesalpiniaceae	kagadéga	Tamakouma	Le, Ro	Dec	Bat, Dri	EP, CH-WI, HA-CL
Diospyros mespiliformis Hochst ex A. DC	Ebenaceae	Gaaka, Gaanka	Sounsoun, Sounsounfi	Le, Ro	Mac, Dec	Bat, Dri	EP, MA-MD, CH-WI, HA-CL
Entada africana Guill. & Perr.	Mimosaceae	Séonego		Ro	Dec	Bat, Dri	EP
Faidherbia albida (Del.) A. Chev.	Mimosaceae	Zaanga	Balanzan, Balãzã	Le, Ro	Dec	Bat, Dri	CH-WI

Table 1. *Cont.*

Scientific Name (Genera and Specie)	Family	Local Name (Mooré)	Local Name (Dioula)	Parts Used	Mode of Preparation	Mode of Administration	Pathologies Treated
Ficus ingens (Miq.) Miq.	Moraceae	Kunkwiga		Ro	Dec	Dri	EP
Ficus iteophylla Miq.	Moraceae	Kunkwi-pèelga	Djetigui faaga, Diatiguifaga	Le, Ro, Ba	Mac, Dec	Bat, Dri	EP, MA-MD, HA-CL
Ficus sycomorus L.	Moraceae	Kankanga	Toro, toro yiri	Le, Ro, Mi	Dec, Tri	Bat, Dri	EP, HA-CL
Ficus vallis-choudae Delile	Moraceae		Torossaba, Toroba	Le	Dec	Bat, Dri	EP
Flueggea virosa (Roxb ex. Willd) Voigt.	Euphorbiaceae	Sugdin-daaga	Balabala, Bala-bala	Le, Ro	Dec	Bat, Dri	CH-WI
Gardenia sp.	Rubiaceae	Subudga, Lambrezunga	Bure, Buré yiri	Wp, Le, St, Ro	Dec, Cal	Bat, Dri	EP, CH-WI, HA-CL
Guiera senegalensis J.F. Gmel	Combretaceae	Wilin-wiiga	Koungouè, Kungouè	Wp, Le, Ro, Mi	Dec, Cal, Tri	Bat, Dri	EP, MA-MD, CH-WI, HA-CL
Hygrophila senegalensis (Nees) T. Anderson	Acanthaceae		Kelebetokala, Klebato-yiri	Le	Mac, Dec	Bat, Dri	EP
Hyptis spicigera Lam.	Lamiaceae	Rung-rungui	Timitimini.	Wp	Dec	Bat, Dri	EP
Indigofera tinctoria L.	Fabaceae	Garga		Le	Tri	Pur	HA-CL
Khaya senegalensis (Desr) A. Juss	Meliaceae	Kuka	Diala, Djala	Le, Ba, Mi	Mac, Dec, Cal, Tri	Bat, Dri, Fum	EP, MA-MD, CH-WI, HA-CL
Lannea acida A. Rich	Anacardiaceae	Labtulga		Le, Ro, Ba	Dec, Tri	Bat, Dri	EP, HA-CL
Leptadenia hastata (Pers.) Decne	Asclepiadaceae	Lelongo	Kosafla	Wp, Le, St, Ro	Dec	Bat, Dri	MA-MD, HA-CL
Mitracarpus villosus (SW.) DC.	Rubiaceae	Yod-pèelga		Wp	Tri	Fum	MA-MD
Mitragyna inermis (Willd) O. Ktze	Rubiaceae	Yiilga	Djou, Diou, Jun, dioum	Wp, Le, Ro	Dec, Tri	Bat, Dri, Fum	EP, MA-MD, HA-CL
Moringa oleifera Lam.	Moringaceae	Arzan-tiiga	Masa yiri	Ro	Dec	Bat, Dri, Fum	MA-MD
Nicotiana rustica L.	Solanaceae	Kinkirs taba, Waamb-tabré	Flavourou	Le	Tri	Fum	HA-CL
Nicotina tabacum L.	Solanaceae	Taba	Kotaba	Le	Cal	Dri, Mas	CH-WI
Ocimum americanum L.	Lamiaceae	Yulin-gnu-raaga	Sukuola	Wp, Le	Dec, Tri	Bat, Fum	EP, HA-CL
Ocimum basilicum L.	Lamiaceae	Yulin-gnuuga	Sukuola-sina	Le	Tri	Fum	HA-CL
Parkia biglobosa (Jacq.) R. BR. ex G. Don. F	Mimosaceae	Roaaga	Nèrè	Le, Ro, Mi	Mac, Dec	Bat, Dri	EP, MA-MD, CH-WI
Pennisetum americanum Stapf	Poaceae	Kazui	Sagnon	Fr	Tri	Pur	EP, CH-WI
Pericopsis laxiflora (BentH ex Bak.) V. Meeawen	Fabaceae	Taankoniliga,	Kolo-kolo, Kolokolo yiri	Le, St	Dec, Tri	Bat, Dri, Fum	MA-MD, HA-CL
Prosopis africana (Guill. Perr. & Rich) Taub.	Mimosaceae	Duanduanga, yamagui	Goulé, Gouélé	Ro, Fr	Dec, Cal	Bat, Dri	CH-WI
Pseudocedrela kotschyi (Schweinf.) Harms	Meliaceae	Siguédré		Le	Dec	Bat, Dri	MA-MD, HA-CL
Saba senegalensis (A. DC) Pichon	Apocynaceae	wèdga	Zaban yiri	Ro	Dec	Bat	HA-CL
Sclerocarya birrea (A. Rich) Hochst	Anacardiaceae	noabga		Le, Ba	Dec	Dri	EP
Scoparia dulcis L.	Scrophulariaceae	Kafremaandé		Wp	Tri	Fum	MA-MD, HA-CL

Table 1. *Cont.*

Scientific Name (Genera and Specie)	Family	Local Name (Mooré)	Local Name (Dioula)	Parts Used	Mode of Preparation	Mode of Administration	Pathologies Treated
Securidaca longepedunculata Fresen	Polygalaceae	Pèlga	Djoro, Diouro	Le, Ro, Ba	Mac, Dec, Cal, Tri	Bat, Dri, Fum, Pur, Mas	EP, MA-MD, CH-WI, HA-CL
Sterculia setigera Del.	Sterculiaceae	Ponsemporgo, Putermuka	Congo-sera, Kongossira	Ro, Mi	Dec	Bat, Dri	EP
Strychnos spinosa Lam.	Loganiaceae	Katrepoaga, Katerpoagha	Kogobaranie, Fouflé barani	Fr	Tri	Ing	CH-WI
Stylosanthes erecta P. Beauv.	Fabaceae	Sakwisabelga		Wp	Cal	Mas	CH-WI
Tamarindus indica L.	Caesalpiniaceae	Pusga	Ntomi, Toni	Le, Ro, Fr, Mi	Mac, Dec, Tri	Bat, Dri, Fum	EP, MA-MD, HA-CL
Vitellaria paradoxa C.F. Gaertn	Sapotaceae	Taanga	Schi yiri, Si yiri	Le, Ro, Mi	Dec, Tri	Bat, Dri, Fum	MA-MD, CH-WI, HA-CL
Vitex doniana Sweet	Verbenaceae	Aadga	Koto	Le, Ro	Dec	Bat, Dri	MA-MD
Ximenia americana L.	Olacaceae	Leenga		Le, Ro	Dec, Cal	Bat, Dri	MA-MD, CH-WI, HA-CL
Zanthoxylum zanthoxyloïdes Lam. Zep et Timl	Rubiaceae	Rapeoka	Wo	Ro, Ba	Tri	Dri, Fum, Mas	EP, MA-MD, HA-CL, IN
Zizyphus mauritiana Lam.	Rhamnaceae	Mugunuga	Tomonon	Le, Ro, Mi	Dec, Tri	Bat, Dri	EP, HA-CL

Part used: Whole plants (Wp); Leaves (Le); Stems (St); *Roots (Ro); Barks (Ba);* Flowers (Fl); *Fruits (Fr);* Mistletoes *(Mi); Bulbs (Bu); Latex (La).* **Mode of preparation:** Maceration (Mac); Decoction (Dec); Calcination (Cal); Trituration (Tri). **Mode of administration:** Bath (Bat); Drink (Dri); Fumigation (Fum); Purging (Pur); Massage (Mas); Ingestion (Ing). **Pathologies:** Epilepsy (EP); Madness or Mental Disorders (MA-MD); Charm or Witchcraft (CH-WI); Hallucination or Consciousness Loss (HA-CL); Insomnia (IN); Nerves diseases (ND).

Table 2. Main plants used, rate and age of TH user, rate of treated diseases and type of use.

Plants	User TH Rate (%)	Average Age of TH	Treated Diseases Rate (%)	Use Alone or Associated
Acacia sieberiana DC.	7.5	45	75	alone
Afzelia africana Smith ex Pers.	11.3	42	75	alone, associated
Allium sativum L.	20.75	57.5	50	associated
Annona senegalensis Pers.	17	55.5	100	alone, associated
Calotropis procera (Ait) Ait. F.	20.75	57	100	alone, associated
Citrus aurantifolia (Christm.) Swingle	7.5	51	75	associated
Daniellia oliveri (Rolfe) Hutch. et Dalz.	19	45.5	75	alone, associated
Datura innoxia Mill.	13.2	60.5	75	alone, associated
Detarium microcarpum Guill. et Perr.	5.7	39	75	associated
Diospyros mespiliformis Hochst ex A. DC.	13.2	39	100	alone, associated
Ficus iteophylla Miq.	7.5	39	75	alone, associated
Guiera senegalensis J.F. Gmel.	13.2	50	100	alone, associated
Khaya senegalensis (Desr) A. Juss	20.75	47	100	alone, associated
Mitragyna inermis (Willd) O. Ktze	7.5	35.5	75	alone, associated
Parkia biglobosa (Jacq.) R. BR. ex G. Don.F	7.5	48	75	alone
Securidaca longepedunculata Fresen	45.3	48	100	alone, associated
Tamarindus indica L.	11.3	46	75	associated
Ximenia americana L.	5.7	46	75	alone, associated
Zanthoxylum zanthoxyloïdes Lam. Zep &Timl	7.5	60	75	alone, associated
Zizyphus mauritiana Lam.	5.7	47	75	alone, associated

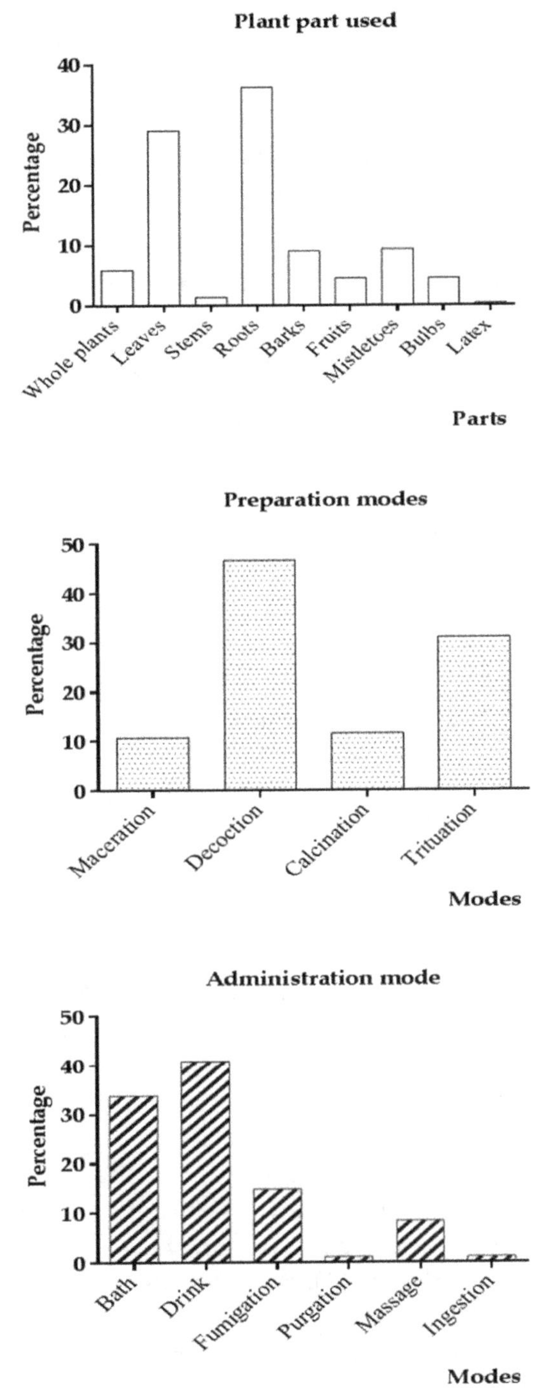

Figure 2. Plant parts used, modes of preparation and administration of remedies.

Table 3. Pathologies treated, traditional healers (TH) rate and medicinal plants used.

Pathologies			Treating TH Rate (%)	Number of Plants Used
English Name	**Local Name (*Mooré*)**	**Local Name (*Dioula*)**		
Epilepsy	*Kisinkindou*	*Cricromansian*	49	31
Hallucination or Consciousness loss	*Ningyilinga, sobgré*	*Djina bana*	79.2	37
Insomnia	*Gueim Baansé*	*Sinõgõtan ya*	3.8	2
Mental disorders or Madness	*Guimdo, Jougkolgo*	*Faatõ ya*	47.2	32
Nerves diseases	*Guiin Baansé*	*Fassadjourou bana*	3.8	1
Witchcraft or Charm diseases	*Rabsgo, Soondo*	*Soubaga ya*	35.8	25

4. Discussion

Traditional medicine practice in Hauts Bassins area is rich and diversified. The most often treated neuropsychiatric disorders are hallucination, epilepsy and mental disorders, respectively treated by 79.2%, 49% and 47.2% of traditional healers (TH). These data correspond to those of other works [7,25,35], which revealed that these pathologies are well-known and treated in the traditional medicine of many African countries.

Sixty-six (66) plant species belonging to various families used in the treatment of neuropsychiatric disorders were listed. This result testifies TH knowledge about plants diversity of this area and their therapeutic virtues. Similar results were observed by previous studies [19,21] which showed that local populations of Burkina Faso were known to profit from the best part of biodiversity in traditional medicine. More than 77% of plants identified are ligneous. This rate could be justified by the relative abundance of these species in the phytogeographical sector of this area, and their availability during all the year. These results were in the same order with those of Traoré's group in the province of Comoé [36], Olivier's group on "Dozo" traditional healers [21] and Zerbo's group in western area [22], which indicates a prevalence of ligneous use in the pharmacopeia of this zone of Burkina Faso. *S. longepedunculata*, *C. procera*, *K. senegalensis*, *A. sativum*, *D. oliveri*, *A. senegalensis* were identified as the main species used and *D. innoxia*, *Z. zanthoxyloïdes* were only used by older TH. They were cited like plant species intervening in the treatment of neuropsychiatric disorders in others African countries [8,35,37]. According to many authors, all these plants have phytochemical components with effects on the nervous system [38,39]. They contain alkaloids, terpenoids, steroids, flavonoids, tannins, saponins and cardiac glycosides (Table 4). These chemical constituents were considered as the main bioactive compounds of medicinal plants [30,40,41]. *C. procera* root bark used in the treatment of anxiety, epilepsy, and madness contain alkaloids such as α-amyrin, β-amyrin, while its leaf and its latex possess cardenolides such as calactin, calotoxin, calotropin and uscharin [42,43].

These chemical contents could be responsible of the traditional use of this plant. Besides, *C. procera* extracts were reported to possess significant anticonvulsant and analgesic properties [42,44]. Tropanic alkaloids as scopolamin, atropin, hyoscianin isolated in *D. innoxia* are known for their anticholinergic effects. They act as acetylcholin antagonists [15]. Scopolamine is an antimuscarinic agent used as analgesic and relaxant [45]. Anticholinergic and antimuscarinic effect of these compounds could explain in part Datura use in mental diseases treatement. Securidine, an alkaloid isolated from *S. longepedunculata* root, has a stimulating effect on the spinal cord. Used in a non-toxic dose, it influenced the function of the autonomic nervous system [46]. Some flavonoids were reported to possess anxiolytic effects and neuroprotective activities; they are capable of binding to GABAA receptors with significant affinity [47]. As examples, 6-methylapigenin is a benzodiazepine binding site ligand and 2S(-)-hesperidin has sedative and sleep-enhancing properties [48]. Quercetin significantly decreased the brain ischemic lesion [49]. Hesperidin was identified in *C. aurantifolia* and *Z. zanthoxyloïdes*, while apigenin was isolated from *S. longepedunculata* and Quercetin in most of plants listed in this study (Table 4).

These bioactive compounds could explain plants efficacy in the treatment of neuropsychiatric diseases [50,51]. Mechanisms through which these compounds act on the central nervous system are various including regulation of neurotransmitters activity [52–54]. However, benefical activities of these plants do not occult their toxic effects. Indeed, they have also cytotoxic and cardiotoxic effects [42]. Securinine in the range 5–30 g/kg act like strychnine, causing spasms and death by respiratory arrest [46]. Tropanic alkaloids are potential neurotoxic agents [15]. Therefore, a controlled use of these plants should be promoted.

Table 4. Phytochemical constituents and pharmacological properties of main plants used.

Plants	Pharmacological Properties	Phytochemical Constituents	Chemical Compounds Identified
Acacia sieberiana DC.	Inhibition of acetylcholinesterase, anti-inflammatory [55].	Alkaloids, cyanogenic glucoside, tannins, terpenoids, Saponins, Flavonoids, essential oils, Cardiac glycosides, steroid, resins [56–58].	Dihydroacacipetalin; acacipetalin [56]. Manganese; calcium; magnesium, cupper, iron, zinc, nickel [57].
Afzelia africana Smith ex Pers.		Alkaloids, tannins, saponins, fiber, flavonoids, cyanides, beta-carotenes, cyanogenic glycosides, terpenoids, steroids, anthocyanins [59–61].	Sodium; potassium; calcium; magnesium; phosphorus; iron; zinc; vitamins A, C, E, B1, B2, B6, B12 [59,62].
Allium sativum L.	Stimulant, antioxydant, anti-inflammatory, antimicrobial, fungicidal, antibacterial, anticancerous, chemopreventive, anti-tumoral, antidiabétic [63–65].	Alkaloids, phenolics, flavonoids, essential oils [64,66,67]	Trisulphide-di-2-propenyl; artumerone; tetrazolo [1,5-b] pyridazine; 2-hydroxyethyl ethyl disulfide; cyclic octa-atomic sulphur [66]. Alliin; allicin [63]. Diallyl trisulfide; diallyl disulfide; methyl allyl trisulfide [65]. Diallyl monosulfide; trisulfide méthyl-2-propenyl; diméthyl tétrasulfide [68].
Annona senegalensis Pers.	Anticonvulsant, anxiolytic, sedative, antibacterial, anti-inflammatory, cytotoxic, antioxydant, anti-nociceptive, antivenenous [15,69].	Alkaloids, flavonoids, saponins, sterols, flavonols, triterpenes, diterpenoids phenols, antraquinones, anthocyanes, coumarines [15,70].	1,2-benzenediol; butylate hydroxytoluene; methylcarbamate; n-hexadecanoique acid; hexadecane; acide oleique; etracosane; 9-octylheptadecane; heneicosane; 13-octadecadien-1-ol; octadecanoique acid; 9,17-octadecandienal; pentadecane; tetratriacontane; squalene [71]. Kaurenoic acid [69]
Calotropis procera (Ait) Ait. F.	Anticonvulsant, analgesic, anti-inflammatory,antitumoral, hepatoprotective, antioxidant, spasmolytic, cytotoxifc, cardio-stimulantg, lipase inhibitory, anti-apoptotic [42,72–74].	Alkaloids, cardenolides, triterpenes, flavonoids, sterols, saponins, diterpenes, resines, tannins, steroides [43,75].	Calactin; calotropagenin; calotropin; calotoxin; uscharin; syriogenin, afrogenin [42,43]. Flavonoid 5-hydroxy-3,7-dimethoxyflavone-4′-O-β-glucopyranoside; 3-O-rutinosides of quercetin; kaempferol; isorhamnetin [75]. Cholin; uscharin; uscharidin; voruscharidin; α-amyrine; β-amyrine [30,76].
Citrus aurantifolia (Christm.) Swingle	Antioxidant, anti-inflammatory, fungicidal, antibactérial [77–79].	Essential oils, glucosides, carotenoïds, flavonoids [67,77].	α-pinene; camphene; sabinene; β-pinene; myrcene; Δ3-carene; limonene; (Z)-β-ocimene; α-terpinene; γ-terpinene ; terpinolene; linalool; citronnelal; isocamphene; borneol; terpinen-4-ol; myrtenal; δ-cadinene; caryophyllen oxide; α-eudesmol; myrcene; p-cymene; benzoic acid; α-cedrene; α-bergamotene; α-bisabolene [77–79]. Hespéridine, vitamine C [67].
Daniellia oliveri (Rolfe) Hutch. et Dalz.	Analgésic, antihistaminic, relaxant, anti-inflammatory, antimicrobial, antidiabetic, antispasmodic, antipyretic, antidiarrhoeal [80–82]	Alkaloids, saponosides, flavonoids, glycosides, diterpenoids, sitosterol, coumarines, antracenosides, tanins, hétérosides cardiotoniques, trierpènes, Sterols [8,81,82].	Rutin; quertcitin-3/-O–methyl–3–O-a-rhamnopyranosyl-($\rightarrow$)-β-D-glucopyranoside (Narcissin); quercitrin; quercimeritrin [80,81].

Table 4. *Cont.*

Plants	Pharmacological Properties	Phytochemical Constituents	Chemical Compounds Identified
Datura innoxia Mill.	Hallucinogen, analgesic, hypnotic, narcotic, anti-cholinergic, antiparkinsonien, sedative, cytotoxic, aphrodisiac, antispasmodic, antiemetic, anti-aflatoxine, anti-bradycardic, anti-inflammatory, anti-dizziness, antitumor [83–85]	Alkaloids tropanics [83,86].	Hyoscyamine; scopolamine; tropinone; tropine; pseudotropine; scopoline; scopine; 3-acetoxytropane; 3-acetoxy-6-hydroxytropane; cuscohygrine; aposcopolamine; 3(α′),6-ditigloyloxytropane; 3(β′),6-ditigloyloxytropane; 3-(′-acetoxytropoyloxy)-tropane; 3,6-Ditigloyloxy-7-hydroxytropane; 7-hydroxyhyoscyamine; 6-hydroxyhyoscyamine; 3-tropoyloxy-6-isovaleroyloxytropane; 6-tigloylhyoscyamine; luteoline [83,85,86].
Detarium microcarpum Guill. et Perr.		Alkaloid, fibers, tannins, saponins, flavonoids, cyanides, beta carotenes, cyanogenic glycosides, terpenoids, steroids, anthocyanines [59,61].	Calcium; phosphorus; iron; zinc; vitamins A, E [59].
Diospyros mespiliformis Hochst ex A. DC.	Antioxydant, astringent, spasmolytic, antibacterial, homeostatic [87].	Alkaloids, polyphenols, flavonoids, anthraquinones, tannins, triterpenes, saponins, saponosides, anthocyanes, anthracenosides, steroids [87,88].	
Ficus iteophylla Miq.	Analgesic, anti-inflammatory, antibacterial [89]	Steroids, furanocoumarines, flavonoids glycosides [80,89]	3β-cholest-5-ene-3, 23diol; 24 ethyl cholest-5-ene- 3β-ol [89].
Guiera senegalensis J.F. Gmel.	Psychoactive, detoxicant, anti-plasmodial, antimicrobial, antifungal, antioxydant, anticancerous, antiviral, [90,91].	Alkaloids, flavonoids, triterpenes, tannins, cardenolides, anthracene, coumarines, sterols, saponosides [91,92].	
Khaya senegalensis (Desr) A. Juss	Anticonvulsant, Anxiolytic, sedative, antioxydant, anti-tumoral, chemopreventive, anti-inflammatory [15,93–95].	Alkaloids, saponins, tannins, triterpenes, flavonoids, glucosides, carbohydrate, phylates, oxalates, triterpenoids [15,94,95].	Gedunin; methyl-angolensate; methyl-6-hydroxyangolensate [96]. Catechin; rutin; quercetin rhamnoside; procyanidins [97]. Fissinolide; 2,6-dihydroxyfissinolide; methyl 3b-acetoxy-6-hydroxy-1-oxomeliac-14-enoate [98]. Magnesium, calcium, potassium, sodium, zinc, iron, manganese, lead, chromium [94].
Mitragyna inermis (Willd) O. Ktze	Anticonvulsant, cardiovascular affects, antibactérial, antiplasmodial, anti-diabetic [99–101].	Alkaloids, polyphenols, sterols, polyterpenes, quinones, tannins, saponins, flavonoids, saponosides [99,100,102].	Rhynchophylline; isorhynchophylline; corynoxeine; isocorynoxeine; ciliaphylline; rhynchociline; isospcionoxeine; 9-methoxy-3-epi-α-yohimbine [103]. 27-nor-terpenoid glucoside [104,105].
Parkia biglobosa (Jacq.) R. BR. ex G. Don. F	Antibacterial, antifungal, antioxidant, antihyperlipidemic, cardioprotective [106–108].	Alkaloids, cardiac glycosides, tannins, steroids, tannins, alkaloids, flavonoids, saponins, terpenes, glycosides [106,109].	

Table 4. *Cont.*

Plants	Pharmacological Properties	Phytochemical Constituents	Chemical Compounds Identified
Securidaca longepedunculata Fresen	Anticonvulsant; antidepressant, anxiolytic, antioxydant, anti-nociceptive, cytotoxic, antivenomous, antibactérial, aphrodisiac, sedative, [110–112]	Alkaloids, saponosides, flavonoids, phenols, xanthones, anthraquinones, essential oils [113–115].	Gallic acide; quercetin; cafeic acid; chlorogenic acid; epicatechin; p-coumaric acid; cinnamic acid; rutin; apigenin [82] Phelandrene; pinene; z-sabinol; limonene; p-cymene [110] Securinin [116,117]. Muchimangine E, muchimangine F [118].
Tamarindus indica L.	Analgesic, antinociceptive, antivenin, hepatoprotective, anti-inflamatory, anti-helminthic, antioxydant, antibacterial [119–121].	Alkaloids, saponins, glycosides, tannins, terpenoids, flavonoids, coumarins, naphthoquinones, anthraquinones, xanthonones [121–124].	C-glycosidesorientin; vitexin; isoorientin; isovitexin; tartaric acid; malic acid [120]. Limonene; methyl salicylate; pyrazine; alkylthiazole; calcium; iron; zinc; vitamins B and C [125].
Ximenia americana L.	Anti-plasmodiale, antioxidant, anticancer, antineoplastic, antitrypanosomal, antirheumatic, antioxidant, analgesic antipyretic [90,126,127].	Alkaloids, anthraquinones, cardiac glycosides, flavonoids, pylobatannins, saponnins, tannins, terpenoids, isoprenoids, triterpenes, sesquiterpenes, quinones [126–128].	Norisoprenoid isophorane; ximenynic acid; methyl-14,14-dimethyl-18-hydroxyheptatracont-27,35-dienoate; dimethyl-5-Methyl-28,29-dihydroxydotriacont-3,14,26-triendioate; 10Z,14E,16E-octadeca-10,14,16-triene-12-ynoic acid, tariric acid; β-sitosterol; oleanene palmitates [127,129,130] .
Zanthoxylum zanthoxyloïdes Lam. Zep &Timl	Antiplasmodial, vasorelaxant, antifungal, antibacterial, inhibition of acetylcholinesterase, antiradical, [131–133].	Alkaloids, tannins [132,134].	Myrcene; germacrene D; limonene, β-caryophyllene; decanal [135]. Acide 3,4-O-divanilloylquinique, acide 3,5-O-divanilloylquinique, acide 4,5-O-divanilloylquinique [136].fagaramide; (+)-sésamine; lupéol; hespéridine; Dihydrochélérythrine; N,N-diméthyllindcarpine; Chélérythrine; Norchélérythrine; 6-(2-oxybutyl) dihydrochélérythrine; 6-hydroxy-dihydrochélérythrine; avicine; arnottianamide [131] .
Zizyphus mauritiana Lam.	Antitumor, antibacterial, antioxidant, antimicrobial, anticancer [137,138].	Alkaloids, flavonoids, triterpenoids, tannins, glycoside, phenol, lignin, saponins [137,139].	2H-1-benzopyran-2-one; 9, stigmasterol; stigmastane-3,6-dione [137]. 3-methyl piperidine; o-methyl delta-tochopherol; octacosane; cyclobarbital; squalene; 2,4-dimethyl; thymol TMS; benzoquinoline; γ-sitosterol; hydroprogesterone [138].

Roots (36.2%) and leaves (29%) were the most used organs for the preparation of remedies. These data are in agreement with those observed by Olivier's group [21] and Kantati's group [35]. That would be explained by the availability of these plant parts at all periods in this region, but their effectiveness would be related to the significant accumulation of chemical compounds in these organs [113,140]. However, roots use should lead to some species disappearance. Thus, conservation measures of those are necessary.

Methods of remedies preparation are similar to those observed in other works. The decoction (46.7%) was the most used, followed by the trituration, calcination and aqueous maceration. These results are comparable to those of Zerbo's group works in Sanan's region and Western area of Burkina Faso [16,22], Adetutu's group in the South-western of Nigeria [141] and Kantati's group in Togo [35]. They noted that these methods were the main ones used by traditional healers in these different areas. In phytochemistry, the decoction is considered to be a method allowing complete extraction of bioactive chemical compounds of plants [142]. The aqueous maceration was quoted as being a good method of alkaloids and polyphenols extraction [142,143]. Likewise, the trituration and the calcination methods allow reducing vegetable material to powder or paste, while preserving bioactive molecules. These data could justify the main use of these modes of preparation.

The majority of drugs are administrated orally (drink, 40.8%), the preferential mode of administration in the traditional medicine [67]. However, some are preferentially used by external ways. That would be related to risks that oral use presents for some plants, because of their toxicity or the specificity of the disease [21]. The nasal way is the third most used mode of administration. It has the advantage of allowing a fast access of the active substances in the brain and their best absorption [144].

Results of the ethnobotanical survey corroborate with previous phytochemical studies about traditional uses of plants listed [7,35] and their psychoactive compounds content [69,91]. Indeed, alkaloids are the most known of molecules possessing psychoactive properties [67,145]. Likewise, some flavonoids, steroids and terpenoids were quoted to have psychoactive effect [47,53,146]. These chemical constituents intervene to disturb neurotransmitters activities. They stimulate, inhibit or block liberation, reception or elimination of neurotransmitters [147,148]. Pharmacological results show that the main plants used possess anticonvulsant, anxiolytic, antispasmodic, antinociceptive, analgesic or sedative properties [44,85,111]. This result could confirm the presence of psychoactive compounds in these plants.

5. Conclusions

This study made it possible to report 66 plant species belonging to 51 genera and 32 families used for the treatment of neuropsychiatric diseases. Roots and leaves were the most organs used, the decoction and the trituration were the principal modes of drug preparation. The administration of remedies was done mainly by oral way. Plants identified were quoted to possess psychoactive properties and some chemical contents which could justify that.

Traditional remedies suggested in this study are a real interest in the fight against neuropsychiatric disorders. Then, further researches will be necessary to identify psychoactive compounds from these plants and their acting mechanisms for neuropsychiatric diseases treatment.

Acknowledgments: The authors wish to thank Sidonie Yabré and traditional healers of "Hauts Bassins" region from Burkina Faso for their availability and assistance during survey.

Author Contributions: M.K. and P.Z. conceived and designed the survey; P.T.K. realized the survey; P.T.K. and M.C. analyzed the data; P.T.K. wrote the paper; P.Z. identified the plant specimen; S.G., M.K. and A.C. corrected the manuscript.

References

1. Hele, B.; Metowogo, K.; Mouzou, A.P.; Tossou, R.; Ahounou, J.; Eklu-Gadegbeku, K.; Dansou, P.; Aklikokou, A.K. Enquête ethnobotanique sur les plantes utilisées dans le traitement traditionnel des contusions musculaires au Togo. *Rev. Ivoir. Sci. Technol.* **2014**, *24*, 112–130. (In French).
2. Organisation Mondiale de la Santé (OMS). *Rapport de l'atelier Interrégional de l'OMS sur l'utilisation de la Médecine Traditionnelle dans les soins de santé Primaires*; OMS: Genève, Suisse, 2009. (In French)
3. Organisation Mondiale de la Santé (OMS). *Projet Zéro de Plan D'action Mondial Sur la Santé Mentale 2013–2020*; OMS: Genève, Suisse, 2012. (In French)
4. Yasamy, M.T.; Maulik, P.K.; Tomlinson, M.; Lund, C.; Van Ommeren, M.; Saxena, S. Responsible Governance for Mental Health Research in Low Resource Countries. *PLoS Med.* **2011**, *8*, 1–6. [CrossRef] [PubMed]
5. Fusar-Poli, P.; Deste, G.; Smieskova, R.; Barlati, S.; Yung, A.R.; Howes, O.; Stieglitz, R.-D.; Vita, A.; McGuire, P.; Borgwardt, S. Cognitive Functioning in Prodromal Psychosis: A meta-analysis. *Arch. Gen. Psychiatry* **2012**, *69*, 562–571. [CrossRef] [PubMed]
6. World Health Organization (WHO). *Mental Health Gap Action Programme: Scaling up Care for Mental, Neurological, and Substance Use Disorders*; WHO: Geneva, Switzerland, 2008.
7. Moshi, M.J.; Kagashe, G.A.B.; Mbwambo, Z.H. Plants used to treat epilepsy by Tanzanian traditional healers. *J. Ethnopharmacol.* **2005**, *97*, 327–336. [CrossRef] [PubMed]
8. Diaby, M.A. Etude de la chimie et des activités biologiques de *Daniellia oliveri* (Rolfe, Hutch et Dalz), une plante utilisée dans la prise en charge de l'épilepsie au Mali. Thèse d'Etat, USTT-B, Bamako, Mali, 2014.
9. Starling, J.; Feijo, I. Schizophrénie et autres troubles psychotiques à début précoce. *IACAPAP E-textb. Child Adolesc. Ment. Health* **2012**, 1–24. (In French).
10. Rey-bellet, P. Quoi de neuf dans le traitement des psychoses. *Curr. Opin. Psychiatry* **2015**, 1–26.
11. World Health Organization (WHO). *Regional Strategy for Mental Health 2000–2010*; WHO: Geneva, Switzerland, 2000.
12. Comité Français d'Education pour la Santé (CFES) et MILDT. *Médicaments Psychoactifs*; EURO RSCG: Puteaux, France, 2000. (In French). Available online: http://perso.mediaserv.net/ganja/sarah/sarah/106_fin.pdf (accessed on 8 October 2016).
13. Fouchey, M. Etat des lieux sur l'industrie du médicament. *Rev. Neuropsychol.* **2010**, 1–8. (In French). Available online: http://psychologie-m-fouchey.psyblogs.net/ (accessed on 8 October 2016).
14. Sobiecki, J.F. A preliminary inventory of plants used for psychoactive purposes in southern African healing traditions. *Trans. R. Soc. S. Afr.* **2002**, *57*, 1–24. [CrossRef]
15. Taïwe, G.S.; Kuete, V. Neurotoxicity and Neuroprotective Effects of African Medicinal Plants. In *Toxicological Survey of African Medicinal Plants*; Elsevier: London, UK, 2014; pp. 423–444.
16. Zerbo, P.; Millogo-rasolodimby, J.; Nacoulma-ouedraogo, O.G.; Van Damme, P. Plantes médicinales et pratiques médicales au Burkina Faso: Cas des Sanan. *Bois Forêts des Tropiques* **2011**, *307*, 41–53. (In French).
17. Millogo, H.; Guissou, I.P.; Nacoulma, O.G.; Traoré, A.S. Savoir traditionnel et médicament traditionnels améliorés. In Proceedings of the Colloque: Développement durable et santé dans les pays du sud, le médicament, de la recherche au terrain, Centre Européen de Santé Humanitaire, Lyon, France, Decembre 2005. (In French)
18. Tapsoba, H.; Deschamps, J.-P. Use of medicinal plants for the treatment of oral diseases in Burkina Faso. *J. Ethnopharmacol.* **2006**, *104*, 68–78. [CrossRef] [PubMed]
19. Dakuyo, V. Contribution à l'étude de la pharmacopée traditionnelle burkinabé: Enquête ethnopharmacologique dans la région des Cascades. Ph.D. Thesis, Université de Ouagadougou, Ouagadougou, Burkina Faso, 2010.
20. Nadembega, P.; Boussim, J.I.; Nikiema, J.B.; Poli, F.; Antognoni, F. Medicinal plants in Baskoure, Kourittenga Province, Burkina Faso: An ethnobotanical study. *J. Ethnopharmacol.* **2011**, *133*, 378–395. [CrossRef] [PubMed]
21. Olivier, M.; Zerbo, P.; Boussim, J.I. Les plantes des galeries forestières à usage traditionnel par les tradipraticiens de santé et les chasseurs Dozo Sénoufo du Burkina Faso. *Int. J. Biol. Chem. Sci.* **2012**, *6*, 2170–2191. (In French). [CrossRef]
22. Zerbo, P.; Compaore, M.; Meda, N.T.R.; Lamien-Meda, A.; Kiendrebeogo, M. Potential medicinal plants used by traditional healers in western areas of Burkina Faso. *World J. Pharm. Pharm. Sci.* **2013**, *2*, 6706–6719.
23. Millogo, A.; Kaboré, J.; Preux, P.-M.; Dumas, M. Traitement des adultes épileptiques en milieu hospitalier à Bobo-Dioulasso (Burkina-Faso). *Epilepsies* **2003**, *15*, 37–40. (In French)

24. Traore, M. Etude du profil et de la prise en charge des cas d'abus de drogues dans la ville de Bobo-Bioulasso (Burkina Baso). Ph.D. Thesis, Université de Ouagadougou, Ouagadougou, Burkina Baso, 2012.
25. Millogo, A.; Ratsimbazafy, V.; Nubukpo, P.; Barro, S.; Zongo, I.; Preux, P. Epilepsy and traditional medicine in Bobo-Dioulasso (Burkina Faso). *Acta Neurol. Scand.* **2004**, *109*, 250–254. [CrossRef] [PubMed]
26. Ministère de l'Economie et du Développement (MED). *Profil des Regions du Burkina Faso: La région des Hauts Bassins*; MED: Ouagadougou, Burkina Faso, 2005. (In French)
27. Fontès, J.; Guinko, S. *CARTE de la Végétation et de L'occupation du Sol du Burkina Faso: Notice Explicative*; Université de Toulouse III: Toulouse, France, 1995. (In French)
28. Institut National de la Statistique et de la Démographie (INSD). *Etat et structure de la population*; INSD: Ouagadougou, Burkina Faso, 2009. (In French)
29. Hutchinson, J.; Dalziel, J.M. *Flora of West Tropical Africa*; The Whitefriars Press: Londre/Tonbridge, UK, 1963.
30. Nacoulma-Ouedraogo, O.G. Plantes médicinales et pratiques médicinales traditionnelles au Burkina Faso: Cas du plateau central. Thèse d'Etat, Université de Ouagadougou, Ouagadougou, Burkina Faso, 1996.
31. Thiombiano, A.; Schmidt, M.; Dressler, S.; Ouédraogo, A.; Hahn, K.; Zizka, G. *Catalogue Des Plantes Vasculaires Du BURKINA Faso.* Conservatoire et jardin botaniques de la ville de genève. 2012. Available online: http://www.worldcat.org/title/ (accessed on 8 October 2016).
32. Kerharo, J.; Bouquet, A. *Plantes Médicinales Et Toxiques De La Côte-d'Ivoire-Haute-Volta. Mission D'étude De La Pharmacopée Indigène En A.O.F*; Editions Vigot Frères: Paris, France, 1950. (In French)
33. Pageard, R. Plantes à brûler chez les Bambara. *J. Soc. Afr.* **1967**, *37*, 87–130. [CrossRef]
34. Moreau, R. *Quelques Plantes de Haute-volta: Leurs noms Vernaculaires en Langues Mossi, dioula, bobo-oulé, Dagari et Peul-wassolo*; Publications des scientifiques de l'IRD: Haute-Volta, French, 1970. (In French)
35. Kantati, Y.T.; Kodjo, K.M.; Dogbeavou, K.S.; Vaudry, D.; Leprince, J.; Gbeassor, M. Ethnopharmacological survey of plant species used in folk medicine against central nervous system disorders in Togo. *J. Ethnopharmacol.* **2016**, *181*, 214–220. [CrossRef] [PubMed]
36. Traoré, A.; Derme, A. I.; Sanon, S.; Gansane, A.; Ouattara, Y.; Nebié, I.; Sirima, S.B. Connaissances ethnobotaniques et pratiques phytothérapeutiques des tradipraticiens de santé de la Comoé pour le traitement du paludisme: Processus d'une recherche scientifique de nouveaux antipaludiques au Burkina Faso. *Ethnopharmacologia* **2009**, *43*, 35–46. (In French).
37. Sobiecki, J.F. A review of plants used in divination in southern Africa and their psychoactive effects. *S. Afr. Humanit.* **2008**, *20*, 333–351.
38. Perveen, T.; Haider, S.; Zubairi, N.A.; Ahmed, W.; Batool, Z.; Begum, S. Effect of herbal combination on biochemical and behavioral responses in rats. *Pak. J. Biochem. Mol. Biol.* **2012**, *45*, 20–22.
39. Sucher, N.J.; Carles, M.C. A pharmacological basis of herbal medicines for epilepsy. *Epilepsy Behav.* **2015**, *52*, 308–318. [CrossRef] [PubMed]
40. Bruneton, J. *Pharmacognosie, Phytochimie, Plantes Médicinales*, 2ème ed.; Tec. et Doc.: Lavoisier, Paris, 1993.
41. Sereme, A.; Millogo-Rasolodimby, J.; Guinko, S.; Nacro, M. Proprietes Therapeutiques Des Plantes a Tanins Du Burkina Faso. *Pharmacopée Méd. Tradit. Afr.* **2008**, *15*, 41–49. (In French).
42. Al-snafi, A.E. The constituents and pharmacological properties of Calotropis procera-an overview. *Int. J. Pharm. Rev. Res.* **2015**, *5*, 259–275.
43. Mohamed, N.H.; Liu, M.; Abdel-mageed, W.M.; Alwahibi, L.H.; Dai, H.; Ahmed, M.; Badr, G.; Quinn, R.J.; Liu, X.; Zhang, L.; et al. Cytotoxic cardenolides from the latex of Calotropis procera. *Bioorg. Med. Chem. Lett.* **2015**, *25*, 4615–4620. [CrossRef] [PubMed]
44. Lima, R.C.D.S.; Silva, M.C.C.; Aguiar, C.C.T.; Chaves, E.M.C.; Dias, K.C.F.; Macêdo, D.S.; Sousa, F.C.F.; Carvalho, K.M.; Ramos, M.V.; Mendes, V.M. Anticonvulsant action of Calotropis procera latex proteins. *Epilepsy Behav.* **2012**, *23*, 123–126. [CrossRef] [PubMed]
45. Steenkamp, P.A.; Harding, N.M.; Van Heerden, F.R.; Van Wyk, B.E. Fatal Datura poisoning: Identification of atropine and scopolamine by high performance liquid chromatography/photodiode array/mass spectrometry. *Forensic Sci. Int.* **2004**, *145*, 31–39. [CrossRef] [PubMed]
46. Maiga, A.; Diallo, D.; Fane, S.; Sanogo, R.; Paulsen, B.S.; Cisse, B. A survey of toxic plants on the market in the district of Bamako, Mali: Traditional knowledge compared with a literature search of modern pharmacology and toxicology. *J. Ethnopharmacol.* **2005**, *96*, 183–193. [CrossRef] [PubMed]
47. Zhang, Z. Therapeutic effects of herbal extracts and constituents in animal models of psychiatric disorders. *Life Sci.* **2004**, *75*, 1659–1699. [CrossRef] [PubMed]

48. Marder, M.; Wasowski, C.; Medina, J.H.; Paladini, A.C. 6-Methylapigenin and hesperidin: New valeriana flavonoids with activity on the CNS. *Pharmacol. Biochem. Behav.* **2003**, *75*, 537–545. [CrossRef]
49. Dajas, F.; Rivera, F.; Blasina, F.; Arredondo, F.; Lafon, L.; Morquio, A.; Heizen, H. Cell Culture Protection and in vivo Neuroprotective Capacity of Flavonoids. *Neurotox. Res.* **2003**, *5*, 425–432. [CrossRef] [PubMed]
50. Lake, J. Natural product-derived treatments of neuropsychiatric disorders: Review of progress and recommendations. *Stud. Nat. Prod. Chem.* **2000**, *24*, 1093–1137.
51. Guenne, S.; Balmus, I.M.; Hilou, A.; Ouattara, N.; Kiendrebéogo, M.; Ciobica, A.; Timofte, D. The relevance of Asteraceae family plants in most of the neuropsychiatric disorders treatment. *Int. J. Phyt.* **2016**, *8*, 176–182.
52. Gurib-Fakim, A. Medicinal plants: Traditions of yesterday and drugs of tomorrow. *Mol. Asp. Med.* **2006**, *27*, 1–93. [CrossRef] [PubMed]
53. Becaud-Boyer, A.-S. *Salvia divinorum*, hallucinogène d'aujourd'hui, outil thérapeutique de demain? Thèse d'Etat, Université Joseph FOURIER, Grenoble, France, 2011.
54. Charlene, B. La soumission chimique. Thèse d'Etat, Université Toulouse III, Toulouse, France, 2013.
55. Eldeen, S.; Mohamed, I. Pharmacological investigation of some trees used in South African traditional medicine. Ph.D. Thesis, University of KwaZulu–Natal, Pietermaritzburg, South Africa, 2005.
56. Seigler, D.S.; Butterfield, C.S.; Dunn, J.E.; Conn, E.E. Dihydroacacipetalin–a new cyanogenic glucoside from Acacia sieberiana var. Woodii. *Phytochemistry* **1975**, *14*, 1419–1420. [CrossRef]
57. Salisu, A.; Ogbadu, G.H.; Onyenekwe, P.C.; Olorode, O.; Ndana, R.W.; Segun, O. Evaluating the Nutritional Potential of Acacia Sieberiana Seeds (Dc) Growing in North West of Nigeria. *J. Biol. Life Sci.* **2014**, *5*, 25–36. [CrossRef]
58. Zeuko´o, M.E.; Jurbe, G.G.; Ntim, P.S.; Ajayi, T.A.; Chuwkuka, J.U.; Dawurung, C.J.; Makoshi, M.S.; Elisha, I.L.; Oladipo, O.O.; Lohlum, A.S. Phytochemical Screening and Antidiarrheal Evaluation of Acetone Extract of A cacia sieberiana var woodii (Fabaceae) stem bark in wistar rats. *Acad. J. Pharm. Pharmacol.* **2015**, *3*, 1–6.
59. Uchenna, A.; Nkiruka, V.; Eze, P. Nutrient and Phytochemical Composition of Formulated Diabetic Snacks Made from Two Nigerian Foods Afzelia africana and Detarium microcarpium Seed Flour. *Pak. J. Nutr.* **2013**, *12*, 108–113. [CrossRef]
60. Olajide, O.B.; Fadimu, O.Y.; Osaguona, P.O.; Saliman, M. Botanical and phytochemical studies of some selected species of leguminoseae of northern nigeria: A study of borgu local government area, niger state. Nigeria. *Analysis* **2013**, *4*, 546–551.
61. Igwenyi, I.O.; Azoro, B.N. Proximate and Phytochemical Compositions of Four Indigenous Seeds Used As Soup Thickeners in Ebonyi State Nigeria. *Food Technol.* **2014**, *8*, 35–40.
62. Egwujeh, S.I.; Yusufu, P.A. Chemical compositions of aril cap of African oak (afzelia africana) seed. *J. Food Sci.* **2015**, *3*, 41–47.
63. Gebreyohannes, G.; Gebreyohannes, M. Medicinal values of garlic: A review. *Int. J. Med. Méd. Sci.* **2013**, *5*, 401–408.
64. Bhandari, S.R.; Yoon, M.K.; Kwak, J. Contents of Phytochemical Constituents and Antioxidant Activity of 19 Garlic (Allium sativum L.) Parental Lines and Cultivars. *Hort. Environ. Biotechnol.* **2014**, *55*, 138–147. [CrossRef]
65. Mallet, A.C.T.; Cardoso, M.G.; Souza, P.E.; Machado, S.M.F.; Andrade, M.A.; Nelson, D.L.; Piccoli, R.H. Chemical characterization of the Allium sativum and Origanum vulgare essential oils and their inhibition effect on the growth of some food pathogens. *Rev. Bras. Plant. Med.* **2014**, *16*, 804–811. [CrossRef]
66. Johnson, O.O.; Ayoola, G.A.; Adenipekun, T. Antimicrobial Activity and the Chemical Composition of the Volatile Oil Blend from Allium sativum (Garlic Clove) and Citrus reticulata (Tangerine Fruit). *Int. J. Pharm. Sci. Drug Res.* **2013**, *5*, 187–193.
67. Yinyang, J.; Mpondo, M.E.; Tchatat, M.; Ndjib, R.C.; Mvogo-Ottou, P.B.; Dibong, S.D. Les plantes à alcaloïdes utilisées par les populations de la ville de Douala (Cameroun). *J. Appl. Biosci.* **2014**, *78*, 6600–6619. [CrossRef]
68. Rainy, G.; Amita, S.; Preeti, M. Study of chemical composition of garlic oil and comparative analysis of co-trimoxazole in response to in vitro antibacterial activity. *Int. Res. J. Pharm.* **2014**, *5*, 1–5.
69. Mustapha, A.A. Annona senegalensis Persoon: A Multipurpose shrub, its Phytotherapic, Phytopharmacological and Phytomedicinal Uses. *Int. J. Sci. Technol.* **2013**, *2*, 862–865.

70. Konate, A.; Sawadogo, W.R.; Dubruc, F.; Caillard, O.; Ouedraogo, M. Phytochemical and Anticonvulsant Properties of Annona senegalensis Pers. (Annonaceae), Plant Used in Burkina Folk Medicine to Treat Epilepsy and Convulsions. *Br. J. Pharmacol. Toxicol.* **2012**, *3*, 245–250.
71. Awa, E.P.; Ibrahim, S.; Ameh, D.A. GC/MS Analysis and antimicrobial activity of Diethyl ether fraction of Methanolic extract from the stem bark of Annona senegalensis pers. *Int. J. Pharm. Sci. Res.* **2012**, *3*, 4213–4218.
72. Ibrahim, S.R.M.; Mohamed, G.A.; Shaala, L.A.; Moreno, L.; Banuls, Y.; Van Goietsenoven, G.; Kiss, R.; Youssef, D.T.A. New ursane-type triterpenes from the root bark of Calotropis procera. *Phytochem. Lett.* **2012**, *5*, 490–495. [CrossRef]
73. Patil, S.G.; Patil, M.P.; Maheshwari, V.L.; Patil, R.H. In vitro lipase inhibitory effect and kinetic properties of di-terpenoid fraction from Calotropis procera (Aiton). *Biocatal. Agric. Biotechnol.* **2015**, *4*, 579–585. [CrossRef]
74. Sayed, A.E.H.; Mohamed, N.H.; Ismail, M.A.; Abdel-mageed, W.M.; Shoreit, A.A.M. Antioxidant and antiapoptotic activities of *Calotropis procera* latex on Catfish (Clarias gariepinus) exposed to toxic 4-nonylphenol. *Ecotoxicol. Environ. Saf.* **2016**, *128*, 189–194. [CrossRef] [PubMed]
75. Nenaah, G.E. Potential of using flavonoids, latex and extracts from Calotropis procera (Ait.) as grain protectants against two coleopteran pests of stored rice. *Ind. Crop. Prod.* **2013**, *45*, 327–334. [CrossRef]
76. Kerharo, J.; Adam, J.G. La Pharmacopée sénégalaise traditionnelle. Plantes médicinales et toxiques. ournal d'agriculture Trop. *Bot. Appl.* **1974**, *21*, 76–77.
77. Jeong-Hyun, L.; Jae-Sug, L. Chemical Composition and Antifungal Activity of Plant Essential Oils against Malassezia furfur. *Kor. J. Microbiol. Biotechnol.* **2010**, *38*, 315–321.
78. Dongmo, P.M.J.; Tchoumbougnang, F.; Boyom, F.F.; Sonwa, E.T.; Zollo, P.H.A.; Menut, C. Antiradical, antioxidant activities and anti-inflammatory potential of the essential oils of the varieties of citrus limon and citrus aurantifolia growing in Cameroon. *J. Asian Sci. Res.* **2013**, *3*, 1046–1057.
79. Ouedrhiri, W.; Bouhdid, S.; Balouiri, M.; Lalami, A.E.O.; Moja, S.; Chahdi, F.O.; Greche, H. Chemical composition of Citrus aurantium L. leaves and zest essential oils, their antioxidant, antibacterial single and combined effects. *J. Chem. Pharm. Res.* **2015**, *7*, 78–84.
80. Ahmadu, A.; Haruna, A.K.; Garba, M.; Ehinmidu, J.O.; Sarker, S.D. Phytochemical and antimicrobial activities of the Daniellia oliveri leaves. *Fitoterapia* **2004**, *75*, 729–732. [CrossRef] [PubMed]
81. Kaboré, A. Activité anthelminthique de deux plantes tropicales testée in vitro et in vivo sur les strongles gastro-intestinaux des ovins de race mossi du Burkina Faso. Thèse de Doctorat, Université Polytechnique de Bobo-Dioulasso, Bobo-Dioulasso, Burkina Faso, 2009.
82. Muanda, F.N.; Dicko, A.; Soulimani, R. Assessment of polyphenolic compounds, in vitro antioxydant and anti-inflammation properties of securidaca longepedunculata root barks. *Comptes Rendus Biol.* **2010**, *333*, 663–669. [CrossRef] [PubMed]
83. SOPCFC (Scientific Opinion of the Panel on Contaminants in the Food Chain). Request from the European Commission Tropane alkaloids (from Datura sp.) as undesirable substances in animal feed. *EFSA J.* **2008**, *691*, 1–55.
84. Mahmood, A.; Mahmood, A.; Mahmood, M. In vitro Biological Activities of Most Common Medicinal Plants of Family Solanaceae. *World Appl. Sci. J.* **2012**, *17*, 1026–1032.
85. Maheshwari, N.O.; Khan, A.; Chopade, B.A. Rediscovering the medicinal properties of Datura sp.: A review. *J. Med. Plant. Res.* **2013**, *7*, 2885–2897.
86. Berkov, S.; Zayed, R. Comparison of Tropane Alkaloid Spectra Between *Datura innoxia* Grown in Egypt and Bulgaria. *Z. Naturforsch. C* **2004**, *59*, 184–186. [CrossRef] [PubMed]
87. Lamien-Meda, A.; Lamien, C.E.; Compaoré, M.M.Y.; Meda, R.N.T.; Kiendrebeogo, M.; Zeba, B.; Millogo, J.F.; Nacoulma, O.G. Polyphenol Content and Antioxidant Activity of Fourteen Wild Edible Fruits from Burkina Faso. *Molecules* **2008**, *13*, 581–594. [CrossRef] [PubMed]
88. Belemtougri, R.G.; Constantin, B.; Cognard, C.; Raymond, G.; Sawadogo, L. Effects of two medicinal plants Psidium guajava L. (Myrtaceae) and Diospyros mespiliformis L. (Ebenaceae) leaf extracts on rat skeletal muscle cells in primary culture. *J. Zhejiang Univ. Sci. B* **2006**, *7*, 56–63. [CrossRef] [PubMed]
89. Abdulmalik, I.A.; Sule, M.I.; Musa, A.M.; Yaro, A.H.; Abdullahi, M.I.; Abdulkadir, M.F.; Yusuf, H. Isolation of Steroids from Acetone Extract of Ficus iteophylla. *Br. J. Pharmacol. Toxicol.* **2011**, *2*, 270–272.
90. Soha, P.M.; Benoit-Vical, F. Are West African plants a source of future antimalarial drugs? *J. Ethnopharmacol.* **2007**, *114*, 130–140. [CrossRef] [PubMed]

91. Somboro, A.A.; Patel, K.; Diallo, D.; Sidibe, L.; Chalchat, J.C.; Figueredo, G.; Ducki, S.; Troin, Y.; Chalard, P. An ethnobotanical and phytochemical study of the African medicinal plant *Guiera senegalensis* J. F. Gmel. *J. Med. Plants Res.* **2011**, *5*, 1639–1651.
92. Ouédraogo, F. Etude in vitro de l'activité antiplasmodiale d'extraits de feuilles, de fleurs et de galles de Guiera senegalensis J. F. Gmel (combretaceae). Thèse Doctorat, Université de Ouagadougou, Ouagadougou, Burkina Faso, 2011.
93. Androulakis, X.M.; Muga, S.J.; Chen, F.; Koita, Y.; Toure, B.; Michael Wargovich, J. Chemopreventive Effects of Khaya senegalensis Bark Extract on Human Colorectal Cancer. *Anticancer Res.* **2006**, *26*, 2397–2406. [PubMed]
94. Idu, M.; Igeleke, C.L. Antimicrobial Activity and Phytochemistry of Khaya senegalensis Roots. *Int. J. Ayurvedic Herb. Med.* **2012**, *2*, 415–422.
95. Wakirwa, J.H.; Idris, S.; Madu, S.J.; Dibal, M.; Malgwi, T. Assessment of the In-vitro antimicrobial potential of Khaya Senegalensis ethanol leaf extract. *J. Chem. Pharm. Res.* **2013**, *5*, 182–186.
96. Nwodo, N.J.; Ibezim, A.; Ntie-Kang, F.; Adikwu, M.U.; Mbah, C.J. Anti-Trypanosomal Activity of Nigerian Plants and Their Constituents. *Molecules* **2015**, *2*, 7750–7771. [CrossRef] [PubMed]
97. Atawodi, S.E.; Atawodi, J.C.; Pala, Y.; Idakwo, P. Assessment of the Polyphenol Profile and Antioxidant Properties of Leaves, Stem and Root Barks Of Khaya senegalensis (Desv.) A.Juss. *Electron. J. Biol.* **2009**, *5*, 80–84.
98. Khalid, S.A.; Friedrichsen, G.M.; Kharazmi, A.; Theander, T.G.; Olsen, C.E.; Christensen, S.B. Limonoids from Khaya senegalensis. *Phytochemistry* **1998**, *49*, 1769–1772. [CrossRef]
99. Zongo, C.; Akomo, E.-F.O.; Sawadogo, A.; Obame, L.C.; Koudou, J.; Traore, A.S. In vitro antibacterial properties of total alkaloids extract from Mitragyna inermis (Will) O. Kuntze, a West African traditional medicinal plant. *Asian J. Plant Sci.* **2009**, *8*, 172–177. [CrossRef]
100. Uthman, G.S.; Gana, G.; Zakama, S. Anticonvulsant Screening of the Ethanol Leaf Extract of Mitragyna inermis (Willd) in Mice and Chicks. *Int. J. Res. Pharm. Biomed. Sci.* **2013**, *4*, 1354–1357.
101. Alowanou, G.G.; Olounlade, A.P.; Azando, E.V.B.; Dedehou, V.F.G.N.; Daga, F.D.; Hounzangbeadote, S.M. A review of Bridelia ferruginea, Combretum glutinosum and Mitragina inermis plants used in zootherapeutic remedies in West Africa: Historical origins, current uses and implications for conservation. *J. Appl. Biosci.* **2015**, *87*, 8003–8014. [CrossRef]
102. Konkon, N.G.; Adjoungoua, A.L.; Manda, P.; Simaga, D.; N'Guessan, K.E.; Kone, B.D. Toxicological and phytochemical screening study of Mitragyna Inermis (willd.) O ktze (Rubiaceae), anti-diabetic plant. *J. Med. Plan. Res.* **2008**, *2*, 279–284.
103. Takayama, H.; Ishikawa, H.; Kitajima, M.; Aimi, N.; Aji, B.M. Anew 9-methoxyyohimbine-type indole alkaloid from Mitragyna inermis. *Chem. Pharm. Bull.* **2004**, *52*, 359–361. [CrossRef] [PubMed]
104. Cheng, Z.H.; Yua, B.Y.; Yang, X.W. 27-Nor-terpenoid glycosides from Mitragyna inermis. *Phytochemistry* **2002**, *61*, 379–382. [CrossRef]
105. Karou, S.D.; Tchacondo, T.; Ilboudo, D.P.; Simpore, J. Sub-saharan Rubiaceae : A review of their traditional uses, phytochemistry and biological activities. *Pak. J. Biol. Sci.* **2011**, *14*, 149–169. [CrossRef] [PubMed]
106. Ajaiyeoba, E.O. Phytochemical antibacterial properties of parkia biglobosa and parkia bicolor leaf extracts. *Afr. J. Riomed. Res.* **2002**, *5*, 125–129. [CrossRef]
107. Bukar, A.; Uba, A.; Oyeyi, T.I. Phytochemical Analysis and Antimicrobial Activity of Parkia Biglobosa (Jacq.) Benth. Extracts Against Some Food – Borne Microrganisms. *Adv. Environ. Biol.* **2010**, *4*, 74–79.
108. Komolafe, K.; Akinmoladun, A.C.; Olaleye, M.T. Methanolic leaf extract of Parkia biglobosa protects against doxorubicin-induced cardiotoxicity in rats. *Int. J. Appl. Res. Nat. Prod.* **2013**, *6*, 39–47.
109. Ezekwe, C.I.; Ada, A.C.; Okechukwu, P.C.U. Effects of Methanol Extract of Parkia biglobosa Stem Bark on the Liver and Kidney Functions of Albino Rats. *Glob. J. Biotechnol. Biochem.* **2013**, *8*, 40–50.
110. Adebiyi, R.A.; Elsa, A.T.; Agaie, B.M.; Etuk, E.U. Antinociceptive and antidepressant like effects of Securidaca longepedunculata root extract in mice. *J. Ethnopharmacol.* **2006**, *107*, 234–239. [CrossRef] [PubMed]
111. Adeyemi, O.O.; Akindele, A.J.; Yemitan, O.K.; Aigbe, F.R.; Fagbo, F.I. Anticonvulsant, anxiolytic and sedative activities of the aqueous root extract of Securidaca longepedunculata Fresen. *J. Ethnopharmacol.* **2010**, *130*, 191–195. [CrossRef] [PubMed]

112. Okomolo, C.M.; Mbafor, J.T.; Bum, E.N.; Kouemou, N.; Kandeda, A.K.; Talla, E.; Dimo, T.; Rakotonirira, A.; Rakotonirira, S.V. Evaluation of the sedative and anticonvulsant properties of three Cameroonnian plant. *Afr. J. Tradit. Complement. Altern. Med.* **2011**, *8*, 181–190. [PubMed]
113. Nébié, R.H.C.; Yaméogo, R.T.; Bélanger, A.; Sib, F.S. Salicylate de méthyle, constituant unique de l'huile essentielle de l'écorce des racines de *Securidaca longepedunculata* du Burkina Faso. *C. R. Chim.* **2004**, *7*, 1003–1006. (In French). [CrossRef]
114. Mitaine-offer, A.; Pénez, N.; Miyamoto, T.; Delaude, C.; Mirjolet, J.; Duchamp, O.; Lacaille-dubois, M. Phytochemistry Acylated triterpene saponins from the roots of *Securidaca longepedunculata*. *Phytochemistry* **2010**, *71*, 90–94. [CrossRef] [PubMed]
115. Sow, P.G. Enquête Ethnobotanique et Ethnopharmacologique des Plantes Médicinales de la pharmacopée Sénégalaise Dans le Traitement des Morsures de Serpents. *Le Pharmacien Hospitalier et Clinicien* **2012**, *47*, 37–41. [CrossRef]
116. Van Wyk, B.E.; Van Oudtshoorn, B.; Gericke, N. *Medicinal Plants of South Africa*, 1st ed.; Briza Publications: Pretoria, South Africa, 2005.
117. Diakité, B. La susceptibilite des larves d'Anopheles gambiae S.L. à des extraits de plantes medicinales du Mali. PhD Thesis, Université de Bamako, Bamako, Mali, 2008.
118. Dibwe, D.F.; Awale, S.; Kadota, S.; Morita, H.; Tezuka, Y. Heptaoxygenated xanthones as anti-austerity agents from Securidaca longepedunculata. *Bioorg. Med. Chem.* **2013**, *21*, 7663–7668. [CrossRef] [PubMed]
119. Bhadoriya, S.S.; Mishra, V.; Raut, S.; Ganeshpurkar, A.; Jain, S.K. Anti-Inflammatory and Antinociceptive Activities of a Hydroethanolic Extract of Tamarindus indica Leaves. *Sci. Pharm.* **2012**, *80*, 685–700. [CrossRef] [PubMed]
120. Tariq, M.; Chaudhary, S.; Rahman, K.; Hamiduddin; Zaman, R.; Shaikh, L. Tamarindus indica: An overview. *J. Biol. Sci. Opin.* **2013**, *1*, 128–131. [CrossRef]
121. Yusha'u, M.; Gabari, D.A.; Dabo, N.T.; Hassan, A.; Dahiru, M. Biological activity and phytochemical constituents of Tamarindus indica stem bark extracts. *Sky J. Microbiol. Res.* **2014**, *2*, 67–71.
122. Doughari, J.H. Antimicrobial Activity of Tamarindus indica Linn. *Trop. J. Pharm. Res.* **2006**, *5*, 597–603. [CrossRef]
123. Kapur, M.A.; John, S.A. Antimicrobial Activity of Ethanolic Bark Extract of Tamarindus indica against some Pathogenic Microorganisms. *Int. J. Curr. Microbiol. Appl. Sci.* **2014**, *3*, 589–593.
124. Ahmed, A.O.E.E.; Ayoub, S.M.H. Chemical composition and antimalarial activity of extracts of Sudanese Tamarindus indica L. (Fabaceae). *Pharma Innov. J.* **2015**, *4*, 90–93.
125. Isha, D.; Milind, P. IMLII: A Craze Lovely. *Int. Res. J. Pharm.* **2012**, *3*, 110–115.
126. Maikai, V.A.; Kobo, P.I.; Maikai, B.V.O. Antioxidant properties of Ximenia Americana. *Afr. J. Biotechnol.* **2010**, *9*, 7744–7746.
127. Monte, F.J.Q.; de Lemos, T.L.G.; de Araújo, M.R.S.; Gomes, E.S. Ximenia americana: Chemistry, Pharmacology and Biological Properties, a Review. 2012. Available online: www.intechopen.com (accessed on 12 December 2016).
128. Araújo, M.R.S.; Assunção, J.C.C.; Dantas, I.N.F.; Costa-Lotufo, L.V.; Monte, F.J.Q. Chemical Constituents of Ximenia americana. *Nat.Prod. Commun.* **2008**, *3*, 857–860.
129. Fatope, M.O.; Adoum, O.A.; Takeda, Y. C18 Acetylenic Fatty Acids of Ximenia americana with Potential Pesticidal Activity. *J. Agric. Food Chem.* **2000**, *4*, 1872–1874. [CrossRef]
130. Saeed, A.E.M.; Bashier, R.S.M. Physico-chemical analysis of Ximenia americana L. oil and structure elucidation of some chemical constituents of its seed oil and fruit pulp. *J. Pharmacogn. Phytother.* **2010**, *2*, 49–55.
131. Kouri, F.C. Investigation phytochimique d'une brosse à dents africaine Zanthoxylum zanthoxyloides (Lam.) Zepernick et Timler (Syn. Fagara zanthoxyloides L.) (Rutaceae). Thèse, Université de Lausanne, Lausanne, Suisse, 2004.
132. Gansane, A.; Sanon, S.; Ouattara, P.L.; Hutter, S.; Olivier, E.; Azas, N.; Traore, A.S.; Guissou, I.P.; Nebie, I.; Sirima, B.S. Antiplasmodial activity and cytotoxicity of semi purified fraction: Zanthoxylum zanthoxyloïdes Lam. Bark of trunk. *Int. J. Pharm.* **2010**, *6*, 921–925. [CrossRef]
133. Ouedraogo, S.; Traore, A.; Lompo, M.; Some, N.; Sana, B.; Guissou, I.P. Vasodilator effect of Zanthoxylum zanthoxyloïdes, Calotropis procera and FACA, a mixture of these two plants. *Int. J. Biol. Chem. Sci.* **2011**, *5*, 1351–1357. [CrossRef]

134. Olounladé, P.A.; Hounzangbé-Adoté, M.S.; Azando, E.V.B.; TAmha, T.B.; Brunet, S.; Moulis, C.; Fabre, N.; Fouraste, I.; Hoste, H.; Valentin, A. Etude in vitro de l'effet des tanins de Newbouldia laevis et de Zanthoxylum zanthoxyloïdes sur la migration des larves infestantes de Haemonchus contortus. *Int. J. Biol. Chem. Sci.* **2011**, *5*, 1414–1422.
135. Affouet, K.M.; Tonzibo, Z.F.; Attioua, B.K.; Chalchat, J.C. Chemical Investigations of Volatile Oils from Aromatic Plants Growing in Côte d'ivoire: *Harisonia abyssinica* Oliv., *Canarium schwerfurthii* Engl. *Zanthoxylum gilletti* (De wild) Waterm. And *Zanthoxylum zanthoxyloides* Lam. *Anal. Chem. Lett.* **2012**, *2*, 367–372.
136. Ouattara, B.; Angenot, L.; Guissou, P.; Fondu, P.; Dubois, J.; Frédérich, M.; Jansen, O.; Van Heugen, J.C.; Wauters, J.N.; Tits, M. LC/MS/NMR analysis of isomeric divanilloylquinic acids from the root bark of Fagara zanthoxyloides Lam. *Phytochemistry* **2004**, *65*, 1145–1151. [CrossRef] [PubMed]
137. Sameera, N.S.; Mandakini, B.P. Investigations into the antibacterial activity of Ziziphus mauritiana Lam. and Ziziphus xylopyra (Retz.) Willd. *Int. Food Res. J.* **2015**, *22*, 849–853.
138. Ashraf, A.; Sarfraz, R.A.; Anwar, F.; Shahid, S.A.; Alkharfy, K.M. Chemical composition and biological activities of leaves of Ziziphus mauritiana l. Native to Pakistan. *Pak. J. Bot.* **2015**, *47*, 367–376.
139. Parmar, P.; Bhatt, S.; Dhyani, D.S.; Jain, A. Phytochemical studies of the secondary metabolites of Ziziphus mauritiana Lam. Leaves. *Int. J. Curr. Pharm. Res.* **2012**, *4*, 153–155.
140. Springer, T.L.; Mcgraw, R.L.; Aiken, G.E.; Michx, L. Variation of Condensed Tannins in Roundhead Lespedeza Germplasm. *Crop Sci.* **2002**, *42*, 2157–2160. [CrossRef]
141. Adetutu, A.; Morgan, W.A.; Corcoran, O. Ethnopharmacological survey and in vitro evaluation of wound-healing plants used in South-western Nigeria. *J. Ethnopharmacol.* **2011**, *137*, 50–56. [CrossRef] [PubMed]
142. Kalla, A. Etude et valorisation des principes actifs de quelques plantes du sud algérien: *Pituranthos scoparius, Rantherium adpressum* et *Traganum nudatum*. Ph.D. Thesis, Université Mentouri-Constantine, Constantine, Algérie, 2012.
143. Feknous, S.; Saidi, F.; Said, R.M. Extraction, caractérisation et identification de quelques métabolites secondaires actifs de la mélisse (*Melissa officinalis* L.). *Nat. Technol.* **2014**, *11*, 7–13.
144. Mohagheghzadeh, A.; Faridi, P.; Shams-ardakani, M.; Ghasemi, Y. Medicinal smokes. *J. Ethnopharmacol.* **2006**, *108*, 161–184. [CrossRef] [PubMed]
145. Ujváry, I. Psychoactive natural products: Overview of recent developments. *Ann Ist Super Sanità* **2014**, *50*, 12–27. [PubMed]
146. Amar, B.M. *La Polyconsommation de Psychotropes et les Principales Interactions Pharmacologiques Associées*; Centre québécois de lutte aux dépendances: Québec, QC, Canada, 2007.
147. Organisation Mondiale de la Santé (OMS). *Neurosciences: Usage de Substances Psychoactives et Dépendance*; OMS: Genève, Suisse, 2004.
148. Stafford, G.I.; Jäger, A.K.; Van Staden, J. African Psychoactive Plants. *Challenges* **2009**, *1021*, 323–346.

5

Angiotensin I-Converting Enzyme (ACE) Inhibitory Activity, Antioxidant Properties, Phenolic Content and Amino Acid Profiles of *Fucus spiralis* L. Protein Hydrolysate Fractions

Lisete Paiva [1], Elisabete Lima [1,2,*], Ana Isabel Neto [3] and José Baptista [1,2]

1 Biotechnology Centre of Azores (CBA), University of Azores, 9501-801 Ponta Delgada, Portugal; lisete.s.paiva@uac.pt (L.P.); jose.ab.baptista@uac.pt (J.B.)
2 Research Center for Agricultural Technology (CITA-A), University of Azores, 9501-801 Ponta Delgada, Portugal
3 Azorean Biodiversity Group, Centre for Ecology, Evolution and Environmental Changes (CE3C), Department of Biology, University of Azores, 9501-801 Ponta Delgada, Portugal; ana.im.neto@uac.pt
* Correspondence: elisabete.mc.lima@uac.pt

Abstract: Food protein-derived hydrolysates with multi-bioactivities such as antihypertensive and antioxidant properties have recently received special attention since both activities can play significant roles in preventing cardiovascular diseases. This study reports, for the first time, the angiotensin I-converting enzyme (ACE)-inhibition and antioxidant properties of ultrafiltrate fractions (UF) with different molecular weight ranges (<1, 1–3 and ≥3 kDa) obtained from *Fucus spiralis* protein hydrolysate (FSPH) digested with cellulase–bromelain. The amino acids profile, recovery yield, protein, peptide and total phenolic contents of these FSPH-UF, and the in vitro digestibility of *F. spiralis* crude protein were also investigated. FSPH-UF ≥3 kDa presented remarkably higher ACE-inhibition, yield, peptide and polyphenolic (phlorotannins) contents. Antioxidant analysis showed that FSPH-UF <1 kDa and ≥3 kDa exhibited significantly higher scavenging of 2,2-diphenyl-1-picrylhydrazyl radical and ferrous ion-chelating (FIC) activity. FSPH-UF ≥3 kDa had also notably higher ferric reducing antioxidant power (FRAP). Strong correlations were observed between ACE-inhibition and antioxidant activities (FIC and FRAP). The results suggest that ACE-inhibition and antioxidant properties of FSPH-UF may be due to the bioactive peptides and polyphenols released during the enzymatic hydrolysis. In conclusion, this study shows the potential use of defined size FSPH-UF for the prevention/treatment of hypertension and/or oxidative stress-related diseases.

Keywords: edible brown algae; protein enzymatic hydrolysate; ultrafiltration; ACE-inhibition; antioxidant properties; phlorotannins; peptide fractions; amino acids composition; marine functional foods; cardiovascular-health

---

1. Introduction

Marine organisms, including macro-algae, are a valuable source of structurally diverse bioactive metabolites with various biological activities due to their living mode in highly competitive and aggressive surroundings, which are very different in many aspects from terrestrial environment, a situation that demands the production of quite specific and potent bioactive molecules. As a result, the importance of these organisms as a natural resource of bioactive compounds, which may lead to the development of new drugs and functional foods or nutraceuticals, is growing rapidly [1].

Macro-algae have been consumed in Asian countries since ancient times and their dietary intake has been shown to decrease blood pressure in humans [2]. However, the angiotensin

I-converting enzyme (ACE) inhibitory activity from macro-algae has not been extensively studied [3]. ACE belongs to the class of zinc metal proteases that catalyzes the conversion of angiotensin I to a potent vasoconstrictor angiotensin II and also promotes the degradation of the vasodilator bradykinin [4]. Therefore, this multifunctional enzyme plays a key role in the control of blood pressure, since the inhibition of its activity leads to a decrease in the angiotensin II concentration and an increase in the bradykinin level, and consequently in the reduction of hypertension that is one of the major causes of chronic diseases and a high risk factor of cardiovascular diseases worldwide [5]. A wide variety of synthetic drugs have been extensively used in treatment of hypertension and most of them have an ACE-inhibitory activity, however, these drugs can cause certain adverse side effects [6]. Therefore, searching for ACE-inhibitors from natural resources, such as marine organisms including macro-algae [3,7–9], has shown a growing interest in the field of nutraceutical, pharmaceutical and functional foods industries. The most commonly studied natural ACE-inhibitors were protein hydrolysates and peptides, however, others molecules that affect the ACE activity include the phorotannins group that are the predominant polyphenols in brown algae, being particularly abundant in Fucaceae [10–13]. In addition to its strong ACE-inhibition, phlorotannins have been recently demonstrated to possess numerous health benefits, including potent antioxidant effects (for a review see [14]). Since functional food products with multi-bioactivities are receiving wider attention, the potential antioxidant of macro-algal protein hydrolysates/peptides with ACE-inhibitory activity has also been investigated [15–17]. In fact, it is well known that natural antioxidants are powerful substances that play an important role against various diseases (atherosclerosis, cancer, chronic inflammation, cardiovascular disorders, hypertension) and ageing process, directly related to oxidative stress [18].

There is substantial scientific evidence that enzymatic hydrolysis of food protein sources is an efficient method to recover potent bioactive peptides that may present lower side effects [1,19]. Furthermore, enzymatic proteolysis can also release other bioactive compounds such as phorotannins bound to proteins, as reported for some brown macro-algae [20].

The Azores Islands (Portugal) being isolated in the middle of Atlantic Ocean and surrounded by waters with low pollution levels [21] is a very promising location to look for new marine ingredients with medicine-like effects in treating or preventing chronic diseases. Traditionally, the Azorean population has gathered seaweeds either as food or for chemicals extraction. The brown seaweed *Fucus spiralis*, which is abundant in the Azorean intertidal zone, is a local delicacy, particularly the frond tips (the receptacles) that are picked and eaten fresh [22]. Previous studies on its nutritional and/or pharmacological value from our research group have reported that *F. spiralis* is a good source of valuable biochemical compounds [23] and its methanol extract could also be a source of powerful ACE-inhibitory phlorotannins with potential impact on human health [9]. *F. spiralis* from other origins have been also demonstrated to possess high antioxidant properties, mainly linked to its phlorotannin content [24–26].

This is, for the best of our knowledge, the first study of *F. spiralis* enzymatic protein hydrolysate as source of compounds with multi-bioactivities for potential use in food and pharmaceutical industries and it was aimed to: (i) optimize the protein extraction process to obtain higher yield of *F. spiralis* protein hydrolysate, (ii) fractionate the cellulase–bromelain protein hydrolysate by ultrafiltration membranes into different molecular weight fractions (<1, 1–3 and $\geq$3 kDa), (iii) evaluate the ultrafiltrate fractions for multifunctional properties in vitro, namely the ACE-inhibitory activity and the antioxidant properties using different assays, such as the scavenging of 2,2-diphenyl-1-picrylhydrazyl radical, the ferrous ion-chelating and the ferric reducing antioxidant power, (iv) determine the amino acids profile, recovery yield, protein, peptide and total phenolic contents of the ultrafiltrate fractions, and (v) evaluate the in vitro digestibility of *F. spiralis* crude protein. The findings of the current study can also contribute to the increasing database of medicinal macro-algae.

2. Results and Discussion

2.1. *F. spiralis* Protein Content and In Vitro Protein Digestibility Evaluation

Results revealed that *F. spiralis* has a protein content of 8.53 ± 0.03% (on a dry basis), which is within the range reported for brown algae (3.0–15.0%) [27]. *F. spiralis* protein digestibility, expressed as a relative percentage of sodium caseinate digestibility normalized at 100%, was 85.95 ± 0.85%. It is well known that amino acid profiles are important in evaluating the proteins quality, and their digestibility is the primary determinant of its amino acid availability, but the in vivo algae protein digestibility is still poorly described. However, the high protein digestibility determined in vitro suggests that *F. spiralis* can be used as a complementary source of food proteins for human and animal nutrition, which according to Fleurence [27], would be a promising way for the exploitation of marine resources in Europe.

2.2. Preparation of *F. spiralis* Protein Hydrolysate (FSPH) and Its Fractionation by Ultrafiltration

In this study, *F. spiralis* protein concentrate after a two steps hydrolysis with a combination of two enzymes (cellulase and bromelain) followed by membrane ultrafiltration yielded three fractions ($Fr_1 < 1$ kDa, 1 kDa $\leq Fr_2 < 3$ kDa and $Fr_3 \geq 3$ kDa) that presented values of 206.28, 53.72 and 703.95 mg/g of dry FSPH, respectively (Table 1). These fractions were assessed for their ACE-inhibitory and antioxidant activities in order to find new marine sources of functional food products with multi-bioactivities for application in food and medicine industries. Indeed, according to some researchers [17,20], enzymatic hydrolysis can enhance the release of ACE inhibitory and antioxidant compounds (such as peptides and polyphenols) from the algal matrix. On the other hand, the use of carbohydrases, such as cellulase that breakdown cellulose and some related polysaccharides [28], can be useful before proteolytic enzymes applications. In fact the results showed that, when cellulase was used before the enzymatic hydrolysis with bromelain, the yield of *F. spiralis* protein concentrate was 1.5-fold increased. The choice of bromelain was based on our previous study [29] that showed the higher proteolytic activity (number of peptides) of bromelain as compared to the other nine commercial proteases tested using *F. spiralis* water extracts.

Table 1. Angiotensin I-converting enzyme (ACE) inhibitory activity, recovery yield, protein and peptide contents of *F. spiralis* protein hydrolysate (FSPH) fractions obtained by ultrafiltration.

Sample	Yield (mg/g of DW FSPH)	ACE-Inhibition		Protein Content (mg/g of DW FSPH)	Peptide Content (mg/g of DW FSPH)
		Percentage	IC_{50} Value (mg/mL)		
$Fr_1 < 1$ kDa	206.28	45.08 ± 0.66 ^{a}	1.850 ± 0.06 ^{b}	123.15 ± 2.78 ^{a}	43.81 ± 2.27 ^{a}
1 kDa $\leq Fr_2 < 3$ kDa	53.72	41.93 ± 1.62 ^{a}	2.000 ± 0.06 ^{b}	336.28 ± 4.96 ^{b}	35.91 ± 1.58 ^{a}
$Fr_3 \geq 3$ kDa	703.95	86.85 ± 1.89 ^{b}	0.500 ± 0.03 ^{a}	474.03 ± 4.44 ^{b}	243.82 ± 2.9 ^{b}

Values are mean ± SD ($n = 3$). Different superscript letters are significantly different ($p < 0.05$). IC_{50} value defined as the concentration which inhibits 50% of the ACE activity (tested concentration = 2 mg/mL). Captopril, used as a positive control for ACE-inhibition, showed an IC_{50} value of 0.163 ng/mL. DW, dry weight.

A two-steps hydrolysis was been previously used by our research group on other macro-algae proteins, to promote the release of low-MW (molecular weight) peptides [3]. Furthermore, this previous report also revealed that bromelain exhibited the highest specificity in the generation of ACE-inhibitory peptides from *Ulva rigida* protein. Other studies on other marine resources, such as different kinds of fish, also showed that bromelain is the most efficient protease tested for the production of protein hydrolysates with higher bioactivities (ACE-inhibitory and/or antioxidant activities) [30–32]. On the other hand, a molecular weight cut-off (MWCO) dialysis of FSPH was further used as means of enhancing its bioactivities, as well as to provide insights into the molecular weight distribution of the bioactive compounds presented in the hydrolysate. Furthermore, it should also be pointed out that the use of bioactive MWCO fractions instead of its purified active constituents for the development of functional foods presents multiple advantages. In fact, besides its low cost production and high production yield, MWCO fractions are formed by sets of compounds which could exhibit different biological activities and may act in synergy to increase its physiological effects on the organism [33]. In addition, the incorporation of protein hydrolysate fractions to foods could confer low cost desirable nutritional and functional properties.

2.3. Protein and Peptide Contents of FSPH Fractions

Protein and peptide contents of FSPH ultrafiltration fractions are also shown in Table 1, being the higher values in Fr_3 (474.03 $\pm$ 4.44 and 243.82 $\pm$ 2.91 mg/g of dry FSPH, respectively). The Fr_1 and Fr_2 presented also a higher value of protein (123.15 $\pm$ 2.78 and 336.28 $\pm$ 4.96 mg/g of dry FSPH, respectively), but only a small content of peptides (43.81 $\pm$ 2.27 and 35.91 $\pm$ 1.58 mg/g of dry FSPH, respectively) as compared to Fr_3.

2.4. Amino Acids Composition of FSPH Fractions

It is known that food protein hydrolysate/fractions containing appropriate amounts of amino acids with strong contribution properties could be potential candidates for use as potent antihypertensive and antioxidant agents [34]. As shown in Table 2, the amino acid's profiles varied among the FSPH ultrafiltration fractions in terms of individual and total amino acid contents. The total amino acid content in Fr_3 was 562.75 mg/g of dry FSPH which is significantly higher than those found in Fr_1 and Fr_2 (196.28 mg/g and 242.48 mg/g of dry FSPH, respectively). All the FSPH fractions showed remarkably higher percentage of the hydrophobic amino acids group (65.4–90.1% of the total amino acids), being valine the major amino acid in all fractions with 79.2%, 86.3% and 42.1% of the total amino acids in Fr_1, Fr_2 and Fr_3, respectively. Glutamic acid, tyrosine, aspartic acid and isoleucine were the other major amino acids in Fr_3, representing 8.2%, 6.8%, 6.7% and 5.8% of the total amino acids, respectively. In fractions Fr_1 and Fr_2, lysine and glutamic acid were the other major amino acids present. The amino acids content of Fr_1 was very similar to that of Fr_2. Overall, the Fr_3 had the highest concentration of aromatic amino acids as well as hydrophobic aliphatic amino acids such as isoleucine, leucine, alanine, methionine and proline that, according to the previous reports [17,33,34], may promote the ACE-inhibitory and antioxidant activities of food protein hydrolysates/fractions.

According to the literature, most seaweeds contains all essential amino acids and some also present high levels of acidic amino acids (8.0–44.0% on a dry basis) and low levels of histidine, threonine, tryptophan, lysine, methionine and cysteine [35]. In our study methionine, threonine and lysine, in which many cereals are deficient [36], were presented in reasonable percentages, particularly in Fr_3 and in Fr_1.

2.5. Total Phenolic Content (TPC) of FSPH Fractions

The TPC was quantified as phloroglucinol equivalents (PE), and the results (Figure 1) revealed that Fr_3 was the one with remarkably higher values (106.83 $\pm$ 0.76 mg PE/g of DW) followed by Fr_2 and Fr_1 with the values of 53.17 $\pm$ 0.76 and 15.00 $\pm$ 0.50 mg PE/g of DW, respectively, suggesting that high-MW phlorotannins are the largest pool of phenolic compounds in *F. spiralis*. On the other hand, the same order was observed for the protein content of FSPH fractions, as previously mentioned, suggesting that the fraction having a high content of protein tended to have a higher TPC. These findings are in accordance with Athukorala and Jeon [37] for the Flavourzyme *Ecklonia cava* hydrolysate fractions.

The TPC values of *F. spiralis* in the present study were higher than the ones reported by Tierney et al. [38] for Irish *F. spiralis*. This fact may be related with differences in the extraction methodology employed. Furthermore, significant intra-species variations of TPC in brown fucoid algae are well documented, showing the effect of several factors such as algae size, age, tissue type and environmental factors, including nutrient availability, light intensity, ultraviolet radiation, salinity, water depth and season [14,39].

Table 2. Amino acid profiles of *F. spiralis* protein hydrolysate fractions (mg amino acids/g of DW FSPH) obtained by ultrafiltration.

Amino Acid (AA)	*F. spiralis* Protein Hydrolysate (FSPH) Fraction		
	$Fr_1 < 1$ kDa	$1\ kDa \leq Fr_2 < 3$ kDa	$Fr_3 \geq 3$ kDa
Alanine	tc	tc	25.34 ± 0.13
Glycine	tc	tc	22.38 ± 0.13
Valine	155.53 ± 2.25	209.37 ± 3.35	236.83 ± 4.65
Threonine	1.22 ± 0.08	1.71 ± 0.03	17.42 ± 0.13
Serine	2.75 ± 0.06	3.18 ± 0.03	19.36 ± 0.16
Leucine	2.24 ± 0.12	2.85 ± 0.05	25.35 ± 0.17
Isoleucine	1.89 ± 0.03	2.84 ± 0.06	32.55 ± 0.43
Proline	1.34 ± 0.05	1.93 ± 0.03	12.47 ± 0.11
Methionine	tc	tc	20.07 ± 0.31
Aspartic acid	3.63 ± 0.07	4.53 ± 0.10	37.53 ± 0.35
Phenylalanine	1.80 ± 0.02	1.49 ± 0.02	15.13 ± 0.15
Glutamic acid	10.40 ± 0.10	7.01 ± 0.22	46.33 ± 0.42
Lysine	15.48 ± 0.20	7.57 ± 0.11	13.82 ± 0.13
Tyrosine	tc	tc	38.17 ± 0.21
Arginine	tc	tc	tc
Histidine	tc	tc	tc
Tryptophan	ND	ND	ND
Total AA	196.28 [a]	242.48 [a]	562.75 [b]
AA distribution (%)			
Hydrophobic	82.94 [a]	90.10 [a]	65.35 [b]
Hydrophilic	15. 04 [a]	7.88 [b]	17.36 [a]
Neutral	2.02 [b]	2.02 [b]	17.29 [a]
Aromatic	0.92 [b]	0.61 [b]	9.47 [a]
Branched-side chains	81.34 [a]	88.69 [a]	52.37 [b]
Negatively charged	7.15 [b]	4.76 [c]	14.90 [a]
Positively charged	7.89 [a]	3.12 [b]	2.46 [b]

Values are mean ± SD ($n = 3$). Means with different superscripts letters in the same row differ significantly ($p < 0.05$). Hydrophobic AA (Ala, Val, Leu, Ile, Pro, Met, Phe). Hydrophilic AA (Asp, Glu, Lys, Arg, His). Neutral AA (Gly, Thr, Ser, Tyr). Aromatic AA (Phe, Tyr). Branched-side chains AA (Val, Leu, Ile). Negatively charged AA (Asp, Glu). Positively charged AA (Lys, Arg, His). Tryptophan is not detected in this methodology. DW, dry weight; ND, not detected; tc, traces.

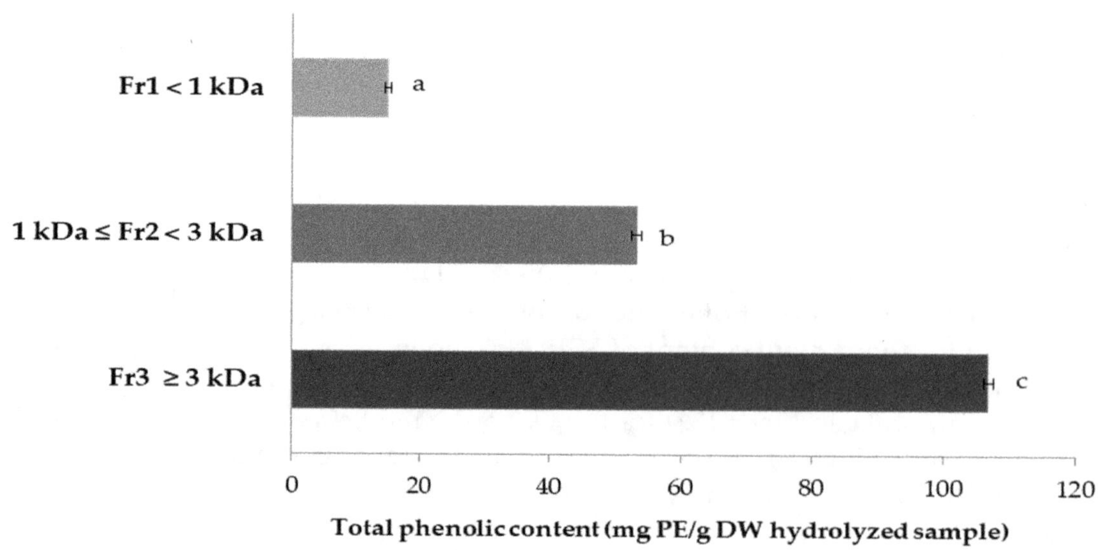

Figure 1. Total phenolic contents (TPC) of *F. spiralis* protein hydrolysate fractions obtained by ultrafiltration (tested concentration 2 mg/mL). Values are mean ± SD ($n = 3$). Different letters are significantly different ($p < 0.05$). Legend: DW, dry weight; PE, phloroglucinol equivalents.

According to the literature, brown macro-algae are a well-known source of phlorotannins, a structurally unique polyphenols that have gathered much attention due to their numerous bioactivities with high commercial interest for pharmaceutical, nutraceutical, cosmetic and especially food industries. Phlorotannins, which have been reported as the only phenolic group detected in some brown algae, such as *Fucus vesiculosus* [14], are highly hydrophilic components with a wide range of molecular sizes ranging between 126 Da and 650 kDa, although they are more commonly found in the 10 to 100 kDa range, particularly in the Fucaceae family [11,25]. Only few reports have focused on phlorotannin profile from *Fucus* spp. Phlorotannins with high degree of polymerization were observed in *F. spiralis* from Canada [40]; this information is important because it is known that ACE-inhibitory and antioxidant activities may depend on the degree of polymerization of phlorotannin derivatives [11,25]. Furthermore, sparse characterization of individual phlorotannin components has been carried out in *F. spiralis* species [9,24,41].

2.6. ACE-Inhibitory Activity of FSPH Fractions

The ACE-inhibition was determined by HPLC-UV method and the results (Table 1) revealed a remarkably higher activity in Fr_3 followed by Fr_1 and Fr_2 with percentage values of 86.85 $\pm$ 1.89%, 45.08 $\pm$ 0.66% and 41.93 $\pm$ 1.62% and IC_{50} values of 0.500 $\pm$ 0.03, 1.850 $\pm$ 0.06 and 2.000 $\pm$ 0.06 mg/mL, respectively. However, all FSPH fractions showed higher IC_{50} values as compared to captopril (0.163 ng/mL), a synthetic ACE-inhibitor used in this study as a positive control. A comparison of the present data with other results is quite difficult due to the lack of literature on ACE-inhibition of *Fucus* spp. protein hydrolysates/fractions, as well as variations in hydrolysis conditions. However, the ACE IC_{50} values obtained in this study (0.500–2.000 mg/mL) were similar to those reported for bromelain–alcalase protein hydrolysate fractions from the sea cucumber *Acaudina molpadioidea* (0.615–1.975 mg/mL) [42]. Furthermore, our values were similar or lower than those described for *Porphyra yezoensis* hydrolysates (1.520–3.210 mg/mL) [7], and are within the range reported for enzymatic hydrolysates from different protein sources (0.20–2.47 mg/mL) with antihypertensive activity in spontaneously hypertensive rats [43].

The difference in the ACE-inhibition among hydrolysate fractions could be related to the differences in amino acid compositions (Table 2) and their sequences, as well as the peptide sizes. Indeed, ACE-inhibitory peptides are usually between 2 and 30 amino acids in size [44]. On the other hand, according to the literature [17,45,46], the presence of aromatic and branched-side chain amino acids (BCAA) in peptides may promote the ACE-inhibition of food protein hydrolysates/fractions. Thus, the results of this study suggested that the relatively good ACE-inhibition (over 40%) of the low-MW FSPH fractions (Fr_1 and Fr_2) can be attributed to the presence of low-MW peptides plus the highest concentration of BCAA. In turn, the Fr_3 was the one with significantly higher aromatic amino acids content that make a substantial contribution to its ACE-inhibition by blocking angiotensin II production, probably due to their high steric properties and low lipophilicity [45]. Furthermore, the remarkably higher ACE-inhibition of Fr_3 could also be due to the contribution of polyphenols (phlorotannins) released during the enzymatic hydrolysis and concentrated in this fraction. In fact, some reports indicate that brown algae might have strong ACE-like inhibitors associated not only with peptides but also with phlorotannins [11,12]. Wijesinghe et al. [12] also reported that the ACE-inhibition may be closely associated with protein-binding abilities of phlorotannins, which are characteristic of all tannins. Indeed, it has been well described that tannins have the ability to form strong complexes with proteins, either reversibly by hydrogen bonding through peptide or amide linkages or irreversibly by covalent condensation, and that polyphenolic compounds inhibit ACE activity through sequestration of the enzyme metal factor (Zn^{2+}) [47]. A previous study by our research group [9] already reported that the strong ACE-inhibition by Azorean *F. spiralis* methanol extract may be due to its rich content of high-MW phorotannins, also concentrated in the MWCO $\geq$3 kDa fraction. Thus, *F. spiralis* phorotannins could be considered as potential phytopharmaceuticals for the development of new ACE inhibitors. On the other hand, it should be also pointed out that for food industry, enzymatic extracts, as obtained in the present study, is safer for consumers than organic solvent extracts, since the enzymatic method does not utilizes any organic solvent or other toxic chemicals.

2.7. Antioxidant Activities of FSPH Fractions

2.7.1. 2,2-Diphenyl-1-picrylhydrazyl (DPPH) Free Radical Scavenging Activity (FRSA) Assay

The scavenging activity of DPPH free radicals had been used extensively to determine the antioxidant power of bioactive natural products. The results revealed that FRSA increased with increasing FSPH fraction concentration (Figure 2). At the highest concentration of 200 µg/mL the Fr_1 presented the highest FRSA value (86.03 ± 0.25%), followed by Fr_3 (80.50 ± 0.53%) whereas the Fr_2 presented the lowest value (32.73 ± 0.32%); furthermore, the FRSA of Fr_1 was comparable to that of the commercial antioxidant butylated hydroxytoluene (BHT). Tierney et al. [38] reported a lower value (6.18 ± 2.16%, the reciprocal of the IC_{50}) of FRSA for the fraction with a MW of 3 kDa obtained from Irish *F. spiralis* hydrolysate digested with carbohydrase Viscozyme. These results may suggest that the enzymatic method used in the present study was more effective for the generation of antioxidant hydrolysates from *F. spiralis*. Several studies have also shown that, generally, low-MW hydrolysate fractions have higher DPPH radical scavenging activity than in high-MW hydrolysate fractions [48,49]. However, Fr_3 showed an IC_{50} value of 55 µg/mL that is lower than Fr_1 (85 µg/mL). Similar results were reported by Udenigwe et al. [50], who found that the high-MW fractions of flaxseed protein hydrolysate showed better FRSA as compared to the low-MW fractions.

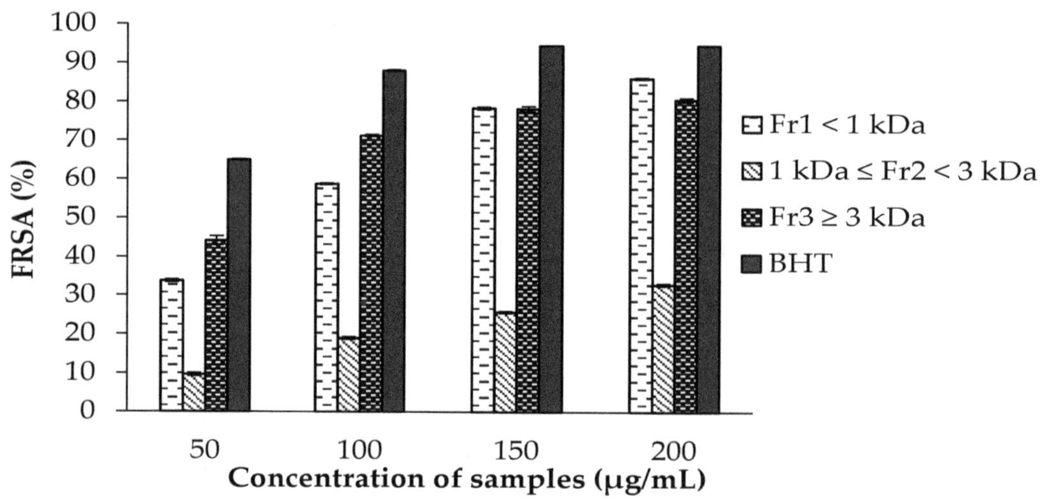

Figure 2. Free radical scavenging activity (FRSA) of *F. spiralis* protein hydrolysate fractions obtained by ultrafiltration. BHT (butylated hydroxytoluene) was used as positive control. Values are mean ± SD (n = 3).

The difference in the FRSA among the hydrolysate fractions might be related not only to their different peptide sizes but also to the differences in the amino acid compositions (Table 2) and their sequences, as well as the synergistic contributions of the active compounds. Indeed, research by Chen et al. [51] and Guo et al. [52] has demonstrated that DPPH radical scavenging activity is related to the amino acids composition. It was reported that aromatic amino acids and hydrophobic aliphatic amino acids (such as alanine, leucine, methionine and valine) play an important role in the DPPH radical scavenging activity [53,54]. Alemán et al. [55] also reports that the presence of those amino acids in a peptide sequence might increase the ability to access and neutralize the reactive free radicals and consequently to enhance the antioxidant activity. In addition, acidic amino acids had showed strong positive effects on scavenging of DPPH and, in contrast, positively-charged amino acids strongly contributed negatively to FRSA [34]. Thus, the lower FRSA IC_{50} value in Fr_3 might be related to the highest content of aromatic, acidic and hydrophobic aliphatic amino acid residues, with exception for valine, as well as to the lowest positively-charged amino acids content. However, the superior TPC of Fr_3 than in low-MW fractions (Fr_1 and Fr_2), as previously mentioned, may suggest that high-MW phlorotannins are the principal contributor to the lower FRSA IC_{50} value observed. Similar results were reported by other researchers, who found that high-MWCO fractions of *Fucus* species, such as *F. vesiculosus* [39] and *F. serrata* [56], had the highest FRSA and phenolic content (phlorotannins). It should also be highlighted that a recent study [26] revealed that phlorotannin-enriched fractions from *F. spiralis* from Peniche (Portugal) have the capacity to inhibit in vitro human cellular damage promoted by reactive oxygen species. Kim et al. [57] also reported that the fraction >30 kDa of the Celluclast enzymatic extract from brown algae *Ecklonia cava* possesses high protective effects against hydrogen peroxide-induced cell damage, attributed to the presence of phlorotannins. As in the present study, this *E. cava* fraction revealed the highest TPC, whereas the lowest content was shown by the fraction <1 kDa.

2.7.2. Ferrous Ion-Chelating (FIC) Activity Assay

Since metal chelating capacity is claimed as one of the important mechanisms of antioxidant activity [58], FIC assay was also chosen to better characterize the antioxidant activity of FSPH fractions. As shown in Figure 3, and in accordance with FRSA results, Fr_3 presented the highest FIC activity ($47.33 \pm 1.15\%$) followed by Fr_1 ($40.28 \pm 1.21\%$), and Fr_2 the lowest value ($28.47 \pm 1.21\%$), but no significant difference was observed between Fr_1 and Fr_3. Similar results were found by Tierney et al. [38] for FIC activity ($50.67 \pm 5.58\%$) in the fraction with MW of 3 kDa from Irish *F. spiralis* Viscozyme hydrolysate. The FSPH Fr_1 and Fr_3 were moderate metal chelating agents as compared to the synthetic antioxidant EDTA, a potent metal-ion chelator used in this study as a positive control.

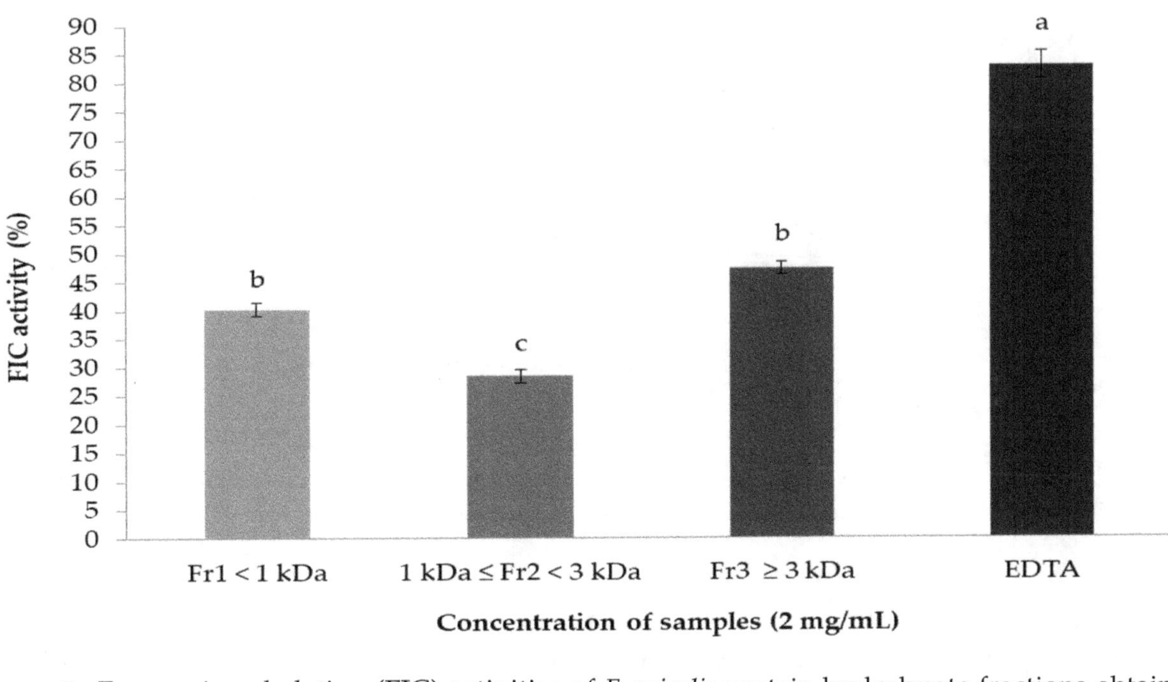

Figure 3. Ferrous ion-chelating (FIC) activities of *F. spiralis* protein hydrolysate fractions obtained by ultrafiltration. EDTA (ethylenediaminetetraacetic acid) was used as positive control. Values are mean ± SD ($n = 3$). Different letters are significantly different ($p < 0.05$).

Most of the reported peptides exhibiting chelating activities were those with low-MW [59], which explains the FIC activity of the lower-MW Fr_1. However, higher FIC activity in some other food hydrolysate fractions is linked to a larger peptide size [60]. Furthermore, peptides with high chelating activities have a high content of acidic amino acids [17]. As shown in Table 2, the Fr_3

had the highest content of negatively charged amino acids followed by Fr_1. On the other hand, Fr_3 presented the highest TPC value, as previously mentioned. Thus, the highest FIC activity of the higher-MW Fr_3 can be attributed to larger size bioactive compounds, such as the large peptides and the high-MW phlorotannins, released during the enzymatic hydrolysis and concentrated in this fraction. Indeed, some studies have demonstrated that polyphenols derived from algae are potent ferrous-ion chelators [61] and that its metal chelating potency is dependent upon their unique phenolic structure and the number and location of the hydroxyl groups [62]. However, to better evaluate the contribution of the polyphenols to the FIC activity of *F. spiralis*, additional research is needed on structural information of the bioactive compounds.

2.7.3. Ferric Reducing Antioxidant Power (FRAP) Assay

The highest FRAP was observed in Fr_3 followed by Fr_1 and Fr_2 fractions (Figure 4) for the higher concentration used (28.41 μg/mL), presenting absorbance values of 0.538, 0.334 and 0.185, respectively. The presence of reducers (antioxidants) causes the conversion of the Fe^{3+}/ferricyanide complex used in this method to the ferrous form. Therefore, by measuring the formation of Perl's Prussian blue at 700 nm, we can monitor the Fe^{2+} concentration, that indicates a higher reducing power, compared to that of BHT, which is known to be a strong reducing agent. The information on FRAP activity is important because the reducing capacity of a compound/fraction may serve as a significant indicator of reductones, that are reported to be terminators of free radicals chain reaction, presents in the samples [63–65].

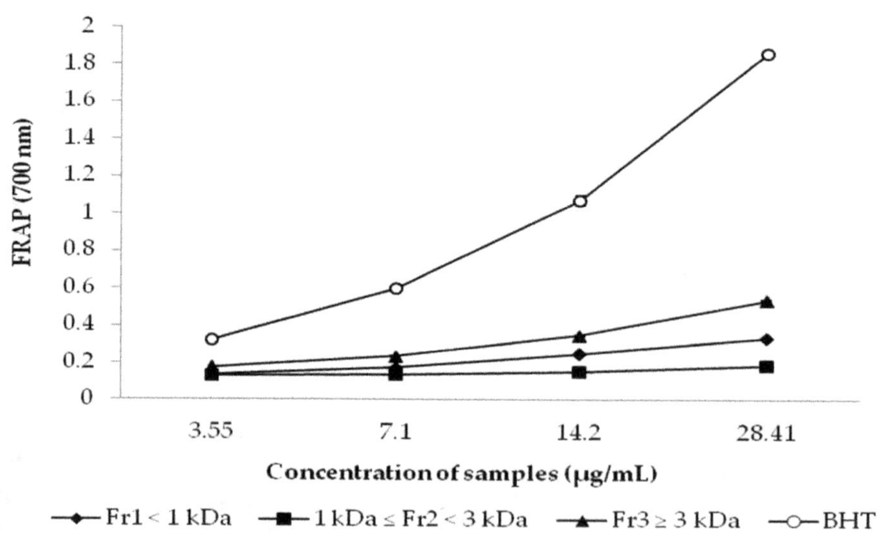

Figure 4. Ferric reducing antioxidant power (FRAP) of *F. spiralis* protein hydrolysate fractions obtained by ultrafiltration. BHT (butylated hydroxytoluene) was used as positive control. Values are mean ± SD (n = 3).

In accordance to the outlined for FRSA and FIC activity results, the highest FRAP of Fr_3 may be due, mainly, to its rich content of high-MW phlorotannins. Our findings are in agreement with previous studies on FRAP of MW-fractionated hydrolysates/extracts from other algae samples, such as the Irish *F. spiralis* [25,38] and other *Fucus* species (*F. vesiculosus* and *F. serrata*) [39,56]. Furthermore, as shown in Table 2, Fr_3 presented the highest content of the amino acids glutamic acid, aspartic acid, glycine, methionine and threonine as well as lysine in lower amount that, based on Udenigwe and Aluko [34], is a type of pattern that could have contributed to the highest FRAP observed in this FSPH fraction. Moreover, other authors observed that higher FRAP in some other food hydrolysate fractions is also linked to a larger size peptide content [60], that is in agreement with our results.

2.8. Pearson Correlation between Parameters

A significant correlation was found to occur among the methods for the antioxidant activities determination in all FSPH fractions (Table 3). FRSA and FIC activity ($r = 0.890$) were strongly correlated as well as FIC activity and FRAP ($r = 0.973$). A moderate correlation was found between FRSA and FRAP ($r = 0.760$). Concerning the correlation between TPC and antioxidant activities, a very weak correlation exists between TPC and FRSA ($r = 0.003$), and a weak correlation between TPC and FIC activity ($r = 0.458$), however, TPC and FRAP were moderately correlated ($r = 0.652$). On the other hand, strong correlations were observed between peptide content and FIC activity or FRAP or TPC ($r = 0.805$, $r = 0.921$ and $r = 0.896$), while the correlation between peptide content and FRSA was weak ($r = 0.446$). These results may reveal that other bioactive compounds such as peptides, in addition to polyphenols (phlorotannins), are contributing to the antioxidant activities of FSPH fractions evaluated by FRSA, FIC activity and FRAP assays. Previous research by Zubia et al. [66] and Vinayak et al. [67] also reported weak correlations ($r = -0.399$ and $r = 0.397$, respectively) between TPC and FRSA of macro-algal extracts. However, it should be noted that individual polyphenols may have a considerable antioxidant potential, but there may be antagonistic or synergistic interactions between phenolic and non-phenolic compounds that may affect the bioactivity [68]. Concerning the FIC activity, the correlations observed in the present study may suggest that polyphenols (phlorotannins) are not the principal chelators in some of FSPH fractions and that others compounds such as peptides, which are also recognized as effective chelating agents [69], may be the main contributors to the observed activities. Research by Wang et al. [48,58] has reported the absence of clear correlations between TPC and FIC ability of macro-algal extracts.

Table 3. Correlation matrix of the studied parameters (Pearson correlations coefficients).

	FRSA	FIC Activity	FRAP	Total Phenolic	ACE-Inhibition	Peptide Content
FRSA	1	-	-	-	-	-
FIC activity	0.890	1		-	-	-
FRAP	0.760	0.973	1	-	-	-
Total phenolic	0.003	0.458	0.652	1	-	-
ACE-inhibition	0.660	0.822	0.932	0.883	1	-
Peptide content	0.446	0.805	0.921	0.896	1	1

FRSA, free radical scavenging activity; FIC, ferrous ions (Fe^{2+}) chelating; FRAP, ferric reducing antioxidant power; ACE, angiotensin I-converting enzyme.

As for ACE-inhibitory activity, a perfect correlation was observed between ACE-inhibition and peptide content ($r = 1$) and strong correlations were observed between ACE-inhibition and FIC activity ($r = 0.822$), between ACE-inhibition and FRAP ($r = 0.932$), and between ACE-inhibition and TPC ($r = 0.883$). Only the correlation between ACE-inhibition and FRSA was moderate ($r = 0.660$). These findings suggest that either some peptides, which are recognized as effective ACE-inhibitors agents or polyphenols are contributing to the ACE-inhibition observed in all FSPH fractions.

Overall results from this study suggest that ACE-inhibition and antioxidant activities observed in FSPH fractions may be due to the sum of the activities of produced peptides and released polyphenols. However, in order to better understand the contribution of peptides and polyphenols to the aforementioned bifunctional properties, a complete chemical characterization of FSPH fractions should be done in future.

3. Materials and Methods

3.1. Chemicals and Reagents

Methanol (MeOH) and acetonitrile (ACN) HPLC grade were purchased from Fluka Chemika (Steinheim, Switzerland). Ammonium sulphate, sodium carbonate (Na_2CO_3), sodium phosphate, sodium tetraborate decahydrate, iron (II) chloride, sodium hydroxide (NaOH), ethanol, phenol and

85% phosphoric acid were from E. Merck (Darmstadt, Germany). Acetyl chloride and isobutanol were purchased from Alltech Associates (Deerfield, IL, USA). Amino acids standard mixture and sequanal grade 6 N HCl were purchased from Pierce Chemicals (Rockford, IL, USA). Sodium chloride (NaCl), ethyl acetate, heptafluorobutyric anhydride (HFB-IBA), sodium caseinate, 2-mercaptoethanol, brilliant Blue G-250, albumin from bovine serum (BSA), potassium ferricyanide, iron (III) chloride, ferrozine, trichloroacetic acid (TCA), trizma base, zinc chloride, hippuric acid (HA), hippuryl-L-histidyl-L-leucine (HHL), Folin–Ciocalteu reagent (FCR), phloroglucinol, butylated hydroxytoluene (BHT), ethylenediaminetetraacetic acid (EDTA), 2,2-diphenyl-1-picrylhydrazyl (DPPH), hydrochloric acid (HCl), glutathione, *O*-phthaldialdehyde (OPA), β-mercaptoethanol, sodium dodecyl sulphate, angiotensin I-converting enzyme (ACE) from porcine kidney, bromelain (B4882), cellulase from *Aspergillus niger* (C1184), chymotrypsin (C9381), peptidase (P7500) and trypsin (T8003) were obtained from Sigma-Aldrich (St. Louis, MO, USA). Ultrafiltration membrane system and membranes were purchased from Millipore Co (Bedford, MA, USA).

3.2. Collection and Preparation of *F. spiralis* Sample

F. spiralis Linnaeus (Ochrophyta, Phaeophyceae) sample was collected in January 2013 from the littoral of São Miguel Island of Azores Archipelago (37°40′ N and 25°31′ W), Portugal, and a voucher specimen was prepared (voucher number AZB, SMG-13-04) and deposited in the Herbarium AZB—Ruy Telles Palhinha of the Department of Biology at the University of Azores. Within 24 h of collection, *F. spiralis* sample was first washed in seawater followed by distilled water to remove encrusting material, epiphytes and salts, and then air-dried and stored in an air-tight container in a freezer (−80 °C) for not more than 6 months until further analysis. Prior to the analytical procedures, the sample was defrosted and dried at 40–45 °C for 48 h (avoiding overheating that could lead to oxidation), and then was grounded into a fine powder of 0.5 mm particle size, re-dried at 40 °C and stored in the dark under N_2 in a desiccator at a refrigerated temperature of 4–5 °C.

3.3. Extraction of Protein from *F. spiralis*

The protein of *F. spiralis* was extracted according to the method described by Wong et al. [70] with slight modifications. Five grams of sample powder were suspended in deionized water (1:10 *w*/*v*) to induce cell lysis by osmotic shock that facilitated subsequent protein extraction. The suspension was gently stirred overnight at 35 °C, which was found to be the optimal temperature for macro-algae protein solubility. After incubation, the suspension was centrifuged at 10,000× *g* and 4 °C for 20 min. The supernatant was collected and the pellet was re-suspended in deionized water with 0.5% 2-mercaptoethanol (*v*/*v*) being the pH adjusted to 12.0 with 1 M NaOH. The solution was gently stirred at room temperature for 2 h before centrifugation under the same conditions as above. The second supernatant was collected and combined with the first one. The combined supernatant was stirred at 4 °C and the pH was adjusted to 7.0 before precipitation with ammonium sulphate. The extraction method mentioned above was repeated three times on the residue. The combined supernatant was precipitated by slowly adding ammonium sulphate, with stirring, until 85% saturation (60 g/100 mL) and allowed to stand for 30 min. Then the solution (precipitated protein) was removed by centrifugation at 10,000× *g*, 4 °C for 20 min. The pellet obtained was dialyzed against distilled water until the total dissolved solutes of dialysate, measured by its conductivity, was similar to that of the distilled water. The retentate containing the protein concentrate of *F. spiralis* was lyophilized in a freeze-drier and stored at −20 °C until required. The protein content was determined by Bradford method [71] using BSA as the calibration standard.

3.4. In Vitro *F. spiralis* Protein Digestibility Evaluation

The in vitro digestibility of *F. spiralis* protein concentrate suspension was determined using a freshly prepared multiproteolytic enzyme solution (trypsin, chymotrypsin and peptidase), according to Paiva et al. [72], in order to reproduce the actual digestion environment in vivo. Fifty milliliters of aqueous protein suspension (6.25 mg protein/mL) in glass distilled water were adjusted to pH 8.0, while stirring in a 37 °C water bath. The multi-enzyme solution [1.6 mg/mL trypsin (10,000 BAEE units/mg protein), 3.1 mg/mL chymotrypsin (80 units/mg solid) and 1.3 mg peptidase/mL (50–100 units/g solid)] was maintained in an ice bath and adjusted to pH 8.0. Five milliliters of the multi-enzyme solution were then added to the protein suspension and the pH change in the mixture, caused by the enzymatic digestion, was measured after exactly 10 min. Sodium caseinate was used as control and the in vitro protein digestibility of the algae was expressed as a relative percentage to that of the sodium caseinate normalized at 100%.

3.5. Preparation of F. spiralis Protein Hydrolysate (FSPH)

The enzymatic reaction of the *F. spiralis* protein concentrate was carried out using two enzymes, cellulase followed by bromelain. One gram of protein concentrate sample was suspended and homogenized in 10 mL of ice-cold distilled water and each enzyme (substrate/enzyme ratio to 100:1, *w*/*w*) was individually added to the homogenate. For the enzymatic reaction was used cellulase at 50 °C and pH 4.5 (adjusted with 0.1 M HCl) followed by bromelain at 37 °C and pH 7.0 (adjusted with 0.5 M NaOH). The hydrolytic reaction was carried out for 20 h and after this period, the digestion solution was boiled for 10 min in order to inactivate the enzymes. The protein hydrolysate solution was centrifuged at 3000× *g* for 15 min, filtered through 0.45 μm filters, lyophilized in a freeze-drier and stored at −20 °C for further analysis.

3.6. Fractionation of FSPH by Ultrafiltration

The digested FSPH with cellulase and bromelain enzymes was further fractionated in a cell dialyzer system through three different ultrafiltration membranes with molecular weight cut-off (MWCO) of 1 and 3 kDa to obtain ultrafiltrates ($Fr_1 < 1$ kDa, 1 kDa $\leq Fr_2 <$ 3 kDa and $Fr_3 \geq$ 3 kDa). All the pooled FSPH fractions were lyophilized in a freeze-drier and assayed for ACE-inhibitory and antioxidant activities. The recovery yield of the ultrafiltration fractions was calculated using the gravimetric method.

3.7. Protein and Peptide Contents Analysis of FSPH Fractions

The protein content was determined by Bradford method [71] using BSA as the calibration standard and its peptide content was measured by OPA method [73] using glutathione as the calibration standard, according to Ghanbari et al. [46].

3.8. Amino Acids Composition of FSPH Fractions

The amino acids composition of FSPH fractions was determined according to Paiva et al. [3]. The dried FSPH fractions (0.5 mg) were placed in a small reaction vials, exposed to a stream of dry nitrogen, then capped and submitted to an acid hydrolysis at 100 °C for 24 h with 100 μL 6 N HCl containing 0.1% phenol for tyrosine protection. After cooling until room temperature, the samples were evaporated under a stream of dry nitrogen and then derivatized slowly by adding the mixture of acetyl chloride:isobutanol (1.25:5 mL, *v*/*v*, the reagent was obtained by adding the acetyl chloride to isobutanol precooled to −20 °C) and heating at 100 °C for 60 min. Next, the sample vials were opened and the mixtures exposed to a stream of dry nitrogen to remove excess reagent. After cooling in an ice bath, the samples were supplemented with 200 μL of acetonitrile and 50 μL of the derivatization reagent HFB-IBA, and heated again at 100 °C for 15 min. After evaporation of the excess reagent at 115 °C under a stream of dry nitrogen and cooling to room temperature, samples were dissolved in 300 μL of ethyl acetate and an aliquot (1 μL) was used for GC analysis. The GC analysis was performed using a Bruker GC model 450-GC gas chromatograph equipped with a split/splitless injector and a flame ionization detector (FID) using a wall-coated open tubular (WCOT) fused silica AT-Amino acid capillary column (25 m × 0.53 mm i.d., 1.2 μm film thickness) from Heliflex/Alltech (San Jose, CA, USA). The temperature started at 60 °C for 3 min, programmed at a rate of 4 °C/min to 210 °C and then held at this temperature for further 20 min. The injector and detector temperatures were held constants at 260 °C and 280 °C, respectively. Helium was the carrier gas at a flow rate of 28 cm/s.

3.9. *Total Phenolic Content (TPC) Determination of FSPH Fractions*

TPC was determined according to the method of Waterhouse [74] with slight modifications. An aliquot of 100 μL of FSPH fraction (2 mg/mL) was mixed with 1500 μL of distilled water and 100 μL of 2N FCR, homogenized in a vortex for 15 s and placed in dark for 3 min. Then, 300 μL of 10% Na_2CO_3 (*w*/*v*) was added to the mixture, homogenized and incubated for 5 min at 50 °C. The Abs values were measured at 760 nm. A blank sample was prepared by replacing the sample with Milli-Q water. The phloroglucinol (a basic structural unit of phlorotannins) was used as a standard and the results are expressed as mg of phloroglucinol equivalents (PE) per gram of dried FSPH fraction. A calibration curve was prepared using a concentration range of 50–300 μg/mL.

3.10. *ACE-Inhibitory Activity Determination of FSPH Fractions*

The determination of ACE-inhibitory activity was performed in vitro by RP-HPLC adapted from the spectrophotometric method described by Cushman and Cheung [75] with slight modifications [3]. This method is based on the liberation of hippuric acid from hippuryl-L-histidyl-L-leucine (Hip-His-Leu) catalyzed by ACE. For the assay, 42.5 μL of the sample solution (2 mg/mL) was pre-incubated at 37 °C for 5 min with 10 μL ACE (0.6 mU/mL) enzyme. The mixture was subsequently incubated at the same temperature for 60 min with 20 μL of the substrate (5 mM HHL in 10 μM zinc chloride containing 100 mM sodium trizma base and 300 mM NaCl at pH 8.3). The reaction was terminated by adding 12.5 μL of 5 M HCl. The percentage of ACE-inhibition was determined by an HPLC system from Waters equipped with a 626 pump and 600S controller coupled to a 486 tunable UV detector. An aliquot of 20 μL from the reaction mixture was analyzed on a reverse-phase Ultrasphere ODS analytical column (25 cm × 4.6 mm i.d., 5 μm particle size) (Beckman Coulter, Miami, FL, USA) using an isocratic elution of MeOH: ACN: 0.1% HCl (25:25:50, *v*/*v*/*v*) at a constant flow-rate of 0.6 mL/min and HA and HHL were detected by UV at 228 nm. The average value from three determinations at each concentration was used to calculate the ACE-inhibition (%) rate as follows: % ACE-inhibition = $[B - A/B - C] \times 100$, where A is the absorbance (Abs) of HA generated in the presence of ACE-inhibitor, B the Abs of HA generated without ACE-inhibitor and C the Abs of HA generated without ACE (corresponding to HHL autolysis in the course of enzymatic assay). The IC_{50} value (mg/mL) was defined as the concentration of inhibitor required to reduce the HA peak by 50% (corresponding to 50% inhibition of ACE activity). The captopril was used as a positive control for ACE-inhibition.

3.11. *Antioxidant Activity Assays on FSPH Fractions*

3.11.1. DPPH Free Radical Scavenging Activity (FRSA) Assay

The FRSA of FSPH fractions was determined according to the method of Molyneux [76] with slight modifications. The FRSA of each FSPH fraction was tested by measuring their ability to quench DPPH. The DPPH, a stable free radical, is reduced changing the purple color of the DPPH radical solution to a bright yellow in the presence of antioxidants that possess hydrogen-donating or chain-breaking properties and the intensity of this can be monitored spectrophotometrically [77]. An aliquot of 250 μL of FSPH fraction with various concentrations (or BHT) was added to 250 μL of 100 mM DPPH solution. BHT was used as reference sample and a mixture without FSPH sample or BHT was used as the control. The Abs was measured at 517 nm after 30 min in the dark. The FRSA of FSPH fractions was calculated as a percentage of DPPH decoloration using the following equation: % FRSA = $(1 - Abs_{sample}/Abs_{control}) \times 100$.

3.11.2. Ferrous Ion-Chelating (FIC) Activity Assay

Chelating ability of FSPH fractions was determined according to the modified method of Wang et al. [58], by measuring the inhibition of the Fe^{2+}–ferrozine complex formation. An aliquot of 100 μL of each FSPH fraction (concentration 2 mg/mL) was mixed with 135 μL of methanol plus 5 μL of 2 mM $FeCl_2$. The reaction was initiated by the addition of 10 μL of 5 mM ferrozine. After 10 min at room temperature, the Abs was determined at 562 nm. Methanol instead of ferrozine solution was used as a sample blank, which is used for error correction because of unequal color of the sample solutions. Methanol instead of sample solution was used as a control. Results are expressed as relative iron chelating activity compared with the unchelated (without ferrozine) Fe^{2+} reaction, and EDTA was used as reference standard. A lower Abs indicated a better FIC ability. The FIC ability was calculated as follows: % FIC ability = $[A_0 - (A_1 - A_2)]/A_0 \times 100$, where A_0 was the Abs of the control, A_1 was the Abs of the sample or standard and A_2 was the Abs of the blank.

3.11.3. Ferric Reducing Antioxidant Power (FRAP) Assay

The FRAP of FSPH fractions was determined according to the method of Oyaizu [78], and evaluated on the basis of their abilities to reduce Fe^{3+} complex to Fe^{2+}. An increased Abs value indicates an increased reducing power of the hydrolysate fractions. Each fraction (concentration range 12.5–100 μg/mL) in methanol (0.4 mL) was mixed with 0.4 mL of 300 mM of phosphate buffer (pH 6.6) plus 0.4 mL of potassium ferricyanide (1%, *w*/*v*) and the mixture was incubated at 50 °C for 20 min. After cooling down, 0.4 mL of TCA (10%, *w*/*v*) was added, and the mixture was centrifuged at 3000× *g* for 10 min. The upper layer (1 mL) was mixed with 1 mL of deionized water plus 0.2 mL of $FeCl_3$ (0.1% *w*/*v*), and the Abs was measured at 700 nm against a blank. The blank solution contained pure methanol instead of the methanolic FSPH fraction. BHT was used for comparison.

3.12. Statistical Analysis

All determinations were performed at least in triplicate and the results were expressed as means ± standard deviations (SD). The statistics analysis was performed using SPSS 17.0 (version 17, SPSS Inc., Chicago, IL, USA) and one-way analysis of variance test (ANOVA) was carried out to assess for any significant differences between the means. Differences between means at the 5% ($p < 0.05$) level were considered significant. Correlations between the parameters evaluated were obtained using Pearson's correlation coefficient (r).

4. Conclusions

Algae remain a relatively untapped source of compounds with ACE-inhibitory and antioxidant activities. To the best of our knowledge, this study revealed, for the first time, that enzymatic hydrolysate fractions with the aforementioned bifunctional properties could be efficiently generated from *F. spiralis* protein hydrolyzed by the cellulase–bromelain enzymes. The fraction with MW ≥3 kDa, obtained from this hydrolysate using ultrafiltration membranes, showed significantly higher recovery yield, ACE-inhibition and ferric reducing antioxidant power than the other fractions, and also showed strong scavenging of DPPH radical and ferrous ions (Fe^{2+}) chelating activity. The significant bioactivity of this fraction can be attributed to the high concentration of the potent active peptide sequences (even though the fraction contains peptides relatively large in size) and phenolic compounds (high-MW phlorotannins). Although additional research is needed on structural information of the bioactive compounds, overall results from this study indicate that the produced *F. spiralis* protein hydrolysate fractions can be promising natural sources to develop functional food ingredients for controlling hypertension and/or oxidative stress, the two major causes of cardiovascular diseases. However, in vivo studies are also needed to verify their physiological effects.

Acknowledgments: This study was financially supported by cE3c funding (Ref: UID/BIA/00329/2013). Lisete Paiva was supported by a doctoral grant (Ref: M3.1.2/F/014/2011) awarded by FRC (Fundo Regional da Ciência).

Author Contributions: Lisete Paiva designed the research project, performed the experimental work, analyzed the results and wrote the paper. Elisabete Lima, Ana Isabel Neto and José Baptista participated in the supervision process and critically revised the manuscript. All the authors approved the final manuscript.

References

1. Lordan, S.; Ross, R.P.; Stanton, C. Marine bioactives as functional food ingredients: Potential to reduce the incidence of chronic diseases. *Mar. Drugs* **2011**, *9*, 1056–1100. [PubMed]
2. Hata, Y.; Nakajima, K.; Uchida, J.I.; Hidaka, H.; Nakano, T. Clinical effects of brown seaweed, *Undaria pinnatifida* (*wakame*), on blood pressure in hypertensive subjects. *J. Clin. Biochem. Nutr.* **2001**, *30*, 43–53. [CrossRef]
3. Paiva, L.; Lima, E.; Neto, A.I.; Baptista, J. Isolation and characterization of angiotensin I-converting enzyme (ACE) inhibitory peptides from *Ulva rigida* C. Agardh protein hydrolysate. *J. Funct. Foods* **2016**, *26*, 65–76. [CrossRef]
4. Soffer, R.L. Angiotensin-converting enzyme and the regulation of vasoactive peptides. *Annu. Rev. Biochem.* **1976**, *45*, 73–94. [CrossRef] [PubMed]
5. Zhang, Y.; Lee, E.T.; Devereux, R.B.; Yeh, J.; Best, L.G.; Fabsitz, R.R.; Howard, B.V. Prehypertension, diabetes, and cardiovascular disease risk in a population-based sample: The strong heart study. *Hypertension* **2006**, *47*, 410–414. [CrossRef] [PubMed]
6. Andrews, P.R.; Carson, J.M.; Caselli, A.; Spark, M.J.; Woods, R. Conformational analysis and active site modelling of angiotensin-converting enzyme inhibitors. *J. Med. Chem.* **1985**, *28*, 393–399. [CrossRef] [PubMed]
7. Suetsuna, K. Purification and identification of angiotensin I-converting enzyme inhibitors from the red alga *Porphyra yezoensis*. *J. Mar. Biotechnol.* **1998**, *6*, 163–167. [PubMed]
8. Sato, M.; Hosokawa, T.; Yamaguchi, T.; Nakano, T.; Muramoto, K.; Kahara, T.; Funayama, K.; Kobayashi, A.; Nakano, T. Angiotensin I-converting enzyme inhibitory peptides derived from Wakame (*Undaria pinnatifida*) and their antihypertensive effect in spontaneously hypertensive rats. *J. Agric. Food Chem.* **2002**, *50*, 6245–6252. [CrossRef] [PubMed]
9. Paiva, L.; Lima, E.; Neto, A.I.; Baptista, J. Angiotensin I-converting enzyme (ACE) inhibitory activity of *Fucus spiralis* macroalgae and influence of the extracts storage temperature: A short report. *J. Pharm. Biomed. Anal.* **2016**, *131*, 503–507. [CrossRef] [PubMed]
10. Jung, H.A.; Hyun, S.K.; Kim, H.R.; Choi, J.S. Angiotensin-converting enzyme I inhibitory activity of phlorotannins from *Ecklonia stolonifera*. *Fish. Sci.* **2006**, *72*, 1292–1299. [CrossRef]
11. Wijesekara, I.; Kim, S.-K. Angiotensin-I-converting enzyme (ACE) inhibitors from marine resources: Prospects in the pharmaceutical industry. *Mar. Drugs* **2010**, *8*, 1080–1093. [CrossRef] [PubMed]
12. Wijesinghe, W.A.J.P.; Ko, S.-C.; Jeon, Y.-J. Effect of phlorotannins isolated from *Ecklonia cava* on angiotensin I-converting enzyme (ACE) inhibitory activity. *Nutr. Res. Pract.* **2011**, *5*, 93–100. [CrossRef] [PubMed]
13. Olivares-Molina, A.; Fernández, K. Comparison of different extraction techniques for obtaining extracts from brown seaweeds and their potential effects as angiotensin I-converting enzyme (ACE) inhibitors. *J. Appl. Phycol.* **2016**, *28*, 1295–1302. [CrossRef]
14. Catarino, M.D.; Silva, A.M.S.; Cardoso, S.M. Fucaceae: A source of bioactive phlorotannins. *Int. J. Mol. Sci.* **2017**, *18*, 1327. [CrossRef] [PubMed]
15. Harnedy, P.A.; FitzGerald, R.J. Bioactive proteins, peptides and amino acids from macroalgae. *J. Phycol.* **2011**, *47*, 218–232. [CrossRef] [PubMed]
16. Samarakoon, K.; Jeon, Y.-J. Bio-functionalities of proteins derived from marine algae—A review. *Food Res. Int.* **2012**, *48*, 948–960. [CrossRef]
17. Cian, R.E.; Alaiz, M.; Vioque, J.; Drago, S.R. Enzyme proteolysis enhanced extraction of ACE inhibitory and antioxidant compounds (peptides and polyphenols) from *Porphyra columbina* residual cake. *J. Appl. Phycol.* **2013**, *25*, 1197–1206. [CrossRef]

18. Oroian, M.; Escriche, I. Antioxidants: Characterization, natural sources, extraction and analysis. *Food Res. Int.* **2015**, *74*, 10–36. [CrossRef] [PubMed]
19. Korhonen, H.; Pihlanto, A. Food-derived bioactive peptides—Opportunities for designing future foods. *Curr. Pharm. Des.* **2003**, *9*, 1297–1308. [CrossRef] [PubMed]
20. Wijesinghe, W.A.; Jeon, Y.-J. Enzyme-assistant extraction (EAE) of bioactive components: A useful approach for recovery of industrially important metabolites from seaweeds: A review. *Fitoterapia* **2012**, *83*, 6–12. [CrossRef] [PubMed]
21. Neto, A.I.; Brotas, V.; Azevedo, J.M.N.; Patarra, R.F.; Álvaro, N.M.V.; Gameiro, C.; Prestes, A.C.L.; Nogueira, E.M. *Qualidade de Águas Costeiras do Grupo Oriental do Arquipélago dos Açores e Proposta de Monitorização*; Universidade dos Açores: Ponta Delgada, Portugal, 2009.
22. Neto, A.I.; Tittley, I.; Raposeiro, P.M. *Flora Marinha do Litoral dos Açores. Rocky Shore Marine Flora of the Azores*; Secretaria Regional do Ambiente e do Mar: Horta, Portugal, 2005.
23. Paiva, L.; Lima, E.; Patarra, R.F.; Neto, A.I.; Baptista, J. Edible Azorean macroalgae as source of rich nutrients with impact on human health. *Food Chem.* **2014**, *164*, 128–135. [CrossRef] [PubMed]
24. Cerantola, S.; Breton, F.; Ar Gall, E.; Deslandes, E. Co-occurrence and antioxidant activities of fucol and fucophlorethol classes of polymeric phenols in *Fucus spiralis*. *Bot. Mar.* **2006**, *49*, 347–351. [CrossRef]
25. Tierney, M.S.; Smyth, T.J.; Rai, D.K.; Soler-Vila, A.; Croft, A.K.; Brunton, N. Enrichment of polyphenol contents and antioxidant activities of Irish brown macroalgae using food-friendly techniques based on polarity and molecular size. *Food Chem.* **2013**, *139*, 753–761. [CrossRef] [PubMed]
26. Pinteus, S.; Silva, J.; Alves, C.; Horta, A.; Fino, N.; Inês Rodrigues, A.; Mendes, S.; Pedrosa, R. Cytoprotective effect of seaweeds with high antioxidant activity from the Peniche coast (Portugal). *Food Chem.* **2017**, *218*, 591–599. [CrossRef] [PubMed]
27. Fleurence, J. Seaweed proteins: Biochemical nutritional aspects and potential uses. *Trends Food Sci. Technol.* **1999**, *10*, 25–28. [CrossRef]
28. Quiroz-Castañeda, R.E.; Folch-Mallol, J.L. Hydrolysis of biomass mediated by cellulases for the production of sugars. In *Sustainable Degradation of Lignocellulosic Biomass-Techniques, Applications and Commercialization*; Chandel, A.K., da Silva, S.S., Eds.; InTech North America: New York, NY, USA, 2013.
29. Paiva, L.; Lima, E.; Neto, A.I.; Baptista, J. Screening for angiotensin I-converting enzyme (ACE) inhibitory activity of enzymatic hydrolysates obtained from Azorean macroalgae. *Arquipél. Life Mar. Sci.* **2015**, *32*, 11–17.
30. Elavarasan, K.; Kumar, V.N.; Shamasundar, B.A. Antioxidant and functional properties of fish protein hydrolysates from fresh water carp (*Catla catla*) as influenced by the nature of enzyme. *J. Food Process. Preserv.* **2014**, *38*, 1207–1214. [CrossRef]
31. Gajanan, P.G.; Elavarasan, K.; Shamasundar, B.A. Bioactive and functional properties of protein hydrolysates from fish frame processing waste using plant proteases. *Environ. Sci. Pollut. Res.* **2016**, *23*, 24901–24911. [CrossRef] [PubMed]
32. Auwal, S.M.; Zarei, M.; Abdul-Hamid, A.; Saari, N. Optimization of bromelain-aided production of angiotensin I-converting enzyme inhibitory hydrolysates from stone fish using response surface methodology. *Mar. Drugs* **2017**, *15*, 104. [CrossRef] [PubMed]
33. Chalé, F.G.H.; Ruiz, J.C.R.; Fernández, J.J.A.; Ancona, D.A.B.; Campos, M.R.S. ACE inhibitory, hypotensive and antioxidant peptide fractions from *Mucuna pruriens* proteins. *Process Biochem.* **2014**, *49*, 1691–1698. [CrossRef]
34. Udenigwe, C.C.; Aluko, R.E. Chemometric analysis of the amino acid requirements of antioxidant food protein hydrolysates. *Int. J. Mol. Sci.* **2011**, *12*, 3148–3161. [CrossRef] [PubMed]
35. Fleurence, J. Seaweed proteins. In *Proteins in Food Processing*; Yada, R.Y., Ed.; Woodhead Publishing Limited: Cambridge, UK, 2004; pp. 197–213.
36. Ge, Y.; Sun, A.; Ni, Y.; Cai, T. Study and development of a defatted wheat germ nutritive noodle. *Eur. Food Res. Technol.* **2001**, *212*, 344–348. [CrossRef]
37. Athukorala, Y.; Jeon, Y.J. Screening for angiotensin I-converting enzyme inhibitory activity of *Ecklonia cava*. *J. Food Sci. Nutr.* **2005**, *10*, 134–139. [CrossRef]
38. Tierney, M.S.; Soler-vila, A.; Croft, A.K.; Hayes, M. Antioxidant activity of the brown macroalgae *Fucus spiralis* Linnaeus harvested from the west coast of Ireland. *Curr. Res. J. Biol. Sci.* **2013**, *5*, 81–90.

39. Wang, T.; Jónsdóttir, R.; Liu, H.; Gu, L.; Kristinsson, H.G.; Raghavan, S.; Ólafsdóttir, G. Antioxidant capacities of phlorotannins extracted from the brown algae *Fucus vesiculosus*. *J. Agric. Food Chem.* **2012**, *60*, 5874–5883. [CrossRef] [PubMed]
40. Steevensz, A.J.; MacKinnon, S.L.; Hankinson, R.; Craft, C.; Connan, S.; Stengel, D.B.; Melanson, J.E. Profiling phlorotannins in brown macroalgae by liquid chromatography-high resolution mass spectrometry. *Phytochem. Anal.* **2012**, *23*, 547–553. [CrossRef] [PubMed]
41. Ferreres, F.; Lopes, G.; Gil-Izquierdo, A.; Andrade, P.B.; Sousa, C.; Mouga, T.; Valentão, P. Phlorotannin extracts from Fucales characterized by HPLC-DAD-ESI-MS^n: Approaches to hyaluronidase inhibitory capacity and antioxidant properties. *Mar. Drugs* **2012**, *10*, 2766–2781. [CrossRef] [PubMed]
42. Zhao, Y.; Li, B.; Dong, S.; Liu, Z.; Zhao, X.; Wang, J.; Zeng, M. A novel ACE inhibitory peptide isolated from *Acaudina molpadioidea* hydrolysate. *Peptides* **2009**, *30*, 1028–1033. [CrossRef] [PubMed]
43. Hong, L.G.; Wei, L.G.; Liu, H.; Hui, S.Y. Mung-bean protein hydrolysates obtained with Alcalase exhibit angiotensin I-converting enzyme inhibitory activity. *Food Sci. Technol. Int.* **2005**, *11*, 281–287.
44. Wilson, J.; Hayes, M.; Carney, B. Angiotensin-I-converting enzyme and prolyl endopeptidase inhibitory peptides from natural sources with a focus on marine processing by-products. *Food Chem.* **2011**, *129*, 235–244. [CrossRef]
45. Segura-Campos, M.R.; Peralta-González, F.; Castellanos-Ruelas, A.; Chel-Guerrero, L.A.; Betancur-Ancona, D.A. Effect of *Jatropha curcas* peptide fractions on the angiotensin I-converting enzyme inhibitory activity. *Biomed. Res. Int.* **2013**. [CrossRef] [PubMed]
46. Ghanbari, R.; Zarei, M.; Ebrahimpour, A.; Abdul-Hamid, A.; Ismail, A.; Saari, N. Angiotensin-I converting enzyme (ACE) inhibitory and anti-oxidant activities of sea cucumber (*Actinopyga lecanora*) hydrolysates. *Int. J. Mol. Sci.* **2015**, *16*, 28870–28885. [CrossRef] [PubMed]
47. Liu, J.-C.; Hsu, F.-L.; Tsai, J.-C.; Chan, P.; Liu, J.Y.; Thomas, G.N.; Tomlinson, B.; Lo, M.-Y.; Lin, J.-Y. Antihypertensive effects of tannins isolated from traditional Chinese herbs as non-specific inhibitors of angiotensin converting enzyme. *Life Sci.* **2003**, *73*, 1543–1555. [CrossRef]
48. Wang, T.; Jónsdóttir, R.; Kristinsson, H.G.; Hreggvidsson, G.O.; Jónsson, J.O.; Thorkelsson, G.; Ólafsdóttir, G. Enzyme-enhanced extraction of antioxidant ingredients from red algae *Palmaria palmata*. *LWT—Food Sci. Technol.* **2010**, *43*, 1387–1393. [CrossRef]
49. Fan, J.; He, J.; Zhuang, Y.; Sun, L. Purification and identification of antioxidant peptides from enzymatic hydrolysates of Tilapia (*Oreochromis niloticus*) frame protein. *Molecules* **2012**, *17*, 12836–12850. [CrossRef] [PubMed]
50. Udenigwe, C.C.; Lu, Y.-L.; Han, C.-H.; Hou, W.-C.; Aluko, R.E. Flaxseed protein-derived peptide fractions: Antioxidant properties and inhibition of lipopolysaccharide-induced nitric oxide production in murine macrophages. *Food Chem.* **2009**, *116*, 277–284. [CrossRef]
51. Chen, H.-M.; Muramoto, K.; Yamauchi, F.; Fujimoto, K.; Nokihara, K. Antioxidative properties of histidine-containing peptides designed from peptide fragments found in the digests of a soybean protein. *J. Agric. Food. Chem.* **1998**, *46*, 49–53. [CrossRef] [PubMed]
52. Guo, H.; Kouzuma, Y.; Yonekura, M. Structures and properties of antioxidative peptides derived from royal jelly protein. *Food Chem.* **2009**, *113*, 238–245. [CrossRef]
53. Rajapakse, N.; Mendis, E.; Jung, W.-K.; Je, J.-Y.; Kim, S.-K. Purification of a radical scavenging peptide from fermented mussel sauce and its antioxidant properties. *Food. Res. Int.* **2005**, *38*, 175–182. [CrossRef]
54. Nimalaratne, C.; Bandara, N.; Wu, J. Purification and characterization of antioxidant peptides from enzymatically hydrolyzed chicken egg white. *Food Chem.* **2015**, *188*, 467–472. [CrossRef] [PubMed]
55. Alemán, A.; Pérez-Santín, E.; Bordenave-Juchereau, S.; Arnaudin, I.; Gómez-Guillén, M.C.; Montero, P. Squid gelatin hydrolysates with antihypertensive, anticancer and antioxidant activity. *Food Res. Int.* **2011**, *44*, 1044–1051. [CrossRef]
56. Heffernan, N.; Smyth, T.J.; Soler-Villa, A.; Fitzgerald, R.J.; Brunton, N.P. Phenolic content and antioxidant activity of fractions obtained from selected Irish macroalgae species (*Laminaria digitata*, *Fucus serratus*, *Gracilaria gracilis* and *Codium fragile*). *J. Appl. Phycol.* **2015**, *27*, 519–530. [CrossRef]
57. Kim, K.N.; Heo, S.-J.; Song, C.B.; Lee, J.; Heo, M.S.; Yeo, I.K.; Kang, K.; Hyun, J.W.; Jeon, Y.-J. Protective effect of *Ecklonia cava* enzymatic extracts on hydrogen peroxide-induced cell damage. *Process Biochem.* **2006**, *41*, 2393–2401. [CrossRef]

58. Wang, T.; Jónsdóttir, R.; Ólafsdóttir, G. Total phenolic compounds, radical scavenging and metal chelation of extracts from Icelandic seaweeds. *Food Chem.* **2009**, *116*, 240–248. [CrossRef]
59. Torres-Fuentes, C.; Alaiz, M.; Vioque, J. Affinity purification and characterisation of chelating peptides from chickpea protein hydrolysates. *Food Chem.* **2011**, *129*, 485–490. [CrossRef]
60. Girgih, A.T.; Udenigwe, C.C.; Aluko, R.E. In vitro antioxidant properties of hemp seed (*Cannabis sativa* L.) protein hydrolysate fractions. *J. Am. Oil Chem. Soc.* **2011**, *88*, 381–389. [CrossRef]
61. Senevirathne, M.; Kim, S.-H.; Siriwardhana, N.; Ha, J.-H.; Lee, K.-W.; Jeon, Y.-J. Antioxidant potential of *Ecklonia cava* on reactive oxygen species scavenging, metal chelating, reducing power and lipid peroxidation inhibition. *Rev. Agaroquim. Tecnol. Aliment.* **2006**, *12*, 27–38.
62. Santoso, J.; Yoshie-Stark, Y.; Suzuki, T. Anti-oxidant activity of methanol extracts from Indonesian seaweeds in an oil emulsion model. *Fish. Sci.* **2004**, *70*, 183–188. [CrossRef]
63. Duh, P.-D. Antioxidant activity of burdock (*Arctium lappa* Linné): It's scavenging effect on free radical and active oxygen. *J. Am. Oil Chem. Soc.* **1998**, *75*, 455–461. [CrossRef]
64. Chandini, S.-K.; Ganesan, P.; Bhaskar, N. In vitro antioxidant activities of three selected brown seaweeds of India. *Food Chem.* **2008**, *107*, 707–713. [CrossRef]
65. Ganesan, P.; Kumar, C.S.; Bhaskar, N. Antioxidant properties of methanol extract and its solvent fractions obtained from selected Indian red seaweeds. *Bioresour. Technol.* **2008**, *99*, 2717–2723. [CrossRef] [PubMed]
66. Zubia, M.; Fabre, M.S.; Kerjean, V.; Lann, K.L.; Stiger-Pouvreau, V.; Fauchon, M.; Deslandes, E. Antioxidant and antitumoural activities of some Phaeophyta from Brittany coasts. *Food Chem.* **2009**, *116*, 693–701. [CrossRef]
67. Vinayak, R.C.; Sabu, A.S.; Chatterji, A. Bio-prospecting of a few brown seaweeds for their cytotoxic and antioxidant activities. *Evid. Based Complement. Altern. Med.* **2011**. [CrossRef] [PubMed]
68. Babbar, N.; Oberoi, H.S.; Uppal, D.S.; Patil, R.T. Total phenolic content and antioxidant capacity of extracts obtained from six important fruit residues. *Food Res. Int.* **2011**, *44*, 391–396. [CrossRef]
69. Pal, R.; Rai, J.P. Phytochelatins: Peptides involved in heavy metal detoxification. *Appl. Biochem. Biotechnol.* **2010**, *160*, 945–963. [CrossRef] [PubMed]
70. Wong, K.H.; Cheung, P.C.K.; Ang, P.O., Jr. Nutritional evaluation of protein concentrates isolated from two red seaweeds: *Hypnea charoides* and *Hypnea japonica* in growing rats. *Hydrobiologia* **2004**, *512*, 271–278. [CrossRef]
71. Bradford, M.M. A rapid and sensitive method for the quantitation of microgram quantities of protein utilizing the principle of protein-dye binding. *Anal. Biochem.* **1976**, *72*, 248–254. [CrossRef]
72. Paiva, L.; Lima, E.; Neto, A.I.; Massimo, M.; Baptista, J. Nutritional and functional bioactivity value of selected Azorean macroalgae: *Ulva compressa*, *Ulva rigida*, *Gelidium microdon*, and *Pterocladiella capillacea*. *J. Food Sci.* **2017**, *82*, 1757–1764. [CrossRef] [PubMed]
73. Church, F.C.; Swaisgood, H.E.; Porter, D.H.; Catignani, G.L. Spectrophotometric assay using *O*-phthaldialdehyde for determination of proteolysis in milk and isolated milk proteins. *J. Dairy Sci.* **1983**, *66*, 1219–1227. [CrossRef]
74. Waterhouse, A.L. Determination of total phenolics. In *Current Protocols in Food Analytical Chemistry*; Wrolstad, R.E., Ed.; John Wiley & Sons: New York, NY, USA, 2002.
75. Cushman, D.W.; Cheung, H.S. Spectrophotometric assay and properties of the angiotensin-converting enzyme of rabbit lung. *Biochem. Pharmacol.* **1971**, *20*, 1637–1648. [CrossRef]
76. Molyneux, P. The use of the stable free radical diphenylpicrylhydrazyl (DPPH) for estimating antioxidant activity. *Songklanakarin J. Sci. Technol.* **2004**, *26*, 211–219.
77. Corrêa, A.P.; Daroit, D.J.; Coelho, J.; Meira, S.M.; Lopes, F.C.; Risso, P.H.; Brandelli, A. Antioxidant, antihypertensive and antimicrobial properties of ovine milk caseinate hydrolyzed with a microbial protease. *J. Sci. Food Agric.* **2011**, *91*, 2247–2254. [CrossRef] [PubMed]
78. Oyaizu, M. Studies on products of browning reactions: Antioxidative activities of products of browning reaction prepared from glucosamine. *Jpn. J. Nutr.* **1986**, *44*, 307–315. [CrossRef]

6

Inhibitory Growth of Oral Squamous Cell Carcinoma Cancer via Bacterial Prodigiosin

Ming-Fang Cheng [1,2], Chun-Shu Lin [3], Yu-Hsin Chen [4,5], Ping-Jyun Sung [4,5,6], Shian-Ren Lin [4], Yi-Wen Tong [4] and Ching-Feng Weng [4,5,*]

1 Department of Pathology, Tri-Service General Hospital, National Defense Medical Center, Taipei 10086, Taiwan; drminfung@gmail.com
2 Division of Histology and Clinical Pathology, Hualian Army Forces General Hospital, Hualien 97144, Taiwan
3 Department of Radiation Oncology, Tri-Service General Hospital, National Defense Medical Center, Taipei 10086, Taiwan; Chunshulin@gmail.com
4 Department of Life Science and Institute of Biotechnology, National Dong Hwa University, Hualien 97401, Taiwan; 810013103@gms.ndhu.edu.tw (Y.-H.C.); pjsung@nmmba.gov.tw (P.-J.S.); d9813003@gms.ndhu.edu.tw (S.-R.L.); mecurry@gmail.com (Y.-W.T.)
5 Graduate Institute of Marine Biotechnology, National Dong Hwa University, Pingtung 94450, Taiwan
6 National Museum of Marine Biology and Aquarium, Pingtung 94450, Taiwan
* Correspondence: cfweng@gms.ndhu.edu.tw

Abstract: Chemotherapy drugs for oral cancers always cause side effects and adverse effects. Currently natural sources and herbs are being searched for treated human oral squamous carcinoma cells (OSCC) in an effort to alleviate the causations of agents in oral cancers chemotherapy. This study investigates the effect of prodigiosin (PG), an alkaloid and natural red pigment as a secondary metabolite of *Serratia marcescens*, to inhibit human oral squamous carcinoma cell growth; thereby, developing a new drug for the treatment of oral cancer. In vitro cultured human OSCC models (OECM1 and SAS cell lines) were used to test the inhibitory growth of PG via cell cytotoxic effects (MTT assay), cell cycle analysis, and Western blotting. PG under various concentrations and time courses were shown to effectively cause cell death and cell-cycle arrest in OECM1 and SAS cells. Additionally, PG induced autophagic cell death in OECM1 and SAS cells by LC3-mediated P62/LC3-I/LC3-II pathway at the in vitro level. These findings elucidate the role of PG, which may target the autophagic cell death pathways as a potential agent in cancer therapeutics.

Keywords: prodigiosin; marine viva; autophage; oral squamous cell carcinoma

---

1. Introduction

Oral cancer is the main cause of cancer death in males in Taiwan and is ranked the fourth leading cause of death overall. Oral cancer mortality and incidence data show that men with oral cancer increases annually. This trend derives from men smoking cigarettes, drinking alcohol, and chewing betel nut. Surprisingly, when a human subject has all three of these habits, the relative risk of oral cancer increases by 122.8 times [1]. Oral squamous cell carcinoma (OSCC) is common in both genders, followed by verrucous carcinoma, undifferentiated carcinoma, and small salivary adenocarcinoma. OSCC is a common type of head and neck cancer [2], excluding oropharynx and hypopharynx. OSCC is locally destructive, may invade the soft tissue and bone, and can be extended to nerves, lymphatic system, and blood vessels. Through these mechanisms, it can spread throughout the body and cause cervical lymph nodes metastasis and distant metastasis [3]. To avoid burdens of the chemotherapy agent in cancer patients, the inductions of cell apoptosis and autophagy are taken firstly into consideration during therapy regimen. This theme is becoming the critical standard for anti-cancer drug discovery.

Autophagy has been shown to be an intracellular degradation process in eukaryotic cells in response to stress, including starvation, clearing damaged proteins and organelles, and promoting cell survival [4,5]. Furthermore, autophagy occurs in multiple processes including nucleation, expansion, and maturation/retrieval to exert the effects of either autophagic cell death or cytoprotection [6]. Currently, two pathways have been investigated to associate with the regulation of autophagy in mammalian cells including the PI3K Class III/Akt/mTOR/p70S6K signaling pathway and the Ras/Raf/MEK/ERK1/2 pathway [7,8]. The ERK1/2 pathway could positively activate autophagy, whereas the Akt/mTOR pathway might suppress autophagy. These signaling pathways could be activated in numerous tumors and are thought to trigger the autophagy and oncogenesis [9]. The stimulation of mTOR protein level is a central regulator of autophagy [10]. Moreover, Akt was associated with cell survival and its expression could down-regulate the LC3-II expression; thereby, suppressing autophagy [11–13]. The amount of LC3-II is demonstrated to correlate well with the amount of autophagosomes [1,14].

Prodigiosin (PG, PubChem CID: 5377753), an alkaloid and natural red pigment, that is a secondary metabolite of *Serratia marcescens*. It is characterized by a common pyrrolyl pyrromethene skeleton [15,16]. Bacterial PGs and their synthetic derivatives have antimicrobial (bactericidal and bacteriostatic) [17–20], antimalarial [17,18,21], and antitumor [17,18,22–24] properties. Additionally, they have been shown to be effective apoptotic agents against various cancer cell lines [25], with multiple cellular targets, including multi-drug resistant cells with little or no toxicity towards normal cell lines, and induce apoptosis in T and B lymphocytes [26,27]. Moreover, PG and its structural analogue (compound R) have induced the expression of p53 target genes accompanied by cell-cycle arrest and apoptosis in p53-deficient cancer cells [28]. PG could be effective as a potential inhibitor compound against COX-2 protein, and can be applied as an anti-inflammatory drug [29]. In melanoma cells, PG activates the mitochondrial apoptotic pathway by disrupting an anti-apoptotic member of the BCL-2 family-MCL-1/BAK complexes by binding to the BH3 domain [30]. Additionally, PG exerts nearly identical cytotoxic effects on the resistant cells in comparison to their parental lines, revealing that this pro-apoptotic agent acts independently on the overexpression of multi-drug resistance transporters-MDR1, BCRP, or MRP [31]. Mechanistically, PG engages the IRE1-JNK and PERK-eIF2α branches of the UPR signaling to up-regulate CHOP, which in turn mediates BCL-2 suppression to induce cell death in multiple human breast carcinoma cell lines [32].

Anti-cancer chemical drugs for oral cancer include 5-FU, cisplatin, paclitaxel, and Ufur. Nonetheless, these chemotherapy drugs always induce side effects, such as nausea, vomiting, loss of appetite, decreased immunity, and adverse effects of oral ulcers. Recently, many natural sources [33–37] and traditional medicinal herbs [38–40] have been studied on OSCC in an effort to mitigate the abovementioned problems, however the solicitation remains incompletely explored. The present study investigated whether PG could have benefits to cause the inhibiting growth of human gingival squamous carcinoma cells (OECM-1) and human tongue cancer (SAS) cell lines by 3-(4,5-Dimethylthiazol-2-yl)-2,5-diphenyltetrazolium bromide (MTT) assay, flow cytometry assay, Western blotting and autophagosome formation assay.

2. Results and Discussion

2.1. *Effect of Prodigiosin on the Cell Viability of Oral Cancer Cells*

To determine the cytotoxicity of PG in normal cell, normal mouse hepatocyte FL83B cell line was examined. The cell viability of FL83B with various concentration of PG treatment was found no significant cytotoxicity of PG treatment except less cytotoxicity at 25 μM (Figure 1A). In addition, SAS and OECM1 cells were initially treated with 0.1, 0.5, 1.0, and 5.0 μM of PG for 24 h to measure cell viability for the cytotoxic effect of PG. The viable SAS and OECM1 cells were significantly decreased after PG treatment in a dose-dependent manner (Figure 1B,C). The values of IC_{50} on OECM1 and SAS cells were also determined at the concentrations of 1.59 ± 0.77 and 3.25 ± 0.49 μM of PG, respectively.

This result indicated that the low concentration of PG elicits the cytotoxicity of OSCC as compared to the untreated cells. Previous reports have demonstrated that PG could cause cell death via apoptotic cell death in several tumors, including human leukemia cells, melanoma, neuroblastoma, colorectal cancer, and breast cancer [32,41,42]. PG and its structural analogue (compound R) are also proven to induce cell-cycle arrest by the expression of p53 target genes in p53-deficient cancer cells [28]. Additionally, as p53 tumor suppressor integrated multiple stress signals, serial anti-proliferative responses would occur to induce apoptosis [43]. In this study, firstly, we presented the inhibitory growth role of PG in human oral squamous cell carcinoma cells in vitro and loss of cell viability was initially found in OECM1 and SAS cells with a dose-dependent fashion after 24 h incubation of PG (Figure 1). Moreover, the IC_{50} of PG on OECM1 and SAS cells were in the low and potential extent.

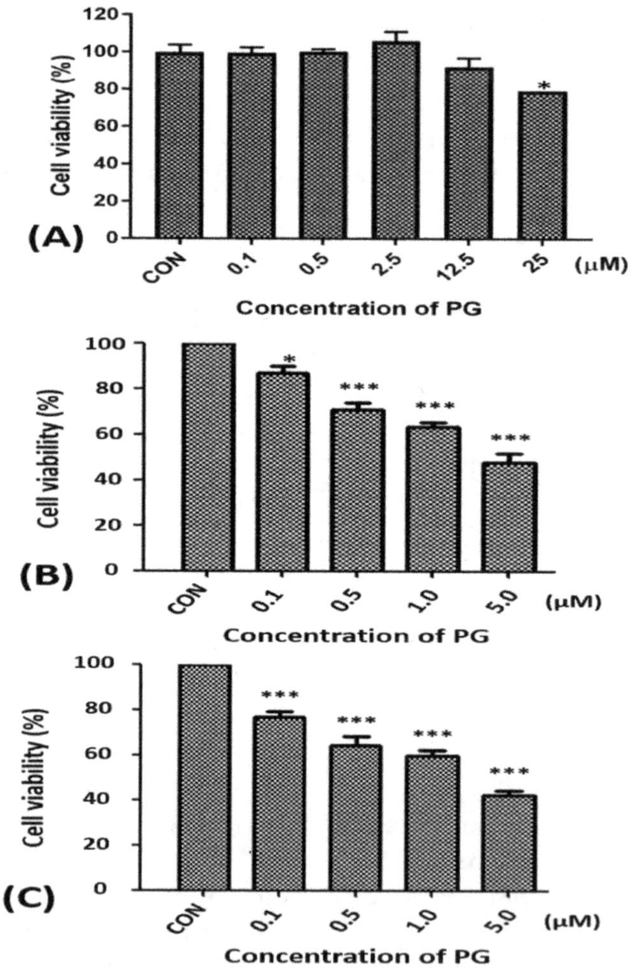

Figure 1. Alterations of the cell viability of FL83B, SAS, and OECM1 cells after prodigiosin treatment. (**A**) FL83B cells were incubated with 0.1 to 25 μM of prodigiosin (PG) for 24 h, (**B**) SAS and (**C**) OECM1 cells were incubated with 0.1, 0.5, 1.0, and 5.0 μM of PG for 24 h, and cell viability was determined by 3-(4,5-Dimethylthiazol-2-yl)-2,5-diphenyltetrazolium bromide (MTT) assay. The data are shown as the mean ± SEM of three independent experiments. * $P < 0.05$; *** $P < 0.001$ when compared with the untreated controls (0 μM).

2.2. *Effect of Prodigiosin on the Cell Cycle of Oral Cancer Cells*

Obviously, cell cycle of SAS cells after 12 and 24 h of PG treatments showed different pattern. In 12 h treatments of PG, sub-G_1 and S phase of SAS cells were not significantly different and G_0/G_1 phase of SAS cells raised from 40.3 ± 3.3% to 51.4 ± 1.2% ($P < 0.05$). G_2/M phase of SAS cells was decreased from 32.4 ± 2.9% to 27.2 ± 0.7% ($P < 0.05$). In 24 h treatments of PG, S phase of SAS cells was still not significantly different but sub-G_1 and G_0/G_1 phase of SAS cells were elevated from 0.9 ± 0.3% to 2.5 ± 0.7% and 42.1 ± 2.7% to 54.0 ± 3.7%, respectively ($P < 0.05$). G_2/M phase of SAS cells was also decreased from 36.6 ± 2.1% to 26.3 ± 3.2% ($P < 0.05$; Table 1).

As SAS cells, sub-G_1 phase of OECM1 cells in 12 h treatments of PG were not significantly different but G_0/G_1 phase of OECM1 cells was significantly increased from 50.9 ± 1.7% to 63.3 ± 0.4% ($P < 0.05$). S and G_2/M phase of OECM1 cells were decreased from 16.6 ± 1.0% to 10.5 ± 0.2% and 32.1 ± 0.4% to 25.7 ± 0.8%, respectively ($P < 0.05$). In 24 h treatments of PG, sub-G_1 phase of OECM1 cells was not significantly different but G_2/M phase of OECM1 cells was decreased from 36.9 ± 3.1% to 18.7 ± 3.3%, respectively ($P < 0.05$). G_0/G_1 and S phase of OECM1 cells were increased from 47.9 ± 2.3% to 61.8 ± 0.4% and 14.0 ± 1.6% to 18.4 ± 2.6%, respectively ($P < 0.05$; Table 2). The above results indicated that PG might inhibit cell growth via arresting cell cycle in G_0/G_1 phase. The protein level of cyclin D1 was analyzed to ensure the hypothesis of cell cycle arrest. Cyclin D1 in two cell lines was significantly decreased after 0.5 and 1.0 μM of PG treatments, which was consistent with the result of cell cycle analysis ($P < 0.05$; Figure 2A,B). These findings indicated that PG could induce cell cycle arrest and delay cell cycle progression, which attributed to inhibitory growth effects of PG in oral cancer cells. In addition, the cell cycle distribution after PG stimulation was observed to arrest in G_0/G_1 phase of SAS cells with various concentrations of PG treatment for 12 h, and in G_0/G_1 phase of OECM1 cells with various concentrations of PG treatment for 12 and 24 h. The findings demonstrated that PG could induce type II program (autophagy) cell death in these cancer cells in a time- and dose-dependent manner. Moreover, there was no significant change of sub-G_1 level in OECM1 and SAS cells after 24 h treatment of PG. We also discovered GFP-LC3 puncta formation in PG-treated OECM1 and SAS cells, which indicated an increase of autophagosome formation in two oral cancer cells (data not shown).

Table 1. Prodigiosin mediated cell cycle distribution in SAS cells.

Cell	Dosage (μM)	Sub G_1 (%)	G_0/G_1 (%)	S (%)	G_2/M (%)
12 h	0	2.2 ± 0.8	40.3 ± 3.3	25.2 ± 4.4	32.4 ± 2.9
	0.1	1.7 ± 0.8	45.3 ± 4.1 *	23.2 ± 0.2	29.9 ± 0.9
	0.5	1.0 ± 0.2	51.2 ± 1.9 *	21.1 ± 2.8	26.6 ± 0.7 *
	1.0	1.4 ± 0.7	51.4 ± 1.2 *	20.0 ± 2.7	27.2 ± 0.2 *
24 h	0	0.9 ± 0.3	42.1 ± 2.7	20.4 ± 2.7	36.6 ± 2.1
	0.1	1.4 ± 0.2	39.7 ± 2.2	25.0 ± 2.0	33.9 ± 3.6
	0.5	1.7 ± 0.3 *	51.7 ± 3.2 *	20.9 ± 0.8	25.7 ± 2.5 *
	1.0	2.5 ± 0.7 *	54.0 ± 3.7 *	17.0 ± 0.7	26.3 ± 3.2 *

SAS cells were treated with 0.1, 0.5, and 1.0 μM of prodigiosin (PG) for 12 and 24 h, respectively, and stained with propidium iodide. The results are shown as the mean ± SEM of three independent experiments. * $P < 0.05$, compared with the untreated control (0 μM).

Table 2. Prodigiosin mediated cell cycle distribution in OECM1 cells.

Cell	Dosage (μM)	Sub G_1 (%)	G_0/G_1 (%)	S (%)	G_2/M (%)
12 h	0	0.5 ± 0.1	50.9 ± 1.7	16.6 ± 1.0	32.1 ± 0.4
	0.1	0.5 ± 0.2	52.3 ± 0.5	17.0 ± 0.5	30.2 ± 2.2
	0.5	0.4 ± 0.1	63.2 ± 0.6 **	12.2 ± 0.2 *	24.1 ± 1.3 *
	1.0	0.4 ± 0.1	63.3 ± 0.4 **	10.5 ± 0.2 *	25.7 ± 0.8 *
24 h	0	1.2 ± 0.2	47.9 ± 2.3	14.0 ± 1.6	36.9 ± 3.1
	0.1	1.1 ± 0.1	50.9 ± 3.8	21.9 ± 2.9 *	26.1 ± 1.6 *
	0.5	1.4 ± 0.1	60.2 ± 2.5 *	19.8 ± 3.1 *	18.7 ± 2.3 **
	1.0	1.2 ± 0.1	61.8 ± 0.4 *	18.4 ± 2.6 *	18.7 ± 3.3 **

OECM1 cells were treated with 0.1, 0.5, and 1.0 μM of prodigiosin (PG) for 12 and 24 h, respectively, and stained with propidium iodide. The results are shown as the mean ± SEM of three independent experiments. * $P < 0.05$ and ** $P < 0.01$, compared with the untreated control (0 μM).

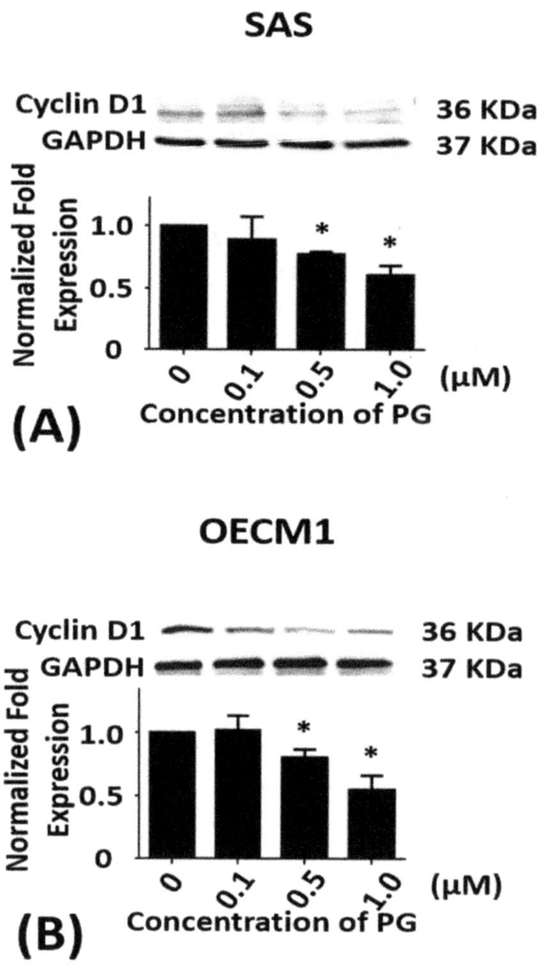

Figure 2. Altered protein levels of cyclin D1 of SAS and OECM1 cells treated with prodigiosin. SAS and OECM1 cells were treated with 0.1, 0.5, and 1.0 μM of prodigiosin (PG) for 24 h and lysed in RIPA buffer for Western blotting. Protein level of cyclin D1 in SAS (**A**) and OECM1 (**B**) cells were shown as the mean ± SEM of three independent experiments. Protein levels were represented as ratio of band intensity to untreated control, which were normalized via internal control GAPDH. * $P < 0.05$ when compared with the untreated control (0 μM).

2.3. Effects of Prodigiosin on AMPKα, PI3K Class III and Akt Protein Levels in Oral Cancer Cells

Cumulative studies have shown that autophagy is mediated by numerous signaling pathway including PI3K/Akt/mTOR [7,8], AMPK/mTOR/Ulk1 [44,45], and Beclin-1 [46]. To evaluate whether PG-induced cell death was related to autophagy, the autophagy-related protein levels of AMPKα, PI3K Class III, Akt, mTOR, Beclin-1, P62, LC3-I, and LC3-II in SAS and OECM1 cells were determined by Western blotting analysis. Compared with the untreated controls, the protein levels of AMPKα in SAS cells exhibited significant differences at 1.0 μM of PG treatment ($P < 0.05$; Figure 3A) while the protein levels of AMPKα in OECM1 cells showed no significant differences in various concentrations of PG treatment (Figure 3B).

When compared with the untreated control, the protein levels of PI3K class III in SAS cells showed no significance (Figure 3C). While the protein levels of PI3K class III in OECM1 cells were markedly down-regulated in 0.5 and 1.0 μM of PG treatments ($P < 0.05$; Figure 3D). The protein level of Akt in SAS and OECM1 cells were evaluated with 0.1, 0.5, and 1.0 μM of PG for 24 h treatments, the results revealed no significant alteration when compared with the untreated controls except significant decrease in 1.0 μM of PG in SAS cells (Figure 3E,F).

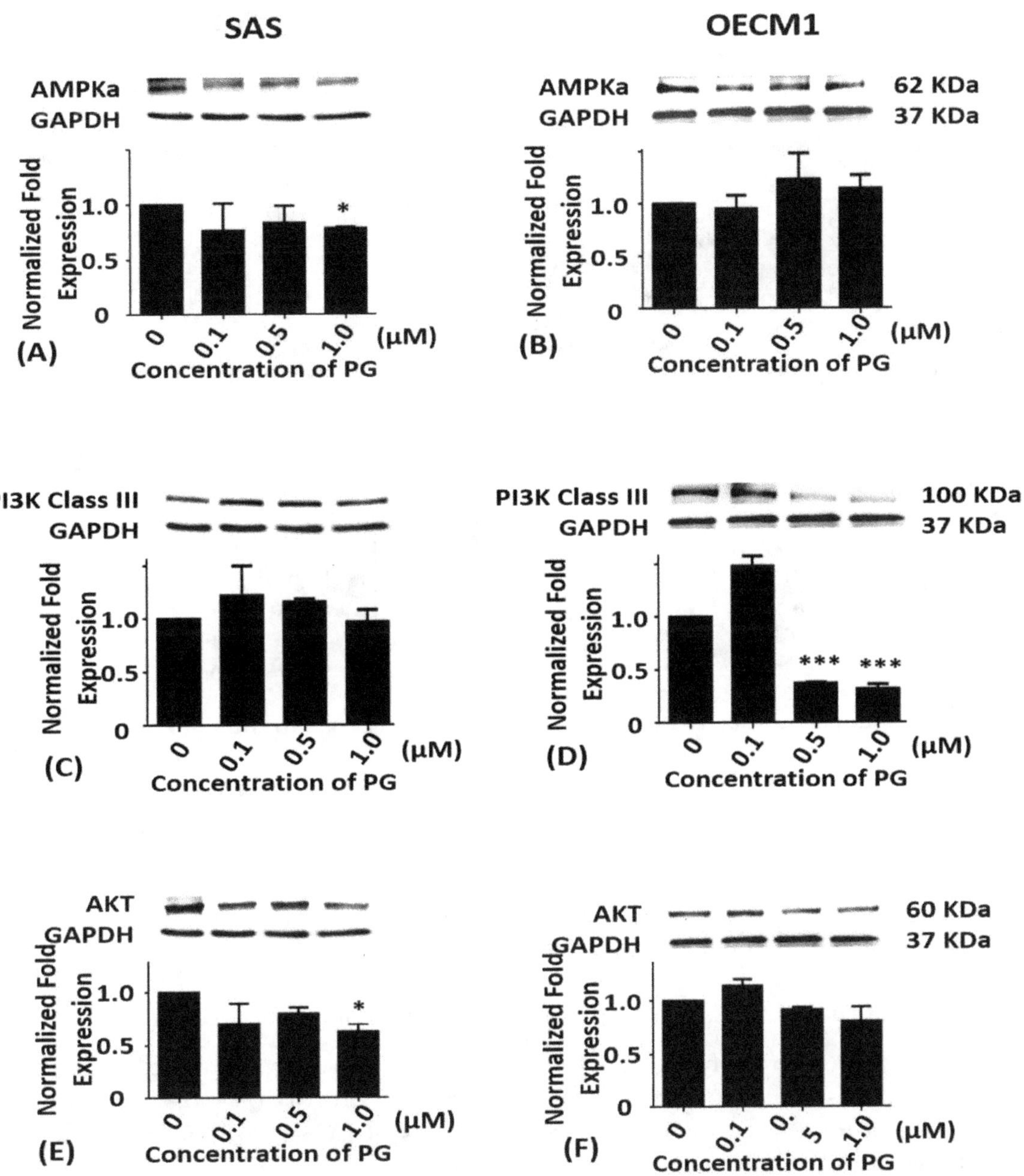

Figure 3. Altered protein levels of AMPKα, PI3K class III, and Akt of SAS and OECM1 cells treated with prodigiosin. SAS and OECM1 cells were treated with 0.1, 0.5, and 1.0 μM of prodigiosin (PG) for 24 h and lysed in RIPA buffer for Western blotting. Protein levels of AMPKα (**A**,**B**), PI3K class III (**C**,**D**), and Akt (**E**,**F**) were shown as the mean ± SEM of three independent experiments. Protein levels were represented as ratio of band intensity to untreated control which were normalized via internal control GAPDH. * $P < 0.05$ and *** $P < 0.001$ when compared with the untreated control (0 μM).

2.4. *Effects of Prodigiosin on mTOR and Beclin-1 Protein Levels in Oral Cancer Cells*

SAS and OECM1 cells were incubated with 0.1, 0.5, and 1.0 μM of PG treatment for 24 h. As compared with the untreated controls, the protein levels of mTOR in SAS cells were significantly decreased in 1.0 μM of PG treatment ($P < 0.05$; Figure 4A). The protein levels of mTOR in OECM1 cells were also reduced in 0.5 and 1.0 μM of PG treatments ($P < 0.05$; Figure 4B). After treatment with 0.1, 0.5, and 1.0 μM of PG for 24 h, the protein levels of Beclin-1 were significantly decreased in 1.0 μM of PG treatment in SAS and OECM1 cells when compared with the untreated controls ($P < 0.05$; Figure 4C,D).

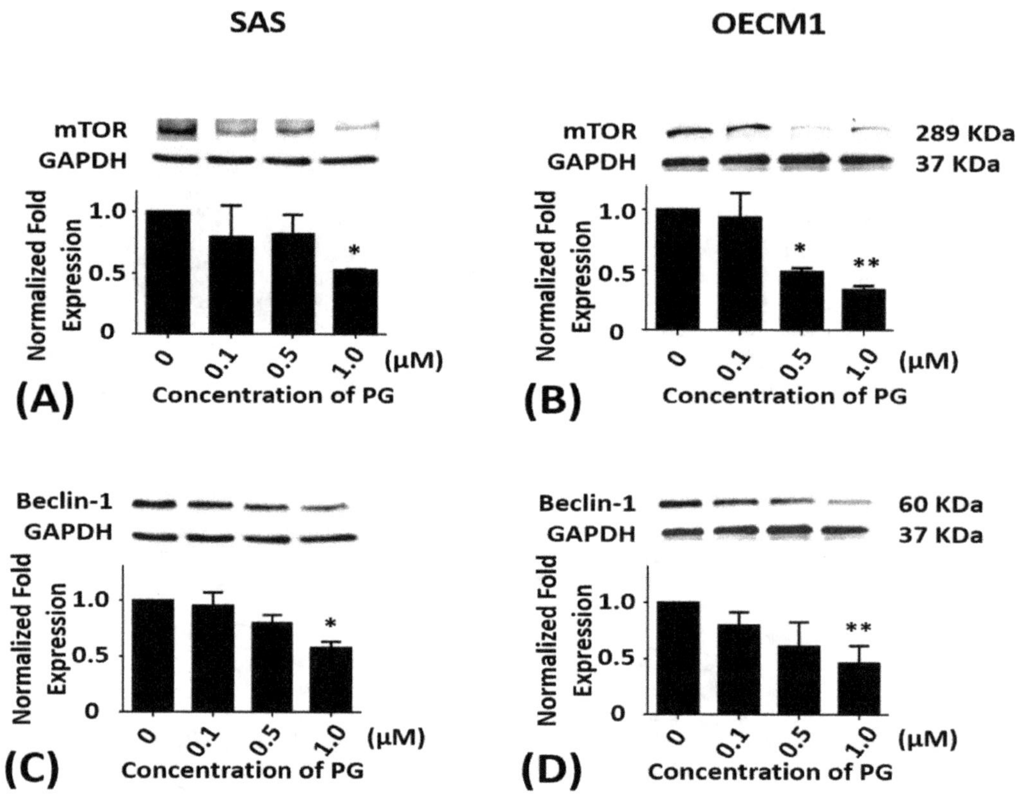

Figure 4. Altered protein levels of mTOR and Beclin-1 of SAS and OECM1 cells treated with prodigiosin. SAS and OECM1 cells were treated with 0.1, 0.5, and 1.0 μM of prodigiosin (PG) for 24 h and lysed in RIPA buffer for Western blotting. Protein levels of mTOR (**A**,**B**) and Beclin-1 (**C**,**D**) were shown as the mean ± SEM of three independent experiments. Protein levels were represented as ratio of band intensity to untreated control which were normalized via internal control GAPDH. * $P < 0.05$ and ** $P < 0.01$ when compared with the untreated controls (0 μM).

2.5. Effects of Prodigiosin on P62, LC3-I and LC3-II Protein Levels in Oral Cancer Cells

Additionally, the P62 protein levels in SAS and OECM1 cells were significantly elevated in 1.0 μM of PG treatments as compared with the untreated controls ($P < 0.05$; Figure 5A,B). When compared with the untreated controls, the protein levels of LC3-I in SAS and OECM1 cells were elevated in 1.0 μM of PG treatments ($P < 0.05$; Figure 5C). The protein levels of LC3-I in OECM1 showed a significant increase in various concentrations of PG for 24 h treatment ($P < 0.05$; Figure 5D). The protein levels of LC3-II were markedly up-regulated in SAS cells with various concentrations of PG treatment for 24 h as compared with the untreated controls ($P < 0.05$; Figure 5E). While the protein levels of LC3-II also revealed a large increase in OECM1 cells with 0.5 and 1.0 μM of PG treatment for 24 h as compared with the untreated controls ($P < 0.05$; Figure 5F). These Western-blotting findings showed that autophagic cell death could be induced by PG treatment in oral cancer cells, which might occur through different signal pathways. Remarkably, the increase of P62, LC3-I, and LC3-II levels in the present study is associated with numerous investigations. Two carbazole alkaloids derived from *Murraya koenigii* (L.) Sprengel (Rutaceae) leaves, mahanine and isomahanine, resulted in increased accumulation of p62/sequestosome1 (p62/SQSTM1), with coordinated expression of LC3-II and cleaved caspase-3, suggesting inhibition of autophagic flux associated with carbazole alkaloid-induced apoptosis in the OSCC cell line CLS-354 [40]. Protein levels of LC3-II and p62 in human breast cancer cell lines MCF-7 and MDA-MB-231 are induced by ramalin that derived from the Antarctic lichen *Ramalina terebrata* [47]. One more recent report has demonstrated the autophagic cell death of $HepG_2$ by dehydroepiandrosterone treatment and also via an increase of JNK-mediated P62 expression [48]. Nutrient depletion has augmented OSCC cell autophagy via increase of p62, LC3-II/LC3-I ratio, and GFP-LC3 levels in time-course patterns from 6 to 48 h when the inhibition of autophagy caused apoptosis in OSCC cells [49]. In study of anticancer effect of ursolic acid in apoptosis-resistant colorectal cancer, JNK signaling pathway has been triggered and further activated P62 expression [50]. Resveratrol can enhance autophagy via increase of JNK-mediated P62 expression and AMPK activation in chronic myelogenous leukemia cells [51,52]. Conversely, isomahanine, a carbazole alkaloid, obviously induces autophagic flux as shown by an increase in punctate GFP-LC3 and the LC3-II/LC3-I ratio with a concomitant p62 level decrease in multidrug-resistant human oral squamous cell carcinoma cells [53]. Treatment with grape seed extract and resveratrol in 4-nitroquinoline-1-oxide (4NQO)-induced tongue tumorigenesis of C57BL/6 mice, that decrease of autophagy flux marker p62 is observed [54]. Human lung cancer tissues that experienced chemotherapy shows an increase of LC3-I to LC3-II conversion and decrease of p62/sequestosome1 as compared with chemo-naïve cancer tissue as well as A549 cell [55]. Sunitinib, an oral multitargeted receptor tyrosine kinase inhibitor with antiangiogenic and antitumor activity that mainly targets vascular endothelial growth factor receptors, significantly increases the levels of LC3-II, concomitant with a decrease of p62 in rat pheochromocytoma PC12 cells [56]. Interestingly, the signaling of P62 seems to be a biphasic response for the induction of autophagy.

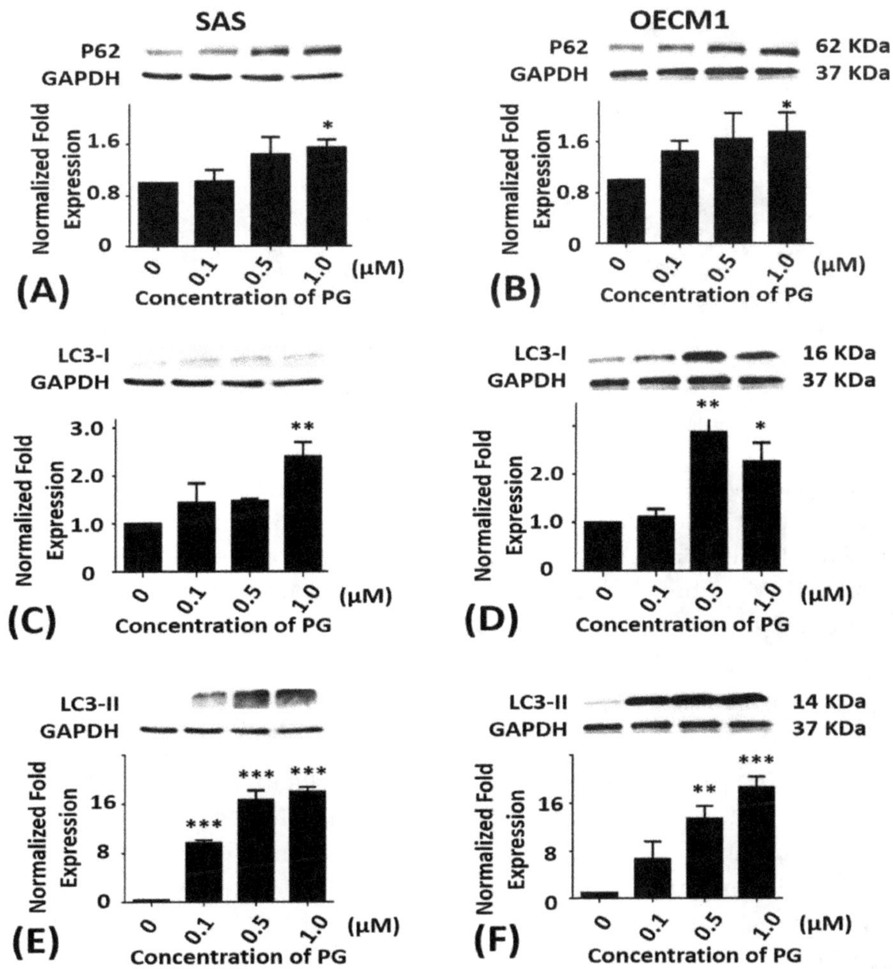

Figure 5. Altered protein levels of P62, LC3-I, and LC3-II of SAS and OECM1 cells treated with prodigiosin. SAS and OECM1 cells were treated with 0.1, 0.5, and 1.0 μM of prodigiosin (PG) for 24 h and lysed in RIPA buffer for Western blotting. Protein levels of P62 (**A**,**B**), LC3-I (**C**,**D**), and LC3-II (**E**,**F**) were shown as the mean ± SEM of three independent experiments. Protein levels were represented as ratio of band intensity to untreated control which were normalized via internal control GAPDH. * $P < 0.05$, ** $P < 0.01$, and *** $P < 0.001$ when compared with the untreated controls (0 μM).

2.6. Phosphorylated Protein Levels of mTOR, Akt, and Ribosomal Protein S6 after PG Treatment

Previous studies have been shown that Akt and mTOR phosphorylation would be reduced while autophagy activation. Moreover, mTOR dephosphorylation reduced downstream protein p70S6K activation and finally inhibited ribosomal protein S6 (rpS6) phosphorylation [57–59]. Consequently, mTOR, Akt and rpS6 phosphorylation could be a marker of autophagy activation. After treatment of 1 μM PG, mTOR, Akt, and rpS6 phosphorylation in both SAS and OECM1 cells were significantly decreased (Figure 6). According to these results, PG could not only reduce mTOR and Akt protein expression, but also inhibit the phosphorylations of mTOR and Akt.

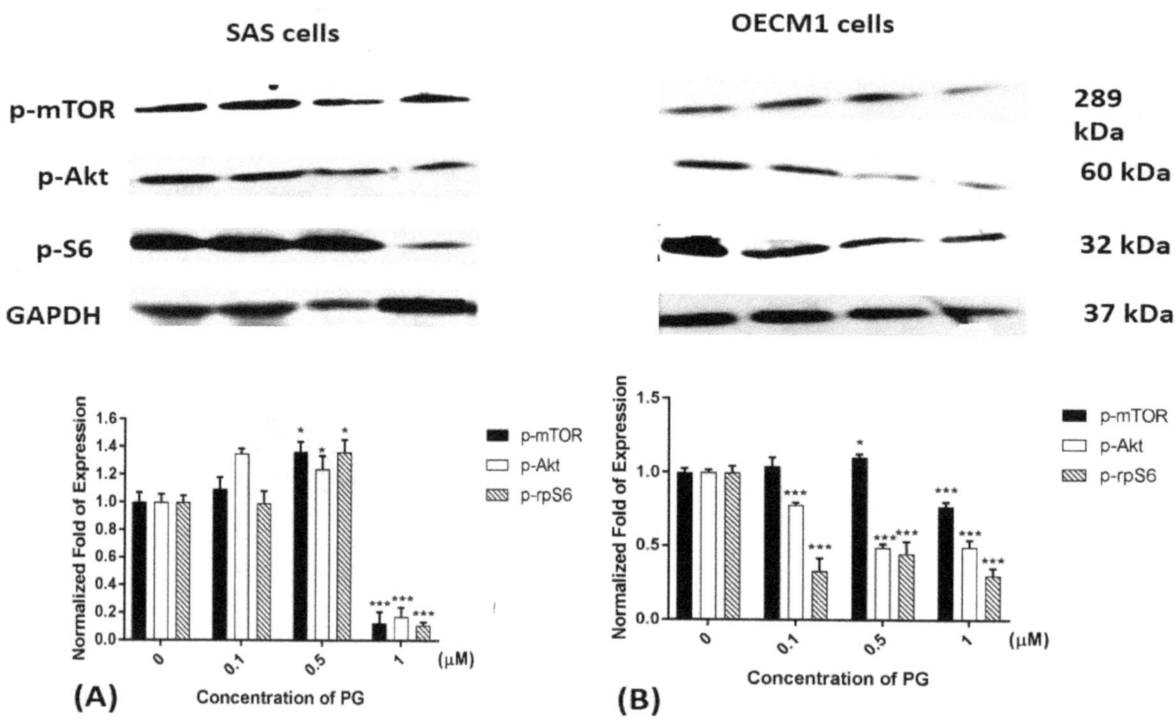

Figure 6. Altered protein levels of p-mTOR, p-Akt, and p-rpS6 of (**A**) SAS and (**B**) OECM1 cells treated with prodigiosin. SAS and OECM1 cells were treated with 0.1, 0.5, and 1.0 μM of prodigiosin (PG) for 24 h and lysed in RIPA buffer for Western blotting. Protein levels of p-mTOR, p-Akt, and p-rpS6 were shown as the mean ± SEM of three independent experiments. Protein levels were represented as ratio of band intensity to untreated control which were normalized via internal control GAPDH. * $P < 0.05$ and *** $P < 0.001$ when compared with the untreated controls (0 μM).

2.7. Effect of Prodigiosin on Autophagosome Formation in Oral Cancer Cells

For evaluating whether autophagy appeared in oral cancer cells after PG treatment, the expressions of LC3-II in autophagosome in SAS and OECM1 cells were further observed via immunofluorescence. During the cascade of autophagy signal pathways, LC3-II can anchor on the autophagosome, and its amount is correlated well with the numbers of autophagosomes [8,14]. Two oral cancer cells were incubated with 0.4 μM PG and 0.4 μM PG plus 5 mM of autophagic inhibitor 3-methyladenine (3MA) for 24 h when compared with the untreated control cells. The results illustrated that increased LC3 puncta cells were significantly increased by presenting numerous autophagosomes in SAS and OECM-1 treated with PG and decreased by the application of 3MA. Figure 7A,B showed the quantitative representations of autophagosome formation in SAS and OECM1 cells ($P < 0.05$). Furthermore, in order to prove PG-induced OSCC cells death was caused by autophagy, cell viability of two OSCC cells were tested after PG treatment with or without 1 mM and 5 mM of 3MA. The data illustrated that cell viability of PG combined with 1 mM 3MA in two cell lines were significantly higher than that of PG alone. However, cell viability of PG combined with 5 mM 3MA was significantly lower than that of PG alone. Meanwhile, 1 and 5 mM of 3MA could increase two cell lines growth (Figure 7C). Previous study has been demonstrated biphasic function of 3MA in cell autophagy. In nutrient-rich environment, 3MA would promote the autophagy [60], which might explain the decrease of cell viability after treatment of 5 mM 3MA plus PG. Take all above results together, autophagy indeed occurred in oral cancer cells in the induction of PG.

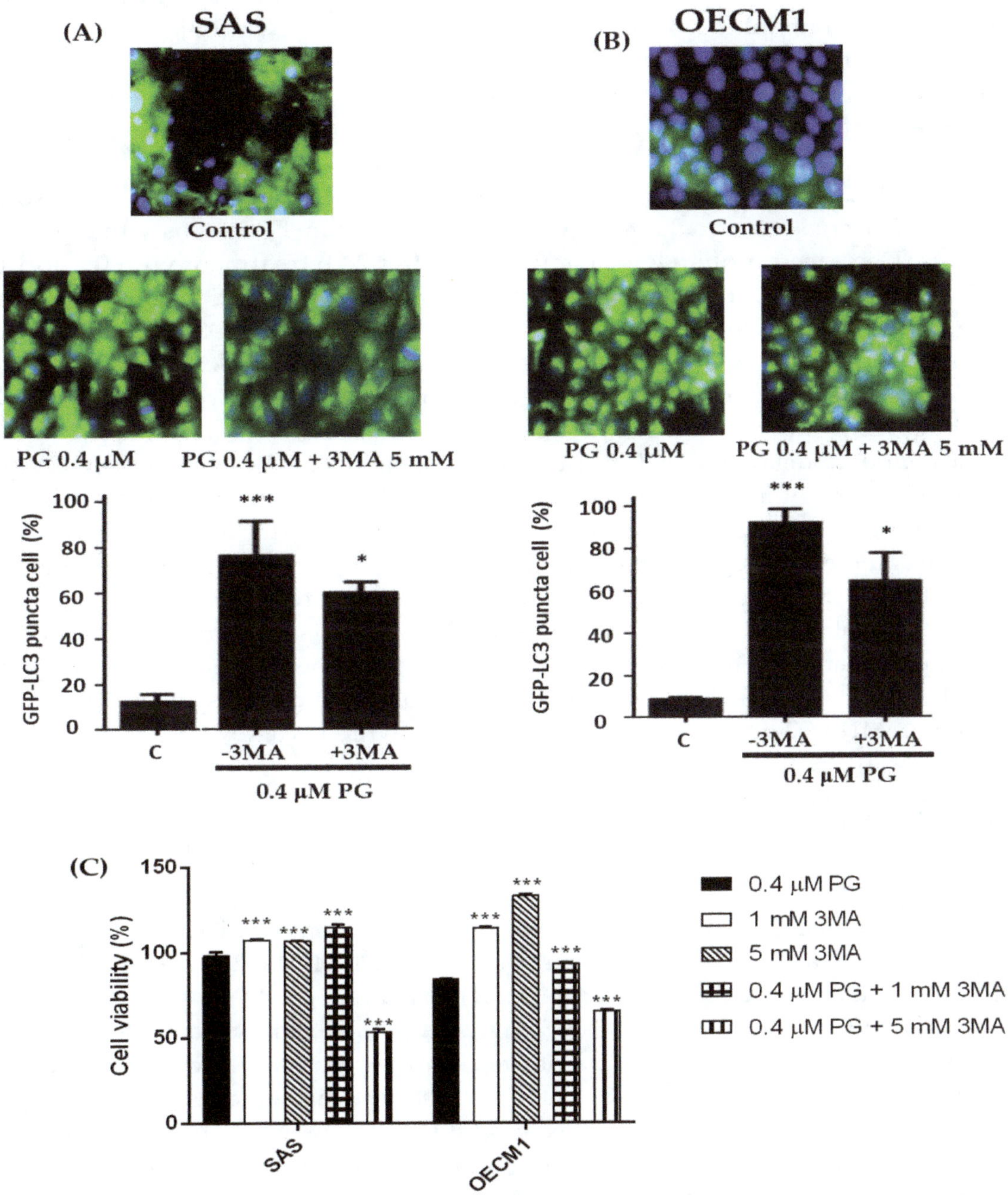

Figure 7. Alterations of autophosome formation of (**A**) SAS and (**B**) OECM1 cells treated with prodigiosin. SAS and OECM1 cells were treated with prodigiosin (PG; 0.1, 0.4, and 1.0 μM) and PG + 3MA (0.4 μM of PG and plus 5 mM of 3MA) for 24 h, followed by staining the autophagosome by LC3 antibody (green) and nucleus by DAPI (blue). The LC3 puncta cells of SAS and OECM1 were observed using fluorescence microscopy and counted the percentage of LC3 positive cell. (**C**) Cytotoxicity of treatment with 0.4 μM of PG + 3MA (1 and 5 mM) in two cell lines was observed by MTT assay. The results were shown as the mean ± SEM of three independent experiments. * $P < 0.05$ and *** $P < 0.001$ when compared with the untreated controls (0 μM).

PG can down-regulate RAD51 expression, and trigger phosphorylation of JNK and p38 MAPK in many human breast carcinoma cell lines, which implicates the cytotoxicity of PG in this cancer [32]. The structural modification of the C-ring of prodigiosenes results in an anti-cancer activity of human K562 chronic myelogenous leukemia cells in both in vitro and in vivo assays [42]. From these data, PGs are thought to play critical roles in cancer therapy via inducing cell death [61]. Recently, PG can induce apoptosis in various cancer cells with low toxicity on normal cells, and PG-induced apoptosis may ascribe to Bcl-2 and survivin inhibition in colorectal cancer (HT-29) cells [62]. In addition, autophagy has been found in squamous cell carcinoma of the head and neck [63]. Increased protein levels of P62 and LC3-II in OSCC tissues have also been reported to correlate with survival, poor prognosis, and advanced stage cancer [64]. In this study, Western blot analyses showed that PG-induced autophagy in OECM1 cells by down-regulation of mTOR, PI3 kinase Class III, and Beclin-1 protein levels while by up-regulation of P62 and LC3 proteins. In SAS cells, PG-induced autophagy was associated with the involvement of decreased signals of mTOR, Akt, and Beclin-1 proteins while increase of P62 and LC3 proteins. Decreased protein level of cyclin D1 after 24 h treatment with 0.5 and 1.0 μM PG was observed in SAS and OECM1 cells (Figure 2), indicating G_0/G_1 checkpoint arrest. Furthermore, marked up-regulation of LC3-I and LC3-II protein levels was exhibited in OSCC cells, and a significant increase was found by presenting numerous autophagosomes in these cancer cells (Figure 7). Thereby, our findings provide the first evidence of increased autophagic signals were involved cell death by PG treatment in OECM1 and SAS cells. These results are consistent with previous findings for cell death of PG induction in melanoma cells of previous report. PG can be a specific mTOR inhibitor in melanoma cells, which might induce a loss of Akt phosphorylation, prevent its activation, and identify a possible new therapeutic option for this cancer [41]. Moreover, Akt is associated with cell survival and its expression could down-regulate the LC3-II expression; thereby, suppressing autophagy [11–13]. The PI3K Class III can be triggered through insulin and insulin-like receptors, for reduction of its signal to Akt; therefore, stimulating the protein level of mTOR, which is a central regulator of autophagy. Subsequently, the activation of mTOR would further suppress the autophagy pathway and induce protein synthesis. In fact, when mTOR is suppressed, autophagy is conversely induced. Autophagy is also promoted by AMP activated protein kinase (AMPK), which is a key energy sensor to maintain energy homeostasis [10].

3. Materials and Methods

3.1. Preparations of Prodigiosin

Vibrio sp. C1-TDSG02-1 was isolated from the sea sediment of Siaogang Harbor at a water depth of 17 m in eastern and southern Taiwan. The strain C1-TDSG02-1 was 99.0% identical with *Vibrio* sp. BL-182 (Genbank accession no. AY663829.1) based on 16S rDNA gene sequence. *Vibrio* sp. C1-TDSG02-1 was cultured in 1.4% soybean flour with 80% sterilized seawater at 25 °C, 5 Lpm (L/min), and pH 7.0–7.5 for 48 h. Extraction of the culture broth (8.0 L) with ethyl acetate (EtOAc, 4 × 8.0 L) yielded 45.7 g of crude extract. The EtOAc layer was separated on silica gel followed by elution chromatography with mixed *n*-hexane/EtOAc (stepwise, pure *n*-hexane, pure EtOAc) to yield 16 sub-fractions. Fraction 6 was chromatographed on silica and eluted using a mixture of *n*-hexane/acetone (stepwise, 10:1, pure acetone) to afford 11 sub-fractions. Sub-fraction 6-5 was chromatographed on silica and eluted using a mixture of *n*-hexane/acetone (4:1) to afford prodigiosin (PG, 1.94 g). The purity of purified PG is 95% confirmed by NMR. Prodigiosin ($C_{20}H_{25}N_3O$; mol. wt.: 323.432 g/mole) was isolated as a red powder that gave an $[M + H]^+$ ion peak at 324 m/z in the ESI/MS. One liter of culture can obtain approximately 1.398 g of PG.

3.2. Cell Cultures

Two human oral squamous carcinoma cell lines (SAS and OECM1) were obtained from Dr. Ta-Chun Yuan of Department of Life Science and Institute of Biotechnology (National Dong-Hwa

University, Hualien, Taiwan). SAS were cultured in Dulbecco's modified Eagle medium (DMEM, Thermo-Fisher, Waltham, MA, USA) supplemented with 5% fetal bovine serum (FBS, Thermo-Fisher), and 1% penicillin/streptomycin (PS, Thermo-Fisher). OECM1 were cultured in Roswell Park Memorial Institute medium 1640 (RPMI 1640) supplemented with 5% FBS and 1% PS. Two cell lines were cultured in CO_2 incubator (Thermo-Fisher) and the culture condition was set up as 37 °C, 5% CO_2. The medium was changed every 2 days, and the cells were detached by 0.25% trypsin/EDTA (Thermo-Fisher) for passage as reached 80–90% confluence. All experiments were obtained within 20 passages concerning uniformity and reproducibility. FL83B (mouse hepatocyte, ATCC CRL-2390) cells were maintained in Kaighn's Modification of Ham's F-12 Medium (F12K, Thermo-Fisher) supplemented with 10% FBS and 1% PS, and incubated at 37 °C with 5% CO_2.

3.3. *Cytotoxicity Assay*

Cytotoxicity was measured by MTT assay. 7×10^3 cells per well of SAS/OECM1 were seeded in 96-well plates and incubated at 37 °C, 5% CO_2 overnight. Then, the cells were treated with various concentrations of PG (0.1, 0.5, 1.0, and 5.0 μM) for 24 h. After treatment, 20 μL per well of 50 mg/mL MTT (Thermo-Fisher) solution was added and incubated at 37 °C for 3 h. As incubation finished, all liquid in wells were replaced to dimethyl sulfoxide and the absorbance at 570 nm was measured by EnSpire Alpha plate reader (Perkin Elmer, Waltham, MA, USA). The absorbance at 570 nm was positively correlated to the number of viable cells so the cell viability was represented as the percentage of absorbance at 570 nm between treated and untreated cells.

3.4. *Cell Cycle Analysis*

A total of 7×10^4 cells of SAS/OECM1 were seeded in 12-well plates and incubated at 37 °C, 5% CO_2 overnight. Then, cells were incubated with 0.1, 0.5, and 1.0 μM of PG for 12 and 24 h. Next, cells were harvested by 0.25% trypsin/EDTA and fixed with 70% ethanol at −20 °C at least 1 h. The fixed cells were washed in cold phosphate buffer saline (PBS) twice, stained with 1 mL staining solution (20 μg/mL of propidium iodide (PI), 0.1% Triton X-100, 0.2 mg/mL RNase) at 37 °C for 30 min, and emission density at 617 nm was analyzed within 10^4 cells for each treatment by Cytomics™ FC500 flow cytometer (Beckman Coulter, Brea, CA, USA).

3.5. *Western Blotting*

A total of 7×10^4 of OECM1 and SAS cell lines were seeded in 12-well plates and cells reached 80% confluence at 37 °C and 5% CO_2. OECM1 and SAS cells were treated with 0.1, 0.5, and 1.0 μM of PG for 24 h. Then, media in wells were removed and washed twice with PBS. Cells in wells were homogenized using RIPA buffer and harvested into a 1.5 mL Eppendorf. The cell lysates were centrifuged at 12,000× *g* at 4 °C for 30 min, and the supernatant was kept at −20 °C until assayed. Interested proteins were separated using sodium dodecyl sulfate polyacrylamide gel electrophoresis and subsequently transferred to PVDF membrane (Millipore, Billerica, MA, USA). The membrane was blocked with 5% non-fat milk or 5% bovine serum albumin (for phosphorylated protein) in TBST saline (20 mM Tris-HCl, pH 7.4, 137 mM NaCl, and 0.05% Tween-20) at room temperature for 1 h, followed by incubation with an appropriate primary antibody at 4 °C overnight. The membrane was washed by TBST saline twice and then incubated with peroxidase conjugated secondary antibody for 1 h. Finally, the membrane was rinsed with ECL reagent (Amershan Bioscience, Little Chalfont, UK) for 1 min and chemiluminescence was collected with a LAS-3000 imager (Fujifilm, Tokyo, Japan). GAPDH was taken as an internal control for normalization. Table 3 shows primary and secondary antibodies used in this study.

Table 3. Primary and second antibodies used in the study.

Antibody	MW(kDa)	Dilution	Sources
mTOR	289	1:1000	Cell Signalling
p-mTOR (Ser2448)	289	1:200	Santa Cruz
PI3K class III	100	1:1000	Cell Signalling
AMPKα	62	1:1000	Cell Signalling
P62	62	1:1000	Cell Signalling
Akt	60	1:1000	Cell Signalling
P-Akt (Ser473)	60	1:200	Santa Cruz
Beclin-1	60	1:1000	Cell Signalling
Cyclin D1	34	1:1000	Cell Signalling
p-Ribosomal protein S6 (Ser235/236)	32	1:200	Santa Cruz
LC3-I	16	1:1000	Cell Signalling
LC3-II	14	1:1000	Cell Signalling
GADPH	37	1:10,000	Cell Signalling
anti-Rabbit (IgG)	-	1:5000	GeneTex
anti-Mouse (IgG)	-	1:10,000	GE

3.6. Autophagosome Formation Analysis

OECM1 and SAS cells were plated into 96-well plates at a cell density of 5×10^3/well. The cells were incubated at 37 °C and 5% CO_2. OECM1 and SAS cells were incubated in 0.4 μM of PG and 0.4 μM of PG plus 5 mM of 3-methyladenine (3MA) for 24 h. Then, cells were fixed with 3.7% formaldehyde/PBS and stained by the Alexa Fluor 488-conjugated anti-LC3-II rabbit antibody (Thermo-Fisher). Images were captured by a Typhoon™ FLA 9000 Biomolecular Imager (GE Healthcare, Little Chalfont, UK). The fluorescence focus units were quantified in each well.

3.7. Statistical Analysis

Data were expressed as mean ± SEM of at least three independent experiments. The results were analyzed by one-way analysis of variance (ANOVA) followed by a Tukey's test. Significant differences ($P < 0.05$) between the means of control and treatment were analyzed. All statistical procedures were performed with GraphPad Prism Ver 5.0 software (GraphPad Software, La Jolla, San Diego, CA, USA).

4. Conclusions

The autophagic mechanism of PG against oral cancer cells was proposed (Figure 8). PG might inhibit cell growth via suppressing the cyclin D1 to cause the arresting cell cycle in G_0/G_1 phase. Furthermore, PG could mediate AMPKα, PI3K class III/Akt signal pathway and directly or indirectly exerts the inhibition of mTOR and Beclin-1 and the induction of p62/LC3 resulting in cell autophagy. In the present study revealed that PG could induce autophagic cell death in human oral cancer cells by LC3-mediated P62/LC3-I/LC3-II pathway in vitro. Our findings elucidated the inhibitory role of PG in this OSCC cancer, which may target the autophagic pathways as a potential agent in cancer therapeutics. Further work in studying anticancer activity of PG should focus on the in vivo test of PG. In a lung cancer xenograft model in vivo studies have demonstrated cancer growth inhibition of tumor growth via cell apoptosis and invasion. Moreover, PG has inhibited RhoA and MMP-2 protein expression in lung cancer 95-D cell line resulting in invasion inhibition [65]. In addition, the activation of p73 and c-Jun-mediated ΔNp73 signaling pathway by PG induced, which can restore p53 tumor suppressor activity in colon cancer [28,66]. In breast cancer, PG could downregulate the Wnt/β-catenin signaling pathway, resulting in the triggered apoptosis process [67]. Based on the present study, this is the first evident that (1) autophagy-induced activity of PG; and (2) growth inhibiting activity of PG in OSCC. This study has confirmed that PG might have a chemotherapeutic potential and promise in treating oral squamous cell carcinoma.

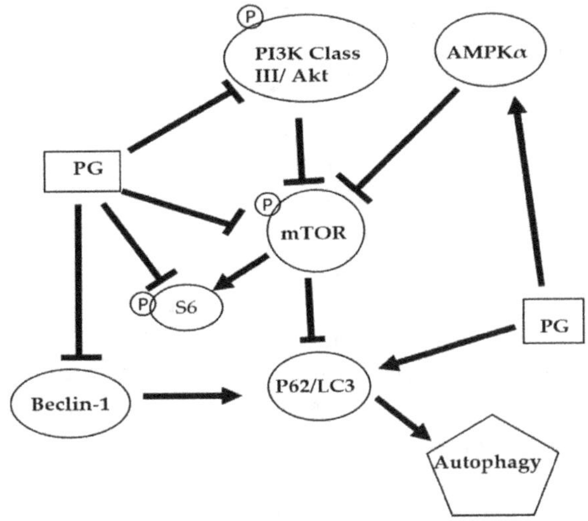

Figure 8. The proposed autophagic mechanism of prodigiosin against oral cancer cells. AMP-activated protein kinase alpha (AMPKα); Mammalian target of rapamycin (mTOR); Microtubule-associated protein 1A/1B-light chain 3 (LC3); Nucleoporin 62 (P62); Phosphoinositide 3-kinase (PI3K); Prodigiosin (PG); Protein kinase B (Akt); and Ribosomal protein S6 (S6)

Acknowledgments: This work was supported by grants from the National Science Council (Ministry of Science and Technology) [Grant 102-2320-B-259-001-3].

Author Contributions: Ming-Fang Cheng, Ping-Jyun Sung and Ching-Feng Weng conceived and designed the experiments. Ming-Fang Cheng, Yi-Wen Tong, Yu-Hsin Chen and Shian-Ren Lin executed the experiments, acquisition and analysis of data. Ming-Fang Cheng, Chun-Shu Lin and Ching-Feng Weng wrote the paper.

References

1. Marques, L.A.; Eluf-Neto, J.; Figueiredo, R.A.; Gois-Filho, J.F.; Kowalski, L.P.; Carvalho, M.B.; Abrahao, M.; Wunsch-Filho, V. Oral health, hygiene practices and oral cancer. *Rev. Saude Publica* **2008**, *42*, 471–479. [CrossRef]
2. Sciubba, J.J. Oral cancer. The importance of early diagnosis and treatment. *Am. J. Clin. Dermatol.* **2001**, *2*, 239–251. [CrossRef] [PubMed]
3. Olsen, S.M.; Moore, E.J.; Koch, C.A.; Kasperbauer, J.L.; Olsen, K.D. Oral cavity and oropharynx squamous cell carcinoma with metastasis to the parotid lymph nodes. *Oral Oncol.* **2011**, *47*, 142–144. [CrossRef] [PubMed]
4. Singletary, K.; Milner, J. Diet, autophagy, and cancer: A review. *Cancer Epidemiol. Biomark. Prev.* **2008**, *17*, 1596–1610. [CrossRef] [PubMed]
5. Wu, J.J.; Quijano, C.; Chen, E.; Liu, H.; Cao, L.; Fergusson, M.M.; Rovira, I.I.; Gutkind, S.; Daniels, M.P.; Komatsu, M.; et al. Mitochondrial dysfunction and oxidative stress mediate the physiological impairment induced by the disruption of autophagy. *Aging* **2009**, *1*, 425–437. [CrossRef] [PubMed]
6. Luo, G.X.; Cai, J.; Lin, J.Z.; Luo, W.S.; Luo, H.S.; Jiang, Y.Y.; Zhang, Y. Autophagy inhibition promotes gambogic acid-induced suppression of growth and apoptosis in glioblastoma cells. *Asian Pac. J. Cancer Prev.* **2012**, *13*, 6211–6216. [CrossRef] [PubMed]
7. Shinojima, N.; Yokoyama, T.; Kondo, Y.; Kondo, S. Roles of the akt/mtor/p70s6k and erk1/2 signaling pathways in curcumin-induced autophagy. *Autophagy* **2007**, *3*, 635–637. [CrossRef] [PubMed]
8. Han, H.Y.; Kim, H.; Jeong, S.H.; Lim, D.S.; Ryu, M.H. Sulfasalazine induces autophagic cell death in oral cancer cells via akt and erk pathways. *Asian Pac. J. Cancer Prev.* **2014**, *15*, 6939–6944. [CrossRef] [PubMed]
9. Ellington, A.A.; Berhow, M.A.; Singletary, K.W. Inhibition of akt signaling and enhanced erk1/2 activity are involved in induction of macroautophagy by triterpenoid b-group soyasaponins in colon cancer cells. *Carcinogenesis* **2006**, *27*, 298–306. [CrossRef] [PubMed]
10. Yao, F.; Lv, Y.C.; Zhang, M.; Xie, W.; Tan, Y.L.; Gong, D.; Cheng, H.P.; Liu, D.; Li, L.; Liu, X.Y.; et al. Apelin-13 impedes foam cell formation by activating class iii pi3k/beclin-1-mediated autophagic pathway. *Biochem. Biophys. Res. Commun.* **2015**, *466*, 637–643. [CrossRef] [PubMed]

11. Sarbassov, D.D.; Guertin, D.A.; Ali, S.M.; Sabatini, D.M. Phosphorylation and regulation of akt/pkb by the rictor-mtor complex. *Science* **2005**, *307*, 1098–1101. [CrossRef] [PubMed]
12. Degtyarev, M.; De Maziere, A.; Orr, C.; Lin, J.; Lee, B.B.; Tien, J.Y.; Prior, W.W.; van Dijk, S.; Wu, H.; Gray, D.C.; et al. Akt inhibition promotes autophagy and sensitizes pten-null tumors to lysosomotropic agents. *J. Cell Biol.* **2008**, *183*, 101–116. [CrossRef] [PubMed]
13. Roy, B.; Pattanaik, A.K.; Das, J.; Bhutia, S.K.; Behera, B.; Singh, P.; Maiti, T.K. Role of pi3k/akt/mtor and mek/erk pathway in concanavalin a induced autophagy in hela cells. *Chem. Biol. Interact.* **2014**, *210*, 96–102. [CrossRef] [PubMed]
14. Song, L.; Ma, L.; Chen, G.; Huang, Y.; Sun, X.; Jiang, C.; Liu, H. Autophagy inhibitor 3-methyladenine enhances the sensitivity of nasopharyngeal carcinoma cells to chemotherapy and radiotherapy. *Zhong Nan Da Xue Xue Bao Yi Xue Ban* **2016**, *41*, 9–18. [PubMed]
15. Chang, C.C.; Chen, W.C.; Ho, T.F.; Wu, H.S.; Wei, Y.H. Development of natural anti-tumor drugs by microorganisms. *J. Biosci. Bioeng.* **2011**, *111*, 501–511. [CrossRef] [PubMed]
16. Marchal, E.; Smithen, D.A.; Uddin, M.I.; Robertson, A.W.; Jakeman, D.L.; Mollard, V.; Goodman, C.D.; MacDougall, K.S.; McFarland, S.A.; McFadden, G.I.; et al. Synthesis and antimalarial activity of prodigiosenes. *Org. Biomol. Chem.* **2014**, *12*, 4132–4142. [CrossRef] [PubMed]
17. Lapenda, J.C.; Silva, P.A.; Vicalvi, M.C.; Sena, K.X.; Nascimento, S.C. Antimicrobial activity of prodigiosin isolated from serratia marcescens ufpeda 398. *World J. Microbiol. Biotechnol.* **2015**, *31*, 399–406. [CrossRef] [PubMed]
18. Wang, Y.; Nakajima, A.; Hosokawa, K.; Soliev, A.B.; Osaka, I.; Arakawa, R.; Enomoto, K. Cytotoxic prodigiosin family pigments from *pseudoalteromonas sp.* 1020r isolated from the pacific coast of Japan. *Biosci. Biotechnol. Biochem.* **2012**, *76*, 1229–1232. [CrossRef] [PubMed]
19. Kimyon, O.; Das, T.; Ibugo, A.I.; Kutty, S.K.; Ho, K.K.; Tebben, J.; Kumar, N.; Manefield, M. Serratia secondary metabolite prodigiosin inhibits pseudomonas aeruginosa biofilm development by producing reactive oxygen species that damage biological molecules. *Front. Microbiol.* **2016**, *7*, 972–987. [CrossRef] [PubMed]
20. Song, Y.; Liu, G.; Li, J.; Huang, H.; Zhang, X.; Zhang, H.; Ju, J. Cytotoxic and antibacterial angucycline- and prodigiosin-analogues from the deep-sea derived *streptomyces sp.* Scsio 11594. *Mar. Drugs* **2015**, *13*, 1304–1316. [CrossRef] [PubMed]
21. Kancharla, P.; Lu, W.; Salem, S.M.; Kelly, J.X.; Reynolds, K.A. Stereospecific synthesis of 23-hydroxyundecylprodiginines and analogues and conversion to antimalarial premarineosins via a rieske oxygenase catalyzed bicyclization. *J. Org. Chem.* **2014**, *79*, 11674–11689. [CrossRef] [PubMed]
22. Perez-Tomas, R.; Vinas, M. New insights on the antitumoral properties of prodiginines. *Curr. Med. Chem.* **2010**, *17*, 2222–2231. [CrossRef] [PubMed]
23. Sam, S.; Sam, M.R.; Esmaeillou, M.; Safaralizadeh, R. Effective targeting survivin, caspase-3 and microrna-16–1 expression by methyl-3-pentyl-6-methoxyprodigiosene triggers apoptosis in colorectal cancer stem-like cells. *Pathol. Oncol. Res.* **2016**, *22*, 715–723. [CrossRef] [PubMed]
24. Yu, C.J.; Ou, J.H.; Wang, M.L.; Jialielihan, N.; Liu, Y.H. Elevated survivin mediated multidrug resistance and reduced apoptosis in breast cancer stem cells. *J. BUON* **2015**, *20*, 1287–1294. [PubMed]
25. Papireddy, K.; Smilkstein, M.; Kelly, J.X.; Shweta; Salem, S.M.; Alhamadsheh, M.; Haynes, S.W.; Challis, G.L.; Reynolds, K.A. Antimalarial activity of natural and synthetic prodiginines. *J. Med. Chem.* **2011**, *54*, 5296–5306. [CrossRef] [PubMed]
26. Chang, C.C.; Wang, Y.H.; Chern, C.M.; Liou, K.T.; Hou, Y.C.; Peng, Y.T.; Shen, Y.C. Prodigiosin inhibits gp91(phox) and inos expression to protect mice against the oxidative/nitrosative brain injury induced by hypoxia-ischemia. *Toxicol. Appl. Pharmacol.* **2011**, *257*, 137–147. [CrossRef] [PubMed]
27. Dalili, D.; Fouladdel, S.; Rastkari, N.; Samadi, N.; Ahmadkhaniha, R.; Ardavan, A.; Azizi, E. Prodigiosin, the red pigment of *serratia marcescens*, shows cytotoxic effects and apoptosis induction in ht-29 and t47d cancer cell lines. *Nat. Prod. Res.* **2012**, *26*, 2078–2083. [PubMed]
28. Hong, B.; Prabhu, V.V.; Zhang, S.; van den Heuvel, A.P.; Dicker, D.T.; Kopelovich, L.; El-Deiry, W.S. Prodigiosin rescues deficient p53 signaling and antitumor effects via upregulating p73 and disrupting its interaction with mutant p53. *Cancer Res.* **2014**, *74*, 1153–1165. [CrossRef] [PubMed]
29. Krishna, P.S.; Vani, K.; Prasad, M.R.; Samatha, B.; Bindu, N.S.; Charya, M.A.; Reddy Shetty, P. In silico molecular docking analysis of prodigiosin and cycloprodigiosin as cox-2 inhibitors. *Springerplus* **2013**, *2*, 172–178. [CrossRef] [PubMed]

30. Hosseini, A.; Espona-Fiedler, M.; Soto-Cerrato, V.; Quesada, R.; Perez-Tomas, R.; Guallar, V. Molecular interactions of prodiginines with the bh3 domain of anti-apoptotic bcl-2 family members. *PLoS ONE* **2013**, *8*, e57562. [CrossRef] [PubMed]
31. Elahian, F.; Moghimi, B.; Dinmohammadi, F.; Ghamghami, M.; Hamidi, M.; Mirzaei, S.A. The anticancer agent prodigiosin is not a multidrug resistance protein substrate. *DNA Cell Biol.* **2013**, *32*, 90–97. [CrossRef] [PubMed]
32. Pan, M.Y.; Shen, Y.C.; Lu, C.H.; Yang, S.Y.; Ho, T.F.; Peng, Y.T.; Chang, C.C. Prodigiosin activates endoplasmic reticulum stress cell death pathway in human breast carcinoma cell lines. *Toxicol. Appl. Pharmacol.* **2012**, *265*, 325–334. [CrossRef] [PubMed]
33. Chang, Y.T.; Huang, C.Y.; Li, K.T.; Li, R.N.; Liaw, C.C.; Wu, S.H.; Liu, J.R.; Sheu, J.H.; Chang, H.W. Sinuleptolide inhibits proliferation of oral cancer ca9–22 cells involving apoptosis, oxidative stress, and DNA damage. *Arch. Oral Biol.* **2016**, *66*, 147–154. [CrossRef] [PubMed]
34. Dai, W.; Sun, C.; Huang, S.; Zhou, Q. Carvacrol suppresses proliferation and invasion in human oral squamous cell carcinoma. *Onco Targets Ther.* **2016**, *9*, 2297–2304. [CrossRef] [PubMed]
35. Kim, D.J.; Lee, J.H.; Park, H.R.; Choi, Y.W. Acetylshikonin inhibits growth of oral squamous cell carcinoma by inducing apoptosis. *Arch. Oral Biol.* **2016**, *70*, 149–157. [CrossRef] [PubMed]
36. Liu, C.M.; Peng, C.Y.; Liao, Y.W.; Lu, M.Y.; Tsai, M.L.; Yeh, J.C.; Yu, C.H.; Yu, C.C. Sulforaphane targets cancer stemness and tumor initiating properties in oral squamous cell carcinomas via mir-200c induction. *J. Formos. Med. Assoc.* **2017**, *116*, 41–48. [CrossRef] [PubMed]
37. Su, N.W.; Wu, S.H.; Chi, C.W.; Liu, C.J.; Tsai, T.H.; Chen, Y.J. Metronomic cordycepin therapy prolongs survival of oral cancer-bearing mice and inhibits epithelial-mesenchymal transition. *Molecules* **2017**, *22*, 629. [CrossRef] [PubMed]
38. Kwak, H.H.; Kim, I.R.; Kim, H.J.; Park, B.S.; Yu, S.B. Alpha-mangostin induces apoptosis and cell cycle arrest in oral squamous cell carcinoma cell. *Evid. Based Complement. Altern. Med.* **2016**, *2016*, e5352412. [CrossRef] [PubMed]
39. Tjioe, K.C.; Tostes Oliveira, D.; Gavard, J. Luteolin impacts on the DNA damage pathway in oral squamous cell carcinoma. *Nutr. Cancer* **2016**, *68*, 838–847. [CrossRef] [PubMed]
40. Utaipan, T.; Athipornchai, A.; Suksamrarn, A.; Jirachotikoon, C.; Yuan, X.; Lertcanawanichakul, M.; Chunglok, W. Carbazole alkaloids from murraya koenigii trigger apoptosis and autophagic flux inhibition in human oral squamous cell carcinoma cells. *J. Nat. Med.* **2017**, *71*, 158–169. [CrossRef] [PubMed]
41. Espona-Fiedler, M.; Soto-Cerrato, V.; Hosseini, A.; Lizcano, J.M.; Guallar, V.; Quesada, R.; Gao, T.; Perez-Tomas, R. Identification of dual mtorc1 and mtorc2 inhibitors in melanoma cells: Prodigiosin vs. Obatoclax. *Biochem. Pharmacol.* **2012**, *83*, 489–496. [CrossRef] [PubMed]
42. Smithen, D.A.; Forrester, A.M.; Corkery, D.P.; Dellaire, G.; Colpitts, J.; McFarland, S.A.; Berman, J.N.; Thompson, A. Investigations regarding the utility of prodigiosenes to treat leukemia. *Org. Biomol. Chem.* **2013**, *11*, 62–68. [CrossRef] [PubMed]
43. Alexandrova, E.M.; Yallowitz, A.R.; Li, D.; Xu, S.; Schulz, R.; Proia, D.A.; Lozano, G.; Dobbelstein, M.; Moll, U.M. Improving survival by exploiting tumour dependence on stabilized mutant p53 for treatment. *Nature* **2015**, *523*, 352–356. [CrossRef] [PubMed]
44. Kim, J.; Kundu, M.; Viollet, B.; Guan, K.L. Ampk and mtor regulate autophagy through direct phosphorylation of ulk1. *Nat. Cell Biol.* **2011**, *13*, 132–141. [CrossRef] [PubMed]
45. Mihaylova, M.M.; Shaw, R.J. The ampk signalling pathway coordinates cell growth, autophagy and metabolism. *Nat. Cell Biol.* **2011**, *13*, 1016–1023. [CrossRef] [PubMed]
46. Funderburk, S.F.; Wang, Q.J.; Yue, Z. The beclin 1-vps34 complex—At the crossroads of autophagy and beyond. *Trends Cell Biol.* **2010**, *20*, 355–362. [CrossRef] [PubMed]
47. Lee, E.; Lee, C.G.; Yim, J.H.; Lee, H.K.; Pyo, S. Ramalin-mediated apoptosis is enhanced by autophagy inhibition in human breast cancer cells. *Phytother. Res.* **2016**, *30*, 426–438. [CrossRef] [PubMed]
48. Vegliante, R.; Desideri, E.; Di Leo, L.; Ciriolo, M.R. Dehydroepiandrosterone triggers autophagic cell death in human hepatoma cell line hepg2 via jnk-mediated p62/sqstm1 expression. *Carcinogenesis* **2016**, *37*, 233–244. [CrossRef] [PubMed]
49. Jiang, L.C.; Xin, Z.Y.; Deborah, B.; Zhang, J.S.; Yuan, D.Y.; Xu, K.; Liu, X.B.; Jiang, H.Q.; Fan, Q.C.; Zhang, B.; et al. Inhibition of autophagy augments apoptosis in human oral squamous cell carcinoma under nutrient depletion. *J. Oral Pathol. Med.* **2015**, *44*, 361–366. [CrossRef] [PubMed]

50. Xavier, C.P.; Lima, C.F.; Pedro, D.F.; Wilson, J.M.; Kristiansen, K.; Pereira-Wilson, C. Ursolic acid induces cell death and modulates autophagy through jnk pathway in apoptosis-resistant colorectal cancer cells. *J. Nutr. Biochem.* **2013**, *24*, 706–712. [CrossRef] [PubMed]
51. Puissant, A.; Auberger, P. Ampk- and p62/sqstm1-dependent autophagy mediate resveratrol-induced cell death in chronic myelogenous leukemia. *Autophagy* **2010**, *6*, 655–657. [CrossRef] [PubMed]
52. Puissant, A.; Robert, G.; Fenouille, N.; Luciano, F.; Cassuto, J.P.; Raynaud, S.; Auberger, P. Resveratrol promotes autophagic cell death in chronic myelogenous leukemia cells via jnk-mediated p62/sqstm1 expression and ampk activation. *Cancer Res.* **2010**, *70*, 1042–1052. [CrossRef] [PubMed]
53. Utaipan, T.; Athipornchai, A.; Suksamrarn, A.; Chunsrivirot, S.; Chunglok, W. Isomahanine induces endoplasmic reticulum stress and simultaneously triggers p38 mapk-mediated apoptosis and autophagy in multidrug-resistant human oral squamous cell carcinoma cells. *Oncol. Rep.* **2017**, *37*, 1243–1252. [PubMed]
54. Shrotriya, S.; Tyagi, A.; Deep, G.; Orlicky, D.J.; Wisell, J.; Wang, X.J.; Sclafani, R.A.; Agarwal, R.; Agarwal, C. Grape seed extract and resveratrol prevent 4-nitroquinoline 1-oxide induced oral tumorigenesis in mice by modulating ampk activation and associated biological responses. *Mol. Carcinog.* **2015**, *54*, 291–300. [CrossRef] [PubMed]
55. Lee, J.G.; Shin, J.H.; Shim, H.S.; Lee, C.Y.; Kim, D.J.; Kim, Y.S.; Chung, K.Y. Autophagy contributes to the chemo-resistance of non-small cell lung cancer in hypoxic conditions. *Respir. Res.* **2015**, *16*, e138. [CrossRef] [PubMed]
56. Ikeda, T.; Ishii, K.A.; Saito, Y.; Miura, M.; Otagiri, A.; Kawakami, Y.; Shimano, H.; Hara, H.; Takekoshi, K. Inhibition of autophagy enhances sunitinib-induced cytotoxicity in rat pheochromocytoma pc12 cells. *J. Pharmacol. Sci.* **2013**, *121*, 67–73. [CrossRef] [PubMed]
57. Huang, S. Inhibition of pi3k/akt/mtor signaling by natural products. *Anticancer Agents Med. Chem.* **2013**, *13*, 967–970. [CrossRef] [PubMed]
58. Park, D.; Jeong, H.; Lee, M.N.; Koh, A.; Kwon, O.; Yang, Y.R.; Noh, J.; Suh, P.-G.; Park, H.; Ryu, S.H. Resveratrol induces autophagy by directly inhibiting mtor through atp competition. *Sci. Rep.* **2016**, *6*, e21772. [CrossRef] [PubMed]
59. Din, F.V.N.; Valanciute, A.; Houde, V.P.; Zibrova, D.; Green, K.A.; Sakamoto, K.; Alessi, D.R.; Dunlop, M.G. Aspirin inhibits mtor signaling, activates amp-activated protein kinase, and induces autophagy in colorectal cancer cells. *Gastroenterology* **2012**, *142*, 1504–1515. [CrossRef] [PubMed]
60. Wu, Y.-T.; Tan, H.-L.; Shui, G.; Bauvy, C.; Huang, Q.; Wenk, M.R.; Ong, C.-N.; Codogno, P.; Shen, H.-M. Dual role of 3-methyladenine in modulation of autophagy via different temporal patterns of inhibition on class i and iii phosphoinositide 3-kinase. *J. Biol. Chem.* **2010**, *285*, 10850–10861. [CrossRef] [PubMed]
61. White, E.; Karp, C.; Strohecker, A.M.; Guo, Y.; Mathew, R. Role of autophagy in suppression of inflammation and cancer. *Curr. Opin. Cell Biol.* **2010**, *22*, 212–217. [CrossRef] [PubMed]
62. Hassankhani, R.; Sam, M.R.; Esmaeilou, M.; Ahangar, P. Prodigiosin isolated from cell wall of *serratia marcescens* alters expression of apoptosis-related genes and increases apoptosis in colorectal cancer cells. *Med. Oncol.* **2015**, *32*, 366–374. [CrossRef] [PubMed]
63. Cosway, B.; Lovat, P. The role of autophagy in squamous cell carcinoma of the head and neck. *Oral Oncol.* **2016**, *54*, 1–6. [CrossRef] [PubMed]
64. Liu, J.L.; Chen, F.F.; Lung, J.; Lo, C.H.; Lee, F.H.; Lu, Y.C.; Hung, C.H. Prognostic significance of p62/sqstm1 subcellular localization and lc3b in oral squamous cell carcinoma. *Br. J. Cancer* **2014**, *111*, 944–954. [CrossRef] [PubMed]
65. Zhang, J.; Shen, Y.; Liu, J.; Wei, D. Antimetastatic effect of prodigiosin through inhibition of tumor invasion. *Biochem. Pharmacol.* **2005**, *69*, 407–414. [CrossRef] [PubMed]
66. Prabhu, V.V.; Hong, B.; Allen, J.E.; Zhang, S.; Lulla, A.R.; Dicker, D.T.; El-Deiry, W.S. Small-molecule prodigiosin restores p53 tumor suppressor activity in chemoresistant colorectal cancer stem cells via c-jun-mediated δnp73 inhibition and p73 activation. *Cancer Res.* **2016**, *76*, 1989–1999. [CrossRef] [PubMed]
67. Wang, Z.; Li, B.; Zhou, L.; Yu, S.; Su, Z.; Song, J.; Sun, Q.; Sha, O.; Wang, X.; Jiang, W.; et al. Prodigiosin inhibits wnt/β-catenin signaling and exerts anticancer activity in breast cancer cells. *Proc. Natl. Acad. Sci. USA* **2016**, *113*, 13150–13155. [CrossRef] [PubMed]

7

Isolation and Cytotoxic Investigation of Flacourtin from *Oncoba spinosa*

Olaoye S. Balogun *, Olukayode S. Ajayi and Olayinka S. Lawal

Department of Chemistry, Obafemi Awolowo University, Ile-Ife 220005, Nigeria; osajayi@oauife.edu.ng (O.S.A.); lawalolayinka@gmail.com (O.S.L.)

* Correspondence: solomonoye@gmail.com or balogunolaoye@oauife.edu.ng

Academic Editor: James D. Adams

Abstract: Background: *Oncoba spinosa,* an endangered medicinal plant whose secondary metabolites have not been extensively profiled, and which is hitherto yet to be examined for cytotoxicity, is being investigated in this study. **Methods:** Leaves of *Oncoba spinosa* (800 g) were extracted with 95% aqueous methanol. The crude extract was partitioned with n-hexane and the resultant defatted extract was extensively chromatographed on silica gel to yield compound **1** which was subjected to spectroscopic analysis. A brine shrimps lethality test was used to establish the cytotoxicity potentials of the isolated compound and the plant extracts. **Results:** Compound **1** was elucidated as flacourtin, 3-hydroxy-4-hydroxymethylphenyl-6-*O*-benzoyl-β-D-glucopyranoside. The LD_{50} values obtained were less than 1000 μg/mL for flacourtin and the plant extracts. **Conclusion:** Flacourtin is being reported for the first time in the *O. spinosa*. The preliminary toxicity assay indicated that flacourtin and the plant extracts were not cytotoxic; thus, the tradomedicinal uses of the plant may portend no danger.

Keywords: *Oncoba spinosa*; Flacourtin; cytotoxicity; Flacourtiaceae; phenolic ester glycoside

---

1. Introduction

O. spinosa is a spiny shrub used for the management of arthritis in southwest Nigeria [1]. The fruit is used for the treatment of anthelminthic, syphilis, wound and sexual impotence [2]. In profiling the chemical constituent of *Oncoba spinosa,* (Flacourtiaceae) five flavonoids, kaempferol, quercetin, apigenin-7-*O*-β-D-glucuronopyranoside, quercetin 3-*O*-β-D-galactopyranoside and quercetin 3-*O*-α-rhamnopyranosyl (1→6) β-D-glucopyranoside have been reported [3]. Flacourtin, a phenolic glycoside ester (3-hydroxy-4-hydroxymethylphenyl-6-*O*-benzoyl-β-D-glucopyranoside) which has been associated with a number of pharmacological activities was first isolated from the bark of a medicinal plant, *Flacourtia indica* (Flacourtiaceae) [4–8], an indigenous medicinal plant widely distributed in India and Bangladesh [9]. Also, Amarasinghe et al. [10] reported isolation of a new glucoside, flacourside, an analog of flacourtin from *Flacourtia indica.* As part of our on-going work on metabolite profiling of indigenous medicinal plants, leaves of *O. spinosa* were collected with the aim of isolating a bioactive compound new to the plant specie.

2. Materials and Methods

2.1. Plant Collection and Purification

Fresh leaves *Oncoba spinosa* were collected at the Botanical Garden University of Ibadan, Oyo State, Nigeria in the month of November, 2014. The plant was identified by the taxonomist and curator, Mr A. Owolabi in the Botanical Garden. A voucher copy of the plant with herbarium number FHI 108806 was deposited at the Forestry Research Institute of Nigeria, Ibadan.

The air-dried and pulverized leaves (800 g) were extracted with 95% aqueous methanol to give a crude extract (140 g). The crude was reconstituted in methanol and defatted with n-hexane to afford 80.60 g of defatted extract. Twenty grams of the defatted extract was chromatographed on silica gel using gradient of dichloromethane and methanol to give a sub-fraction (1.22 g) which was further purified on silica with gradient of hexane, ethyl acetate and methanol. Compound **1** (6 mg) was obtained as an off-white powder which was recrystallized in ethylacetate and thereafter subjected to spectroscopic analysis.

2.2. *Cytotoxicity Assay*

Cytotoxicity of the crude extract, defatted fraction and compound **1** were investigated using brine shrimp lethality assay. A spoonful quantity of the egg of brine shrimps (*Artemia salina* Leach) was sprinkled into a partly covered crucible containing seawater in order to allow partial illumination. The eggs hatched into matured *nauplii* after about 48 h and 10 matured *nauplii* were added to varying concentration of the test samples (1000, 100 and 10 μg/mL). All the experiments were carried out in triplicate and distilled water was used in place of the test samples for negative control. Numbers of survivors were counted after 24 h and the LC_{50} was computed at 95% confidence limit using the Finney program.

3. Results

IR ν_{max} (cm^{-1}): 3000 (ArO–H str), 3050 (Ar–H str), 1710 (C=O str), 1600 (Ar C–C str), 1220 (C–O ester), 1053 (C–O alc).

^{13}C-NMR (MeOD, 75 MHz): δc 134.5 ($C_{-1'}$), 130.7 ($C_{-2'}$ and $C_{-6'}$), 129.7 ($C_{-3'}$ and $C_{-5'}$), 132 ($C_{-5'}$), 150.1 ($C_{-1''}$), 116.3 ($C_{-2''}$), 154 ($C_{-3''}$), 134.1 ($C_{-4''}$), 115.7 ($C_{-5''}$), 119.7 ($C_{-6''}$), 61.1 ($C_{-7''}$), 104.6 (C_{-1}), 75.7 (C_{-2}), 75.2 (C_{-3}), 72.1(C_{-4}), 78.1 (C_{-5}), 64.8 (C_{-6}), 182 (C=O).

^{1}H-NMR (MeOD, 300 MHz): δ 8.05 (2H, m, J_o 7.2 Hz, J_m 1.5 Hz, H_{-2} and H_{-6}), 7.53 (2H, m, $J_{3,2}$ 7.2 Hz, $J_{3,5}$ 7.8 Hz , H_{-3} and H_{-5}), 7.66 (1H, m, J_o 7.5 Hz, J_m 1.5 Hz, H_{-5}), 6.77 (1H, d, J_m 3.0 Hz, $H_{-2''}$), 7.03 (1H, d, J_o 8.7 Hz, $H_{-5''}$), 6.48 (1H, dd, J_o 8.7 Hz, J_m 3.3 Hz, $H_{-6''}$), 4.62 (1H, d, H_{-1}), 3.51 (3H, m, H_{-2}, H_{-3} and H_{-4}), 3.73 (1H, m, $J_{5,6}$ 7.5 Hz, H_{-5}), 4.46 (1H, d, $J_{5,6}$ 7.5 Hz, H_{-6a}), 4.42 (IH, d, $J_{5,6}$ 7.5 Hz, H_{-6b}), 4.72 (H, $H_{-6a''}$), 4.76 (1H, $H_{-6b''}$), 4.95, 4.82 and 4.72 (glucose OH), 4.69 (benzylic OH).

4. Discussion

The NMR spectra of compound **1** showed a pattern characteristic of a phenolic ester glycoside. Clusters of peaks at δ 3.5–5.0 indicated the presence of a sugar moiety while the aromatic region showed the presence of eight protons with *J* values typical of an aromatic system, thus suggesting two substituted benzene rings (Figure 1). The IR spectrum showed absorption bands (cm^{-1}) at 3000 (ArO–H str), 3050 (Ar–H str), 1710 (C=O str), 1600 (Ar C–C str), 1220 (C–O ester), 1053 (C–O alc) and 810 (1,2,4-trisubstituted aromatic). The chemical shift δ 61.1–78.1 ppm in the ^{13}C-NMR spectrum indicated *O*-linked carbons of the sugar moiety and the carbinol carbon of the phenolic aglycone. The anomeric carbon and the carbonyl of ester resonated at δ 104.6 and 182 ppm respectively while the aromatic carbons were observed at δ 115.7–150.1 ppm. The spectrum of ^{1}H NMR indicated a multiplet at δ 3.50 assignable to three methine protons on the glucose moiety and two doublets of carbinol protons at δ 4.46 (1H, d, $J_{5,6}$ 7.5 Hz) and δ 4.42 (IH, d, $J_{5,6}$ 7.5 Hz) coupling with H_{-5} at δ 3.73 ppm (1H, m, $J_{5,6}$ 7.5 Hz). The anomeric proton appeared as a doublet at δ 4.62 ppm indicating an axial position to the pyranose ring.

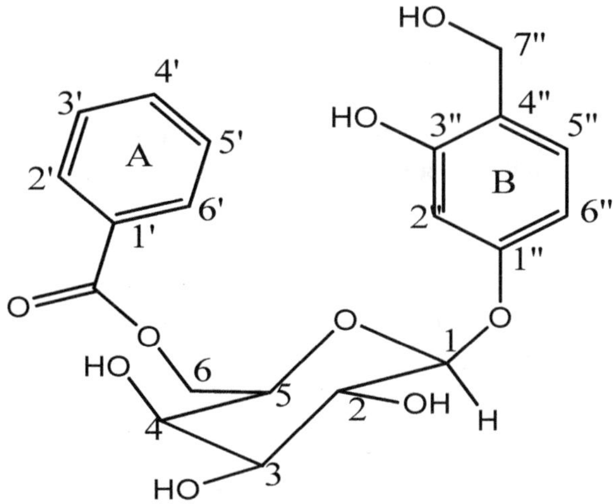

1

Figure 1. Flacourtin.

Three aromatic protons of ring B with *J* values attributable to a 1,2,4-trisubstituted aromatic system showed at δ 7.03, 6.77 and 6.48. The two protons each at ortho and meta position in ring A are in the same chemical environment, thus both protons at ortho position resonated at δ 8.05 with J_o and J_m of 7.2 and 1.5 Hz respectively. Similarly, symmetrical protons at meta positions were observed at δ 7.53 with coupling constant of 7.2 and 7.8 Hz, showing that the protons were doubly ortho-coupled, which connoted that ring A is monosubstituted. All the spectroscopic data and their assignments were in good agreement with the report of Bhaumik et al. [4]. The compound (Figure 1), which was isolated for the first time from leaves of *O. spinosa,* was elucidated as 3-hydroxy-4-hydroxymethylphenyl-6-*O*-benzoyl-β-D-glucopyranoside, previously named flacourtin.

The brine shrimps lethality test indicated that crude extract, methanol fraction and flacourtin had LD_{50} values greater than 1000 μg/mL (Table 1) which implied that they exhibited no cytotoxic activity on the *nauplii*.

Table 1. Cytotoxicity of test samples.

Sample	Crude	n-Hexane Fraction	Defatted Fraction	Flacourtin
LD_{50} (μg/mL)	1203	>10,000	>10,000	>10,000

5. Conclusions

Flacourtin is being reported for the first time in the *O. spinosa*. The preliminary toxicity profile as indicated by brine shrimp lethality test showed that the compound and the plant extracts were not cytotoxic; therefore, the tradomedicinal uses of the plant may portend no danger.

Author Contributions: Olaoye S. Balogun conceived and designed the experiment with Olukayode S. Ajayi while Lawal S. Olayinka performed the experiment.

References

1. Gbadamosi, I.T.; Oloyede, A.A. Mineral, proximate and phytochemical components of ten Nigeria medicinal plants used in the management of arthritis. *Afr. J. Pharm. Pharmacol.* **2014**, *8*, 638–643. [CrossRef]
2. Ramzi, A.; Mothana, A.; Kriegisch, S.; Harms, M.; Kristian, W.; Landequist, U. Assessment of Yemeni medinal plant for their in vitro antimicrobial, anticancer, and antioxidant activities. *J. Pharm. Biol.* **2011**, *49*, 200–210.

3. Djoussi, M.G.; Jean, D.M.; David, N.; Jules, R.K.; Leon, A.T.; Dominique, H.; Laurence, V.N. Antimicrobial and antioxidant flavonoids from the leaves of *Oncoba spinosa*. *BMC Complement. Altern. Med.* **2005**, *15*, 134. [CrossRef] [PubMed]
4. Bhaumik, P.K.; Guha, K.P.; Biswas, G.K.; Mukherjee, B. (−)Flacourtin, a phenolic glucoside ester from *Flacourtia indica*. *Phytochemistry* **2005**, *26*, 3090–3091. [CrossRef]
5. Nazneen, M.; Mazid, M.A.; Kundu, J.K.; Bachar, S.C.; Begum, F.; Datta, B.K. Protective effects of *Flacourtia indica* aerial parts extracts against paracetamol-induced hepatotoxiciy in rats. *J. Taibah Univ. Sci.* **2009**, *2*, 1–6. [CrossRef]
6. Saxena, A.; Patel, B.D. In vitro antioxidant activity of methanolic and aqueous extract of *Flacourtia indica* Merr. *Am.-Eurasian J. Sci. Res.* **2010**, *5*, 201–206.
7. Singh, T.S.; Singh, M.; Yadav, D.; Singh, I.; Mansoori, M.H. Antiasthmatic potential of *Flacourtia indica* Merr. *Afr. J. Basic Appl. Sci.* **2011**, *3*, 201–204.
8. Eramma, N.; Gayathri, D. Antibacterial potential and phytochemical analysis of *Flacourtia indica* (Burm.f.) Merr. root extract against human pathogens. *Indo Am. J. Pharm. Res.* **2013**, *3*, 3832–3846.
9. Patro, S.K.; Behera, P.C.; Kumar, P.M.; Sasmal, D.; Padhy, R.K.; Dash, S.K. Pharmacological Review of *Flacourtia sepiaria* (Ruxb.). *Sch. Acad. J. Pharm.* **2013**, *2*, 89–93.
10. Amarasinghe, N.R.; Jayasinghe, L.; Hara, N.; Fujimoto, Y. Flacourside, a new 4-oxo-2-cyclopentenylmethyl glucoside from the fruit juice of *Flacourtia indica*. *Food Chem.* **2007**, *102*, 95–97. [CrossRef]

8

Compounds from *Terminalia mantaly* L. (Combretaceae) Stem Bark Exhibit Potent Inhibition against Some Pathogenic Yeasts and Enzymes of Metabolic Significance

Marthe Aimée Tchuente Tchuenmogne [1], Thierry Ngouana Kammalac [2], Sebastian Gohlke [3], Rufin Marie Toghueo Kouipou [2], Abdulselam Aslan [4], Muslum Kuzu [5], Veysel Comakli [6], Ramazan Demirdag [6], Silvère Augustin Ngouela [1], Etienne Tsamo [1], Norbert Sewald [3], Bruno Ndjakou Lenta [7,*] and Fabrice Fekam Boyom [2,*]

1 Laboratory of Natural Products and Organic Synthesis, Department of Organic Chemistry, Faculty of Science, University of Yaoundé 1, P.O. Box 812, Yaoundé, Cameroon; tch_aimee@yahoo.fr (M.A.T.T.); sngouela@yahoo.fr (S.A.N.); tsamoet@yahoo.fr (E.T.)

2 Antimicrobial & Biocontrol Agents Unit, Laboratory for Phytobiochemistry and Medicinal Plants Studies, Department of Biochemistry, Faculty of Science, University of Yaoundé I, P.O. Box 812, Yaoundé, Cameroon; ngouanathi@yahoo.com (T.N.K.); toghueo.rufin@yahoo.fr (R.M.T.K.)

3 Chemistry Department, Organic and Bioorganic Chemistry, Bielefeld University, P.O. Box 100131, D-33501 Bielefeld, Germany; sebastian.gohlke@uni-bielefeld.de (S.G.); norbert.sewald@uni-bielefeld.de (N.S.)

4 Faculty of Engineering, Department of Industrial Engineering, Giresun University, 28200 Giresun, Turkey; abdulselam@hotmail.de

5 Faculty of Pharmacy, Department of Basic Pharmaceutical Sciences, Agrı Ibrahim Cecen University, 04100 Agri, Turkey; mkuzu@agri.edu.tr

6 School of Health, Department of Nutrition and Dietetics, Agrı Ibrahim Cecen University, 04100 Agri, Turkey; veysel_comakli@hotmail.com (V.C.); r.demirdag@hotmail.com (R.D.)

7 Department of Chemistry, Higher Teacher Training College, University of Yaoundé 1, Yaoundé, Cameroon

* Correspondence: lentabruno@yahoo.fr (B.N.L.); fabrice.boyom@fulbrightmail.org (F.F.B.);

Academic Editor: James D. Adams

Abstract: Background: Pathogenic yeasts resistance to current drugs emphasizes the need for new, safe, and cost-effective drugs. Also, new inhibitors are needed to control the effects of enzymes that are implicated in metabolic dysfunctions such as cancer, obesity, and epilepsy. **Methods:** The anti-yeast extract from *Terminalia mantaly* (Combretaceae) was fractionated and the structures of the isolated compounds established by means of spectroscopic analysis and comparison with literature data. Activity was assessed against *Candida albicans*, *C. parapsilosis* and *C. krusei* using the microdilution method, and against four enzymes of metabolic significance: glucose-6-phosphate dehydrogenase, human erythrocyte carbonic anhydrase I and II, and glutathione *S*-transferase. **Results:** Seven compounds, 3,3′-di-*O*-methylellagic acid 4′-*O*-α-rhamnopyranoside; 3-*O*-methylellagic acid; arjungenin or 2,3,19,23-tetrahydroxyolean-12-en-28-oïc acid; arjunglucoside or 2,3,19,23-tetrahydroxyolean-12-en-28-oïc acid glucopyranoside; 2α,3α,24-trihydroxyolean-11,13(18)-dien-28-oïc acid; stigmasterol; and stigmasterol 3-*O*-β-d-glucopyranoside were isolated from the extract. Among those, 3,3′-di-*O*-methylellagic acid 4′-*O*-α-rhamnopyranoside, 3-*O*-methylellagic acid, and arjunglucoside showed anti-yeast activity comparable to that of reference fluconazole with minimal inhibitory concentrations (MIC) below 32 μg/mL. Besides, Arjunglucoside potently inhibited the tested enzymes with 50% inhibitory concentrations (IC_{50}) below 4 μM and inhibitory constant (Ki) <3 μM. **Conclusions:** The results achieved indicate that further SAR studies will likely identify potent hit derivatives that should subsequently enter the drug development pipeline.

Keywords: *Terminalia mantaly*; Combretaceae; anti-yeast; enzyme inhibitors

1. Introduction

Fungal diseases affect 3–4 million people worldwide every year. Of particular importance, the increasing resistance of pathogenic opportunistic yeasts to current drugs is a serious concern and has attracted the attention of the scientific community. New, safe, and cost-effective drugs of natural or synthetic origin are therefore actively being researched [1]. Recent epidemiological data highlight the increasing burden of pathogenic yeasts on people in poor settings [2–4]. *Candida* species and *Cryptococcus neoformans* are the major pathogenic yeasts and only a few antifungal drugs have been developed so far to treat the invasive infections they cause [5,6]. Medicinal plants have shown credibility as sources of treatment for infectious diseases [7]. In Cameroon, extracts from medicinal plants such as *Terminalia mantaly* (Combretaceae) are widely used by traditional healers to control diverse infections or associated symptoms, including but not limited to dysentery, gastroenteritis, hypertension, diabetes, and oral, dental, cutaneous and genital affections [8]. Previous studies on the extracts of this plant have showed antibacterial and antifungal properties, but their chemical compositions have not yet been determined [9]. However, phytochemical studies of other species of the genus *Terminalia* have reported the presence of flavonoids, terpenoids and their glycosides derivatives, tannins, flavonones and chalcones [10–18]. In spite of the work done on *Terminalia* species, no investigation has been attempted yet on the enzyme inhibition properties of their extracts and constituents targeting glucose-6-phosphate dehydrogenase, carbonic anhydrase and glutathione *S*-transferase.

Glucose-6-phosphate dehydrogenase (G6PD; EC 1.1.1.49) is an enzyme that catalyzes the reaction of glucose-6-phosphate into phosphogluconate, which is the rate-limiting first step of the pentose phosphate pathway. The end products of this pathway are ribose-5-phosphate and NADPH. Ribose-5-phosphate is used in DNA or RNA synthesis in cell reproduction, and NADPH is used as a coenzyme for the enzymes participating in the production of reduced glutathione. Given its role in cell growth, this enzyme is of high importance to mammal cells [19,20]. However, several studies have shown that this enzyme has an important role in the pathology of some diseases like cancer, hypertension, heart failure and type 2 diabetes. G6PD activity increases in cancer cells and its inhibition results in decreased cell proliferation and induction of apoptosis. For example, 6-aminonicotinamide, which is an inhibitor of G6PD, has found use in the therapy of various tumors in the past [21].

The carbonic anhydrase (CA; carbonate hydro-lyase, EC 4.2.1.1) enzyme exists commonly in living organisms, and has various isoenzymes according to conditions and necessities of the medium. It is one of the most studied enzymes and CAI and CAII are the most common isoenzymes [22]. In many physiological and pathological processes, CAs catalyze the conversion of CO_2 to HCO_3^- and H^+. In addition, CA inhibitors may be used in the treatment of various diseases such as oedema, glaucoma, obesity, cancer, epilepsy and osteoporosis [23].

In living cells, the deleterious effects of free radicals and their intermediates are eliminated or minimized by various enzymatic and non-enzymatic defense systems. Enzymatic defense is provided by several enzymes such as glutathione *S*-transferase (GST), glutathione reductase, glutathione peroxidase, superoxide dismutase, and catalase [24]. The GSTs (EC 2.5.1.18) are a group of multifunctional enzymes that play an important role in animal metabolism [25]. GSTs are important for the fight against cancer because of their interactions with carcinogens and chemotherapeutic agents. They are the target of antiasthmatic and antitumor drugs [26]. Production of excessive amounts of GST in mammalian tumor cells leads to resistance to some anticancer drugs and chemical carcinogens [27].

The reduction of drug effects in tumor cells is an important factor limiting the therapeutic efficacy of an antineoplastic agent. Over time, the development of this resistance is associated with glutathione (GSH) and glutathione *S*-transferase (GST) levels in cells and changes in permeability to the drug. In this regard, G6PD, CA I, II or GST inhibitors may be useful because of their several applications, in particular for the treatment of glaucoma, epilepsy, cancer and as diuretics.

In our search for bioactive secondary metabolites from Cameroonian medicinal plants, we have investigated the MeOH extract of the stem bark of *T. mantaly* L. (Combretaceae) that previously showed anti-yeast activity. We report in this paper the inhibitory potential of compounds isolated from this extract against some pathogenic yeasts and some enzymes of metabolic significance.

2. Materials and Methods

2.1. General Experimental Procedures

The physicochemical analyses of the isolated natural products were essentially performed as previously described [28]. Optical rotations were measured on a JASCO digital polarimeter (model DIP-3600, JASCO, Tokyo, Japan). UV spectra were determined on a Spectronic Unicam spectrophotometer (Thermo Scientific, Waltham, MA, USA). IR spectra were determined on a JASCO Fourier transform IR-420 spectrometer (JASCO, Tokyo, Japan). ^{1}H and ^{13}C NMR spectra were run on a Bruker spectrometer (Bruker Corporation, Brussels, Belgium) equipped with 5 mm ^{1}H and ^{13}C probes operating at 500 and 125 MHz, respectively, with Tetramethylsilane (TMS) as internal standard. Silica gel 230–400 mesh (Merck, Bielefeld, Germany) and silica gel 70–230 mesh (Merck) were used for flash and column chromatography while precoated aluminum-backed silica gel 60 F254 sheets were used for TLC. Spots were visualized under UV light (254 and 365 nm) or using MeOH–H_2SO_4 reagent.

2.2. Plant Material

The stem bark of *T. mantaly* (Combretaceae) was collected in Yaoundé, Cameroon in May 2012 and identified at the Cameroon National Herbarium where a voucher specimen is deposited under the reference N° 64212/HNC (*T. mantaly* H. Perrier).

2.3. Microbial Isolates

Yeast isolates were kindly provided by the Laboratory of Clinical Biology, Yaoundé Central Hospital and consisted of clinical isolates of *C. albicans*, *C. krusei* and *C. parapsilosis*. Yeasts were maintained at room temperature and cultured at 37 °C for 24 h on Sabouraud Dextrose Agar (Oxoid, Drongen, Belgium) slants prior to use.

2.4. Plant Extraction and Screening of Anti-Yeast Activity

The harvested *T. mantaly* stem bark was dried at room temperature and ground using a blender. The powdered stem bark (7 kg) was extracted at r.t. with MeOH (48 h). The extract was concentrated under vacuum to afford a dark residue (250 g). Minimal inhibitory concentration (MIC) of the extract was determined according to the CLSI M27-A3 [6] protocol with little modifications. The RPMI 1640 supplemented with 2% glucose was used as culture medium. Briefly for the fungal susceptibility tests, 50 μL of serially two-fold diluted concentrations of the crude extract were added in triplicate wells of a 96-wells microtiter plate. Fifty μL of fungal inocula standardized to a final concentration of 0.5–2.5 × 10^3 CFU/mL were then individually added in each well of the plate. Plant crude extract and the positive control (fluconazole) at concentrations of 0.12 to 64 μg/mL were tested in a final volume of 100 μL. So-prepared plates were incubated at 37 °C for 48 h. MIC value was subsequently determined through macroscopic observation of plate wells, and was defined as the lowest concentration of the inhibitor that allowed no visible growth of the microorganism after overnight incubation compared to the growth control.

2.5. Isolation of Compounds and Screening for Activity

A portion of 180 g of the extract was subjected to medium pressure flash chromatography over silica gel (Merck, 70–230 mesh) using mixtures *n*-hexane-EtOAc of increasing polarity ((70:30)–(0:100)) and EtOAc–MeOH ((95:5)–(50:50)), resulting in the collection of 75 fractions of 500 mL each, which were combined on the basis of TLC analysis to create four fractions labeled T_1–T_4. Fraction T_1 (m = 14.4 g) obtained from the mixtures of *n*-hexane-EtOAc (100:0 to 70:30) was subjected to silica gel column chromatography, eluted with *n*-hexane-EtOAc, and yielded oils stigmasterol (23 mg) and arjungenin (7 mg). From fraction T_2 (m = 60.3 g), eluted with *n*-hexane-EtOAc ((50:50)–(25:75)), stigmasterol 3-*O*-β-D-glucopyranoside (12 mg), arjungenin (17 mg), 2α,3α,24-trihydroxyolean-11,13(18)-dien-28-oic acid (5.0 mg) and arjunglucoside (6 mg) were isolated. Column chromatography of fraction T_3 (m = 55.0 g) on silica gel and eluted with the mixtures of EtOAc–MeOH ((100:0)–(85:15)), yielded 3,3′-di-*O*-methylellagic acid 4′-*O*-α-rhamnopyranoside (32 mg), arjungenin (12.0 mg), arjunglucoside (3.5 mg), 2α,3α,24-trihydroxyolean-11,13(18)-dien-28-oic acid (3.5 mg) and a dark mixture that was subjected to column chromatography on Sephadex LH-20 with MeOH as an isocratic eluent and yielded 3-*O*-methyl ellagic acid (12.5 mg). Fraction T_4 (m = 56.18 g) obtained with the solvent system of EtOAc–MeOH (85:15 to 65:35) was a complex mixture and thus was not studied. All the isolated compounds were screened as described above for anti-yeast activity, and as described below for enzyme inhibition activities.

2.6. Purification of Glucose 6-Phosphate Dehydrogenase and Activity Determination

G6PD was purified from the gill tissue of Lake Van fish according to Kuzu et al. [29], and the enzyme activity was determined spectrophotometrically using a Shimadzu UV-1800 spectrophotometer (Shimadzu, Tokyo, Japan) at 25 °C, according to the method described by Beutler [30] and based on the principle of the reduction of $NADP^+$ to NADPH in the presence of glucose 6-phosphate and absorbance recorded at 340 nm.

2.7. Purification of Carbonic Anhydrase Isoenzymes by Affinity Chromatography and Activity Determination

The purification of hCA I and II isozymes was performed with a simple one step method by a Sepharose-4B anilinesulphanilamide affinity column chromatograph as previously described [31]. Briefly, CNBr activated Sepharose-4B was washed with ddH_2O and tyrosine further attached to the activated gel as a spacer arm and finally diazotized sulphanilamide clamped with tyrosine molecule as ligand. The homogenate was applied to the prepared Sepharose-4B-L-Tyrosine Sulphanilamide affinity column equilibrated with 25 mM Tris–HCl/0.1 M Na_2SO4 (pH 8.7) (Sigma-Aldrich, Taufkirchen, Germany). The affinity gel was washed with 25 mM Tris–HCl/22 mM Na_2SO4 (pH 8.7).

The esterase activity was assessed following the change in absorbance of 4-nitrophenylacetate (NPA) to 4-nitrophenylate ion at 348 nm over a period of 3 min at 25 °C using a Beckman Coulter UV-VIS spectrophotometer (Beckman Coulter, Atlanta, GA, USA) according to the method described by Verpoorte et al. [32].

2.8. Purification of Glutathione S-Transferase Enzyme and Activity Determination

Firstly, heamolysate from human erythrocytes was prepared according to the method of Hunaiti et al. [33]. The prepared heamolysate was directly applied to the glutathione-agarose affinity column and washed with 10 mM KH_2PO_4 and 0.1 M KCl (pH 8.0) (Sigma-Aldrich). The washing procedure was monitored on a spectrophotometer through equal–to–blind absorbance values. After the column was stabilized, the enzyme was purified by gradient elution at +4 °C [24,34]. Elution solvent was prepared from a solvent gradient containing 50 mM Tris–HCl and (1.25–10 mM GSH, pH 9.5). Thereafter, 1-chloro-2,4-dinitrobenzene (Sigma-Aldrich) was used to determine GST enzyme activity. In fact the complex obtained using dinitrobenzene *S*-glutathione (DNB-SG) displays maximum absorbance at 340 nm. Activity measurements were thus carried out using the absorbance increment at this wavelength. [35].

2.9. In Vitro Inhibition and Kinetic Studies

To determine the effects of compounds on enzymes, enzyme activities were measured with saturated substrate concentration and five different inhibitor concentrations. The 50% inhibitory concentrations (IC_{50}) were determined by plotting curves of percent inhibition versus compound concentration. Results are reported as IC_{50} values. Ki constants were calculated using the Cheng-Prusoff equation [36].

3. Results and Discussion

The methanol extract of the stem bark of *T. mantaly* was screened for anti-yeast activity in vitro against three clinical isolates consisting of *C. albicans*, *C. krusei* and *C. parapsilosis*. The crude extract exhibited good activity with MIC values of 24 µg/mL against *C. parapsilosis* and 39 µg/mL against *C. albicans* and *C. krusei* (Table 1).

Table 1. Anti-yeast activity of *Terminalia mantaly* extract and isolates.

Extract/Fractions		*C. parapsilosis*	*C. albicans*	*C. krusei*
		MIC * (µg/Ml ± SD)		
MeOH Extract		24.00 ± 0.21	39.00 ± 0.33	39.00 ± 0.30
Fraction T1		1250.00 ± 1.23	2500.00 ± 0.98	2500.00 ± 1.03
Fraction T2		39.00 ± 0.38	>5000	>5000
Fraction T3		0.16 ± 0.02	0.64 ± 0.12	0.02 ± 0.09
Fraction T4		>5000	>5000	>5000
	Fraction of origin			
3,3′-di-*O*-methylellagic acid 4′-*O*-α-rhamnopyranoside	T3	39.00 ± 0.88 (80.4 µM)	9.70 ± 0.72 (20 µM)	>5000 (10,300 µM)
3-*O*-methyl ellagic acid	T3	78.00 ± 0.92 (247.6 µM)	156.00 ± 1.00 (495 µM)	19.50 ± 0.57 (61.9 µM)
Arjungenin	T1, T2, T3	>5000 (9487 µM)	>5000 (9487 µM)	>5000 (9487 µM)
Arjunglucoside	T2, T3	39.00 ± 0.13 (56.60 µM)	9.70 ± 0.36 (14.07 µM)	312.00 ± 1.04 (452 µM)
2α,3α,24-trihydroxyolean-11, 13(18)-dien-28-oic acid	T1, T3	>5000 (9823 µM)	>5000 (9823 µM)	>5000 (9823 µM)
Fluconazole **		2.00 ± 0.01 (6.53 µM)	8.00 ± 0.25 (26.14 µM)	32.00 ± 0.42 (10.45 µM)

* Plant extracts were tested using the CLSI M27-A3 protocol. Activity was expressed as minimal inhibitory concentration; ** Reference used as positive control. MIC, minimum inhibitory concentration.

The flash chromatography of the crude extract generated four fractions exhibiting varying antifungal activities. As shown in Table 1, fraction T3 was the most active, with activity magnification over 1950 times against *C. krusei* (MIC = 0.02 µg/mL), 150 times against *C. parapsilosis* (MIC = 0.16 µg/mL), and over 60 times against *C. albicans* (0.64 µg/mL), compared to the crude extract (MIC = 24–39 µg/mL). *C. krusei* was the most susceptible isolate to fraction T3. Compounds 3,3′-di-*O*-methylellagic acid-4′-*O*-α-rhamnopyranoside, 3-*O*-methylellagic acid, arjungenin, arjunglucoside, and 2α,3α,24-trihydroxyolean-11,13(18)-dien-28-oic acid that were all found in fraction T3 were also tested for biological activity (Table 1; Figure 1). Overall, they showed drastically reduced potency against the tested yeasts compared to the mother fraction T3, indicating that fractionation has negatively affected the biological activity. Compounds stigmasterol and stigmasterol 3-*O*-β-D-glucopyranoside were not tested due to reduced solubility in the culture medium. Among the tested compounds, 3,3′-di-*O*-methylellagic acid-4′-*O*-α-rhamnopyranoside and arjunglucoside showed the best potency against *C. albicans* with an MIC of 9.7 μg/mL. They also moderately inhibited *C. parapsilosis* with an MIC of 39 μg/mL. In addition, compound 3-*O*-methylellagic acid inhibited *C. krusei* with an MIC of 19.5 μg/mL.

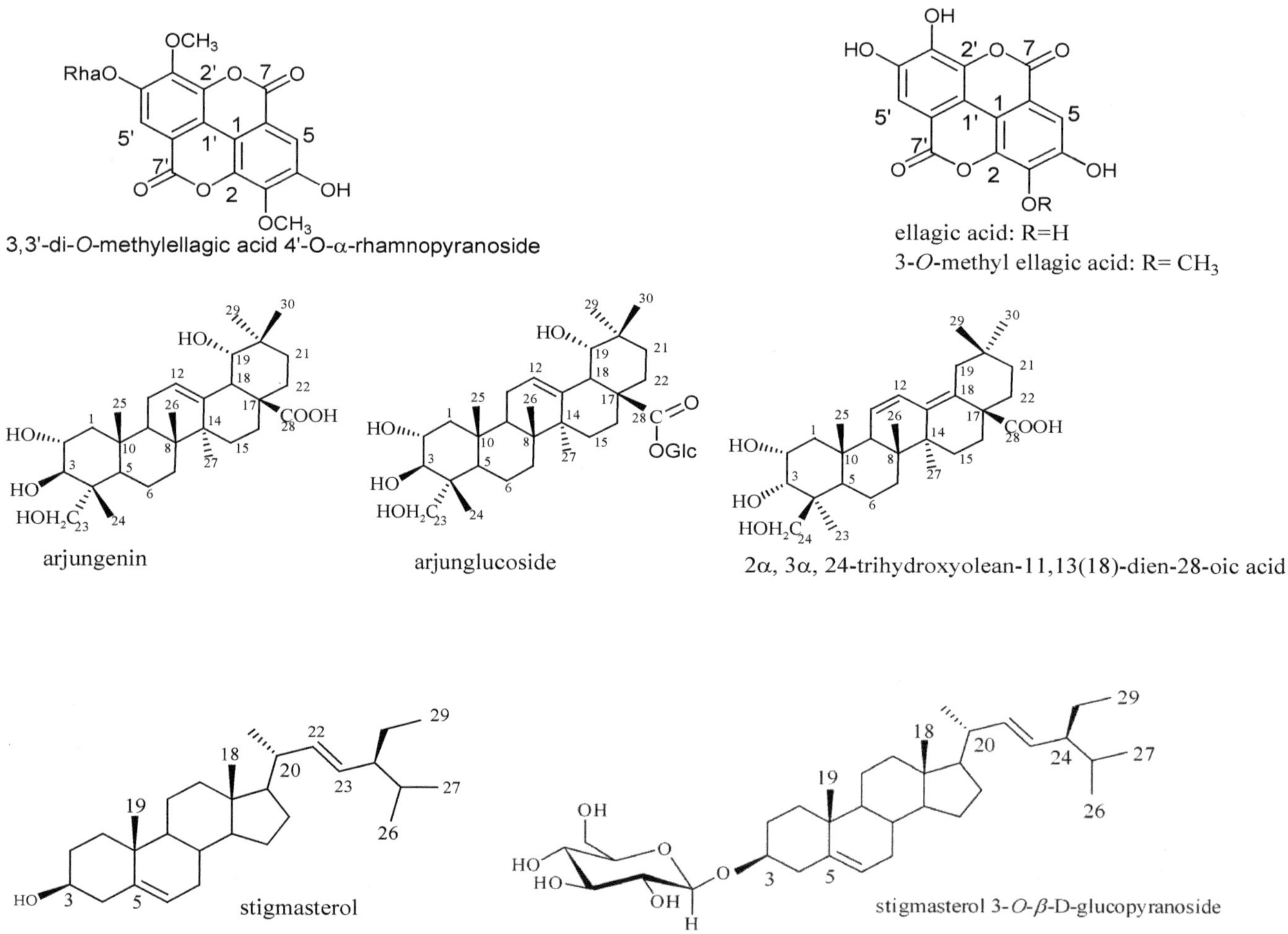

Figure 1. Structures of the isolated compounds from *Terminalia mantaly* (Combretaceae). The isolated compounds were tested against pathogenic yeast isolates and enzymes of metabolic significance. 3,3′-di-*O*-methylellagic acid 4′-*O*-α-rhamnopyranoside: IC_{50} = 39 μg/mL *C. parapsilosis;* 9.7 μg/mL *C. albicans;* >5000 μg/mL *C. krusei;* CAI: IC_{50} = 53.31 μM, Ki = 44.11 μM; CAII: IC_{50} = 69.11 μM, Ki = 55.78 μM; GST: IC_{50} = 63.01 μM, Ki = 42.00 μM. 3-*O*-methyl ellagic acid: IC_{50} = 78 μg/mL *C. parapsilosis;* 156 μg/mL *C. albicans;* 19.5 μg/mL *C. krusei*. arjungenin: *C. parapsilosis, C. albicans, krusei*: IC_{50} > 5000 μg/mL; CAI: IC_{50} = 86.64 μM, Ki = 71.68 μM; GST: IC_{50} = 1.51 μM, Ki = 1.00 μM; arjunglucoside: IC_{50} = 39 μg/mL *C. parapsilosis;* 9.7 μg/mL *C. albicans;* 312 μg/mL *C. krusei;* G6PD: IC_{50} = 1.84 μM, Ki = 0.19 μM; CAI: IC_{50} = 3.28 μM, Ki = 2.72 μM; CAII: IC_{50} = 1.28 μM, Ki = 1.03 μM; GST: IC_{50} = 1.84 μM, Ki = 1.23 μM. 2α,3α,24-trihydroxyolean-11,13(18)-dien-28-oic acid: IC_{50} > 5000 μg/mL *C. parapsilosis, C. albicans, C. krusei.*

4. NMR Spectral Data of the Tested Compounds

The physicochemical profiles of the isolated compounds were acquired following previously described approaches [37–40].

3,3′-di-O-methylellagic acid 4′-O-α-rhamnopyranoside. Yellowish powder; molecular formula $C_{21}H_{18}O_{12}$; ESI-MS: $[M + Na]^+$ *m/z* 485,049 ^{1}H-NMR (300 MHz, DMSO-d_6): δ_H 1.13 (3 H, d, CH_3, H-6″), 3.54 (1 H, q, *J* = 8.0 and 12.0 Hz, H-5″), 4.01 (1 H, t, H-4″), 4.04 (3 H, s, OMe-3), 4.72 (1 H, brd, *J* = 8.0 Hz, H-3″), 4.94 (1 H, brd, *J* = 4.0 Hz, H-2″), 5.47 (1 H, brs, H-1″), 7.52 (1 H, s, H-5), 7.73 (1 H, s, H-5′); ^{13}C-NMR (125 MHz, DMSO-d_6), aglycone moiety: δ_C 113.4 (C-1), 140.5 (C-2), 141.8 (C-3), 153.1 (C-4), 111.9 (C-5), 113.4 (C-6), 159.1 (C-7), 114.7 (C-1′), 136.6 (C-2′), 142.2 (C-3′), 146.9 (C-4′), 112.0 (C-5′), 107.4 (C-6′), 159.1 (C-7′); rhamnose moiety: 100.5 (C-1″), 70.4 (C-2″), 70.5 (C-3″), 72.2 (C-4″), 70.3 (C-5″), 18.3 (C-6″) and 61.4 (C-3, OMe).

3-O-methyl ellagic acid. Yellowish powder; molecular formula $C_{15}H_8O_8$; ESI-MS: $[M - H]^-$ *m/z* 315, ^{1}H-NMR (DMSO-d_6): δ 7.50 (1 H, s, H-5), 7.44 (1 H, s, H-5′), 4.02 (3 H, s, 3-OMe). ^{13}C-NMR (DMSO-d_6): δ 158.9 (C-7), 158.6 (C-7′), 152.2 (C-4), 148.2 (C-4′), 141.7 (C-2), 140.0 (C-3), 139.8 (C-3′), 136.1 (C-2′), 112.4(C-1′), 112.1 (C-6), 111.7 (C-1), 111.3 (C-5), 110.1 (C-5′), 107.2 (C-6′), 60.8 (3-OMe).

Arjungenin or 2,3,19,23-tetrahydroxyolean-12-en-28-oic acid. White powder; molecular formula $C_{30}H_{48}O_6$; ESI-MS: $[M + Na]^+$ *m/z* 527,322. ^{1}H-NMR (300 MHz, DMSO-d_6): δ_H 1.23, 1.09, 0.90, 0.88, 0.84 and 0.65 (each 3 H, s); 2.92 (1 H, brs, H-18); 2.86 (1 H, d, *J* = 8 Hz, H-3) and 3.57 (1 H, m, H-2); 5.23 (1 H, brs, H-12); ^{13}C-NMR (125 MHz; DMSO-d_6): δ_C 16.8, 17.1, 23.9, 24.9, 28.9 and 24.5; 64.3 (C-23), 80.5 (C-3), 179.6 (C-28), 122.6 (C-12); 143.9 (C-13).

Arjunglucoside or 2,3,19,23-tetrahydroxyolean-12-en-28-oïc acid glucopyranoside. White powder; molecular formula $C_{36}H_{58}O_{11}$; ESI-MS: $[M + Na]^+$ *m/z* 689,396; ^{1}H-NMR (300 MHz, DMSO-d_6): δ 1.23, 1.08, 0.89, 0.86, 0.84 and 0.63 (each 3 H, s); between 2.90 and 3.80: glucose moiety with anomeric proton at 5,20 (1 H, d, *J* = 6.9 Hz, H-1′); ^{13}C-NMR (125 MHz; DMSO-d_6): δ 16.9, 24.5, 24.9 and 28.5; glucose moiety: 61.0, 69.9, 72.8, 77.1, 78.2, 94.5; 64.3 (C-23), 67.4 (C-2), 80.4 (C-3), 176.3 (C-28), 122.6 (C-12), 143.7 (C-13).

2α,3α,24-trihydroxyolean-11,13(18)-dien-28-oic acid. Yellowish powder; molecular formula $C_{30}H_{46}O_5$; ESI-MS: $[M + Na]^+$ *m/z* 509,375 (calc. 509,324) for $C_{30}H_{46}NaO_5$); ^{1}H-NMR(400 MHz; pyridin-d_5): δ 1.58; 1.06; 1.05; 1.03; 0.90 and 0.87 (each 3 H, s); 6.62 (1 H, d, *J* = 8.0 Hz, H-11) and 5.81 (1 H, d, *J* = 8.0 Hz, H-12); 4.38 (1 H, ddd, *J* =2.2; 7.6 and 8.9 Hz, H-2); 3.59 (1 H, d, *J* = 7.5 Hz, H-3); 4.43 (1 H, d, *J* = 8.7 Hz, H-24) and 3.75 (1 H, d, *J* = 8,76 Hz, H-24); 2.69 (1 H, d, *J* = 12.4 Hz, H-19) and 2.15 (1 H, d, *J* = 12.4 Hz, H-19); ^{13}C-NMR (125 MHz; pyridin-d_5): δ_C 16.6, 19.5, 19.8, 23.7, 24.0 and 32.1; 65.1 (C-24), 68.4 (C-2), 85.5 (C-3), 178,6 (C-28);136,1 (C-13); 133,3 (C-18); 126,4 (C-12) et 125,9 (C-11).

Apart from the activity profile described above, MIC values for the other tested fractions and compounds were above 39 μg/ml. The activity level of compounds 3,3′-di-*O*-methylellagic acid 4′-*O*-α-rhamnopyranoside and arjunglucoside was comparable to that of the reference drug fuconazole against *C. albicans*, and compound 3-*O*-methylellagic acid showed to be over 1.5 times more active than the same reference drug against *C. krusei*. Based on the basic skeleton of the tested compounds, it is important to notice that one of the most active derivatives, arjunglucoside and the less active compounds, arjungenin and 2α,3α,24-trihydroxyolean-11,13(18)-dien-28-oic acid are all triterpenoids. Preliminary structure-activity relationship (SAR) study clearly indicated that the glycosylation of the acidic function of arjungenin at C-28 is important for activity improvement. The other active compounds 3,3′-di-*O*-methylellagic acid 4′-*O*-α-rhamnopyranoside and 3-*O*-methylellagic acid are ellagic acid derivatives. Previous studies have reported the antifungal activity of ellagic acid against fungal strains *Trichophyton rubrum*, *T. verrucosum*, *T. mentagrophytes*, *T. violaceum*, *T. schoenleinii*, *Microsporum canis*, *C. glabrata*, *C. albicans* and *C. tropicalis* [41]. Also, the observed antifungal potency of compounds 3,3′-di-*O*-methylellagic acid 4′-*O*-α-rhamnopyranoside and 3-*O*-methylellagic acid, respectively glycosylated and methylated derivatives of ellagic acid, highlights the potency of this class of secondary metabolites [41].

Overall, it was observed that fraction T3 exerted the more potent effect against the tested yeasts, far better than the derived compounds. This is an indication that fractionation has declined the anti-yeast activity, emphasizing the relevance of potential synergistic interactions among the components of fraction T3. Moreover, these results indicate future directions in the progression of this fraction to develop a phytodrug against yeasts infections.

Selected isolated compounds were further tested against G6PD, carbonic anhydrase I, II and GST enzymes. The results achieved are shown in Table 2.

The G6PD enzyme was strongly inhibited by the triterpenoid arjunglucoside with IC_{50} value of 1.84 μM and Ki (the inhibitor constant indicating how potent an inhibitor is; or the concentration required to produce half maximum inhibition) value of 0.19 μM. It has been shown that this key metabolic enzyme which catalyzes the first step of the pentose phosphate pathway is expressed abundantly and is very active in human tumors [21]. In contrast, G6PD-deficient tumor cell lines showed relatively slow growth and enhanced apoptosis [42]. Previous studies also reported G6PD inhibitory properties for few compounds such as steroids and derivatives [43,44], chalcones [29], catechin gallates [45], and some phenolic molecules [46]. In this study, the substituted ellagic acid derived compound 3,3′-di-*O*-methylellagic acid 4′-*O*-α-rhamnopyranoside did not show any effect on the G6PD enzyme activity, although Adem et al. [46] had previously reported that ellagic acid inhibited the enzyme with an IC_{50} value of 0.072 mM. The methoxy group in this derivative may hinder the enzyme–inhibitor interaction. Based on the skeletal features of the tested triterpenoids—arjungenin, arjunglucoside, and 2α,3α,24-trihydroxyolean-11,13(18)-dien-28-oic acid—the presence of the hydroxyl group at C-19 and the glycosylation of the C-28 carboxylic group may be both factors of activity improvement. The G6PD inhibitory potential of a terpenoid is reported here for the first time.

Compound arjunglucoside exhibited very good potency against both CAI and CAII enzymes with respective activity parameters of IC_{50} = 3.28 μM and Ki = 2.72 μM; and IC_{50} = 1.28 μM and Ki = 1.03 μM respectively. The other tested compounds including 3,3′-di-*O*-methylellagic acid 4′-*O*-α-rhamnopyranoside and arjungenin were found to be moderately active against CAI and CAII (3,3′-di-*O*-methylellagic acid 4′-*O*-α-rhamnopyranoside) with IC_{50} and Ki values globally above 44 μM. Previous studies by Sarıkaya et al. [47] have indicated that ellagic acid inhibited CAI and CAII with K_i values of 0.207 and 0.146 mM respectively. In the present study, compound 3,3′-di-*O*-methylellagic acid 4′-*O*-α-rhamnopyranoside, a substituted derivative of ellagic acid has exhibited moderate, however highly improved potency toward CAI (K_i = 44.11 μM) and CAII (55.78 μM) enzymes. On the other hand, this substitution has also considerably decreased the activity as observed against the G6PD enzyme. In addition to the established role of CA inhibitors (CAIs) as diuretics and antiglaucoma drugs, it has recently emerged that they could have potential as novel anti-obesity, anticancer and anti-infective drugs [23]. The high inhibitory potency of the triterpenoid arjunglucoside against CAs indicates that it is a promising compound that might be a candidate for the formulation of drugs against CAIs-related diseases.

The screening of 3,3′-di-*O*-methylellagic acid 4′-*O*-α-rhamnopyranoside, arjungenin, and arjunglucoside against GST enzyme showed inhibitory effects. However, the triterpenoids arjungenin, and arjunglucoside exhibited highly potent inhibitory effects (IC_{50} of 1.57 and 1.84 μM respectively; and K_i of 1.00 and 1.23 μM respectively). Compound 3,3′-di-*O*-methylellagic acid 4′-*O*-α-rhamnopyranoside only exerted a moderate inhibitory effect on the enzyme (IC_{50} = 63.01 μM; K_i = 42.00 μM). These results are of higher significance as GST inhibitors are anti-cancer agents [25,26]. Ellagic acid was recently shown to inhibit GSTs A1-1, A2-2, M1-1, M2-2 and P1-1 with IC_{50} values ranging from 0.04 to 5 μM [48]. Preliminary SAR studies indicate that the substitution of ellagic acid at C-3 and C-4′ gave the derivative 3,3′-di-*O*-methylellagic acid 4′-*O*-α-rhamnopyranoside which showed an IC_{50} value of 63.01 μM, thus therefore considerably decreased the activity. The inhibitory effect of this class of secondary metabolite derivatives is reported here for the first time.

Table 2. Inhibitory parameters of isolated compounds against G6PD, CAI, CAII, and GST.

Activity	G6PD				CAI				CAII				GST			
Parameter	1	2	3	4	1	2	3	4	1	2	3	4	1	2	3	4
IC_{50} [a] (μM)	n.a	n.a	n.a	1.84 ± 0.31	53.31 ± 1.09		86.64 ± 0.93	3.28 ± 0.13	69.31 ± 1.13	n.a	n.a	1.03 ± 0.01	63.01 ± 1.15	n.a	1.51 ± 0.78	1.84 ± 0.73
Ki [b] (μM)	n.a	n.a	n.a	0.19 ± 0.03	44.11 ± 1.12		71.68 ± 0.96	2.72 ± 0.64	55.78 ± 0.97	n.a	n.a	1.84 ± 0.11	42.00 ± 1.39	n.a	1.00 ± 0.03	0.19 ± 0.77

Enzymes were expressed and purified, and subsequently assessed for in vitro susceptibility to inhibitors. [a] Serially diluted triplicate concentrations of compounds were tested and activity expressed as 50% inhibitory concentration; [b] Inhibitory constant which is reflective of the binding affinity; the smaller the Ki, the greater the binding affinity and the smaller amount of medication needed in order to inhibit the activity of that enzyme. n.a = non active. 1: 3,3′-di-*O*-methylellagic acid 4′-*O*-α-rhamnopyranoside; 2: 3-*O*-methylellagic acid; 3: arjungenin; 4: arjunglucoside. G6PD, glucose-6-phosphate dehydrogenase; CAI, human erythrocyte carbonic anhydrase I; CAII, human erythrocyte carbonic anhydrase II; GST, glutathione *S*-transferase.

5. Concluding Remarks

The results obtained from the investigation of the methanolic extract of *T. mantaly* stem bark have identified a highly potent anti-yeast fraction T3 that showed to be more promising than subsequently isolated compounds. Overall, the five compounds, 3,3′-di-*O*-methylellagic acid 4′-*O*-α-rhamnopyranoside, arjungenin, arjunglucoside, 2α,3α,24-trihydroxyolean-11,13(18)-dien-28-oic acid, and 3-*O*-methyl ellagic acid were found to be 243 to 31,250 times, 15 to 7,812 times, and 975 to 250,000 times less active than the mother fraction (T3) against *C. parapsilosis*, *C. albicans*, and *C. krusei* respectively. This promising fraction deserves to be further investigated with the ultimate aim of formulating a plant-based drug against yeast infections. Compounds 3,3′-di-*O*-methylellagic acid 4′-*O*-α-rhamnopyranoside and arjunglucoside showed anti-yeast activity close to that of the reference drug fuconazole against *C. albicans*. Moreover, compound 3-*O*-methyl ellagic acid was over 1.5 times more active than fuconazole against *C. krusei*. In addition, two of the islolated compounds, arjungenin and arjunglucoside were found to be very active against enzymes of metabolic significance, namely G6PD (arjunglucoside) and GST (arjungenin and arjunglucoside). Finally, given the anti-yeast potency of these compounds, and also the implication of the tested enzymes in some metabolic dysfunctions of public health significance (cancer, obesity, epilepsy), we envisage further SAR studies to identify potent hit derivatives that should subsequently enter the drug development pipeline.

Acknowledgments: The authors acknowledge the Alexander von Humboldt Foundation for providing a Fellowship to Bruno Ndjakou Lenta at Bielefeld University. Part of this study was supported by equipment from the Seeding Labs' Instrumental Access Grant (SL2012-2) to Fabrice Fekam Boyom.

Author Contributions: N.S., E.T., B.N.L., F.F.B. and S.A.N. designed and supervised the study; M.A.T.T., T.N.K., S.G., R.M.T.K., A.A., M.K., V.C. and R.D. performed the chemical and biological parts of the study and drafted the manuscript; B.N.L. and F.F.B. critically revised the manuscript. All authors agreed on the final version of the manuscript for submission to *Medicines*.

References

1. Arif, T.; Mandal, T.K.; Dabur, R. Natural products: Anti-fungal agents derived from Plants. In *Opportunity, Challenge and Scope of Natural Products in Medicinal Chemistry*; Pandalai, S.G., Ed.; Research Signpost: Trivandrum, India, 2011; pp. 283–311.
2. Nelesh, G. HIV-associated opportunistic fungal infections: A guide to using the clinical microbiology laboratory. *South. Arf. J. HIV Med.* **2007**, *1*, 18–23.
3. Álvaro-Meca, A.; Jensen, J.; Micheloud, D.; Asunción, D.; Gurbindo, D.; Resino, S. Rate of candidiasis among HIV infected children in Spain in the era of highly active antiretroviral therapy (1997–2008). *BMC Inf. Dis.* **2013**, *13*, 1–15. [CrossRef] [PubMed]
4. Brissaud, O.; Guichoux, J.; Harambat, J.; Tandonnet, O.; Zaoutis, T. Invasive fungal disease in PICU: Epidemiology and risk factors. *Ann. Intensiv. Care* **2012**, 2. [CrossRef] [PubMed]
5. Ngouana, K.T.; Krasteva, D.; Drakulovski, P.; Toghueo, K.R.; Kouanfack, C.; Ambe, A.; Reynes, J.; Delaporte, E.; Boyom, F.F.; Mallié, M.; et al. Investigation of minor species *Candida africana*, *Candida stellatoidea*, and *Candida dubliniensis* in the *Candida albicans* complex among Yaoundé (Cameroon) HIV-infected patients. *Mycoses* **2015**, *58*, 33–39. [CrossRef] [PubMed]
6. Ngouana, K.T.; Dongtsa, J.; Kouanfack, C.; Tonfack, C.; Foména, S.; Krasteva, D.; Drakulovski, P.; Aghokeng, A.; Mallié, M.; Delaporte, E.; et al. Cryptoccocal meningitis in Yaoundé (Cameroon) HIV infected patients: Diagnosis, frequency and susceptibility of *Cryptococcus neoformans* isolates to fluconazole. *J. Mycol. Med.* **2015**, *25*, 11–16. [CrossRef] [PubMed]
7. Newman, D.J.; Cragg, G.M. Natural products as sources of new drugs over the last 25 years. *J. Nat. Prod.* **2007**, *70*, 461–477. [CrossRef] [PubMed]
8. Coulibaly, K. Evaluation of the Antifungal Activity of Extracts of Bark of Commercial Species, Category P1 the Forest of Mopri, Tiassalé (Southern Ivory Coast). Master's Thesis, University of Cocody-Abidjan, Abidjan, Côte D'Ivoire, 2006; pp. 23–25.

9. Ngouana, T.K.; Mbouna, C.D.J.; Kuipou, R.M.T.; Tchuenmogne, M.A.T.; Zeuko'o, E.M.; Ngouana, V.; Mallié, M.; Bertout, S.; Boyom, F.F. Potent and Synergistic Extract Combinations from *Terminalia Catappa, Terminalia Mantaly* and *Monodora tenuifolia* against Pathogenic Yeasts. *Medicines* **2015**, *2*, 220–235. [CrossRef]
10. Cock, I. The medicinal properties and phytochemistry of plants of the genus *Terminalia* (Combretaceae). *Inflammopharmacology* **2015**, *23*, 203–229. [CrossRef] [PubMed]
11. Valsaraj, R.; Pushpangadan, P.; Smitt, U.W.; Adsersen, A.; Christensen, S.B.; Sittie, A.; Nyman, U.; Nielsen, C.; Olsen, C.E. New anti-HIV-1, antimalarial and antifungal compounds from *Terminalia bellerica*. *J. Nat. Prod.* **1997**, *60*, 739–742. [CrossRef] [PubMed]
12. Srivastava, S.K.; Srivastava, S.D.; Chouksey, B.K. New constituents of *Terminalia alata*. *Fitoterapia* **1999**, *70*, 390–394. [CrossRef]
13. Conrad, J.; Vogler, B.; Klaiber, I.; Roos, G.; Walter, U.; Kraus, W. Two triterpene esters from *Terminalia macroptera* bark. *Phytochemistry* **1998**, *48*, 647–650. [CrossRef]
14. Conrad, J.; Vogler, B.; Reeb, S.; Klaiber, I.; Papajewski, S.; Roos, G.; Vasquez, E.; Setzer, M.C.; Kraus, W. Isoterchebulin and 4,6-*O*-isoterchebuloyl-D-glucose, Novel Hydrolyzable Tannins from *Terminalia macroptera*. *J. Nat. Prod.* **2001**, *64*, 294–299. [CrossRef] [PubMed]
15. Kandil, F.E.; Nassar, M.I. A tannin anti-cancer promotor from *Terminalia arjuna*. *Phytochemistry* **1998**, *47*, 1567–1568. [CrossRef]
16. Mahato, S.B.; Nandy, A.K.; Kundu, A.H. Pentacyclic triterpenoids sapogenols and their glycosides from *Terminalia bellerica*. *Tetrahedron* **1992**, *48*, 2483–2484. [CrossRef]
17. Singh, D.V.; Verma, R.K.; Singh, C.S.; Gupta, M.M. RP-LC determination of oleane derivatives in *Terminalia arjuna*. *J. Pharm. Biomed. Anal.* **2002**, *28*, 447–452. [CrossRef]
18. Garcez, R.F.; Garcez, S.W.; Santana, A.L.B.D.; Alves, M.M.; Matos, M.F.C.C.; Scaliante, A.M. Bioactive flavonoids and triterpenes from *Terminalia fagifolia* (Combretaceae). *J. Braz. Chem. Soc.* **2006**, *17*, 1223–1228. [CrossRef]
19. Yeh, G.C.; Daschner, P.J.; Lopaczynska, J.; MacDonald, C.J.; Ciolino, H.P. Modulation of glucose-6-phosphate dehydrogenase activity and expression is associated with aryl hydrocarbon resistance in vitro. *J. Biol. Chem.* **2001**, *276*, 34708–34713. [CrossRef] [PubMed]
20. Matsubara, S.; Kato, T.; Oshikawa, K.; Yamada, T.; Takayama, T.; Koike, T.; Sato, I. Glucose-6-phosphate dehydrogenase in rat lung alveolar epithelial cells. An ultrastructural enzyme-cytochemical study. *Eur. J. Histochem.* **2002**, *46*, 243–248. [CrossRef] [PubMed]
21. Preuss, J.; Richardson, A.D.; Pinkerton, A.; Hedrick, M.; Sergienko, E.; Rahlfs, S.; Bode, L. Identification and characterization of novel human glucose-6-phosphate dehydrogenase inhibitors. *J. Biomol. Screen.* **2013**, *18*, 286–297. [CrossRef] [PubMed]
22. Tripp, B.C.; Smith, K.; Ferry, J.G. Mini review: Carbonic anhydrase: New insights for an ancient enzyme. *J. Biol. Chem.* **2001**, *276*, 48615–48618. [CrossRef] [PubMed]
23. Supuran, C.T. Carbonic anhydrases: Novel therapeutic applications for inhibitors and activators. *Nat. Rev. Drug Discov.* **2008**, *7*, 168–181. [CrossRef] [PubMed]
24. Comakli, V.; Ciftci, M.; Kufrevioglu, O.I. Effects of some metal ions on rainbow trout erythrocytes glutathione *S*-transferase enzyme: An in vitro study. *J. Enzyme Inhib. Med. Chem.* **2013**, *28*, 1261–1266. [CrossRef] [PubMed]
25. Mannervik, B.; Danielson, U.H. Glutathione transferases—Structure and catalitic activity. *CRC Crit. Rev. Biochem.* **1988**, *23*, 283–337. [CrossRef] [PubMed]
26. Matshushita, N.; Aritake, K.; Takada, A.; Hizue, M.; Hayashi, K.; Mitsui, K. Pharmacological studies on the novel antiallergenic drug HQL-79: 2. Elucidation of mechanisms for antiallergic and antiasthmatic effects. *Jpn. J. Pharmacol.* **1998**, *78*, 11–22. [CrossRef]
27. Hayes, J.D.; McLellan, L.I.; Stockman, P.K.; Chalmers, J.; Beckett, G.J. Glutathione *S*-transferases in man: The relationship between rat and human enzymes. *Biochem. Soc. Trans.* **1987**, *15*, 721–725. [CrossRef] [PubMed]
28. Mga'ning, B.M.; Lenta, B.N.; Noungoue, D.T.; Antheaume, C.; Fongang, Y.F.; Ngouela, S.A.; Boyom, F.F.; Rosenthal, P.J.; Tsamo, E.; Sewald, N.; et al. Antiplasmodial sesquiterpenes from the seeds of *Salacia longipes* var. *camerunensis*. *Phytochemistry* **2013**, *96*, 347–352. [CrossRef] [PubMed]

29. Kuzu, M.; Aslan, A.; Ahmed, I.; Comakli, V.; Demirdag, R.; Uzun, N. Purification of glucose-6-phosphate dehydrogenase and glutathione reductase enzymes from the gill tissue of Lake Van fish and analyzing the effects of some chalcone derivatives on enzyme activities. *Fish Physiol. Biochem.* **2016**, *42*, 483–491. [CrossRef] [PubMed]
30. Beutler, E. *Red Cell Metabolism: A Manual of Biochemical Methods*, 3rd ed.; Grune and Stratton Inc.: Orlando, FL, USA, 1984; pp. 68–70.
31. Ekinci, D.; Cavdar, H.; Talaz, O.; Sentürk, M.; Supuran, C.T. NO-releasing esters show carbonic anhydrase inhibitory action against human isoforms I and II. *Bioorg. Med. Chem.* **2010**, *18*, 3559–3563. [CrossRef] [PubMed]
32. Verpoorte, J.A.; Mehta, S.; Edsall, J.T. Esterase activities of human carbonic anhydrases B and C. *J. Biol. Chem.* **1976**, *242*, 4221–4229.
33. Hunaiti, A.A.; Soud, M. Effect of lead concentration on the level of glutathione, glutathione *S*-transferase, reductase and peroxidase in human blood. *Sci. Total Environ.* **2000**, *248*, 45–50. [CrossRef]
34. Güvercin, S.; Erat, M.; Sakiroglu, H. Determination of some kinetic and characteristic properties of glutathione *S*-transferase from bovine erythrocytes. *Protein Pept. Lett.* **2008**, *15*, 6–12. [PubMed]
35. Habig, W.H.; Pabst, M.J.; Jakoby, W.B. Glutathione *S*-transferases. The first enzymatic step in mercapturic acid formation. *J. Biol. Chem.* **1974**, *249*, 7130–7139. [PubMed]
36. Cheng, Y.; Prusoff, W.H. Relationship between the inhibition constant (K1) and the concentration of inhibitor which causes 50 per cent inhibition (I50) of an enzymatic reaction. *Biochem. Pharmacol.* **1973**, *22*, 3099–3108. [PubMed]
37. Liu, M.; Katerere, R.D.; Gray, I.A.; Seidel, V. Phytochemistry and antifungal studies on *Terminalia mollis* and *Terminalia brachystemina*. *Fitoterapia* **2009**, *80*, 369–373. [CrossRef] [PubMed]
38. Nandy, A.K.; Podder, G.; Sahu, N.P.; Mahato, S.B. Triterpenoids and their glycosides from *Terminalia bellerica*. *Phytochemistry* **1989**, *28*, 2769–2772. [CrossRef]
39. Jossang, A.; Seuleiman, M.; Maidou, E.; Bodo, B. Pentacyclic triterpenes from *Combretum nigricans*. *Phytochemistry* **1996**, *41*, 591–594. [CrossRef]
40. Kojima, H.; Tominaga, H.; Sato, S.; Ogura, H. Pentacyclic triterpenoids from *Prunella vulgaris*. *Phytochemistry* **1987**, *26*, 1107–1111. [CrossRef]
41. Li, Z.; Guo, X.; Dawuti, G.; Aibai, S. Antifungal activity of ellagic acid in vitro and in vivo. *Phytother. Res.* **2015**, *29*, 1019–1025. [CrossRef] [PubMed]
42. Kuo, W.Y.; Lin, J.Y.; Tang, K. Human glucose-6-phophate dehydrogenase (G6PD). Gene transforms NIH 3T3 cells and induces tumors in nude mice. *Int. J. Cancer* **2000**, *85*, 857–864. [CrossRef]
43. Gupta, S.; Cordeiro, T.A.; Michels, P.A.M. Glucose-6-phosphate dehydrogenase is the target for the trypanocidal action of human steroids. *Mol. Biochem. Parasitol.* **2011**, *176*, 112–115. [CrossRef] [PubMed]
44. Hamilton, M.N.; Dawson, M.; Fairweather, E.E.; Hamilton, S.N.; Hitchin, R.J.; James, I.D.; Jones, D.S.; Jordan, M.A.; Lyones, J.A.; Small, F.H. Novel steroid inhibitors of glucose 6-phosphate dehydrogenase. *J. Med. Chem.* **2012**, *55*, 4431–4445. [CrossRef] [PubMed]
45. Shin, E.S.; Park, J.; Shin, J.M.; Cho, D.; Cho, S.Y.; Shin, D.W.; Ham, M.; Kim, J.B.; Lee, T.R. Cathechin gallates are $NADP^+$-competitive inhibitors of glucose-6-phosphate dehydrogenase and other enzymes that employ $NADP^+$ as a coenzyme. *Bioorg. Med. Chem.* **2008**, *16*, 3580–3586. [CrossRef] [PubMed]
46. Adem, S.; Comakli, V.; Kuzu, M.; Demirdag, R. Investigation of the effects of some phenolic compounds on the Activities of glucose-6-phosphate dehydrogenase and 6-Phosphogluconate dehydrogenase from human erythrocytes. *J. Biochem. Mol. Toxicol.* **2014**, *28*, 510–514. [CrossRef] [PubMed]
47. Beyza, Ö.S.; Gülçin, İ.; Supuran, C.T. Carbonic anhydrase inhibitors: Inhibition of human erythrocyte isozymes I and II with a series of phenolic acids. *Chem. Biol. Drug Des.* **2010**, *75*, 515–520. [CrossRef] [PubMed]
48. Hayeshi, R.; Mutingwende, I.; Mavengere, W.; Masiyanise, V.; Mukanganyama, S. The inhibition of human glutathione *S*-transferases activity by plant polyphenolic compounds ellagic acid and curcumin. *Food Chem. Toxicol.* **2007**, *45*, 286–295. [CrossRef] [PubMed]

9

Methanol Extract from *Anogeissus leiocarpus* (DC) Guill. et Perr. (Combretaceae) Stem Bark Quenches the Quorum Sensing of *Pseudomonas aeruginosa* PAO1

Vincent Ouedraogo and Martin Kiendrebeogo *

Laboratoire de Biochimie & Chimie Appliquées, Université Ouaga 1 Pr. Joseph KI-ZERBO, Ouagadougou, 03 BP 7021, Burkina Faso; vicenteoued@gmail.com
* Correspondence: martinkiendrebeogo@yahoo.co.uk

Academic Editor: James D. Adams

Abstract: Background: Due to its extensive arsenal of virulence factors and inherent resistance to antibiotics, *Pseudomonas aeruginosa* is a threat particularly in immunocompromised patients. Considering the central role of quorum sensing in the production of virulence factors, inhibition of bacterial communication mechanism constitute an opportunity to attenuate pathogenicity of bacteria resistant to available antibiotics. Our study aimed to assess the anti-quorum sensing activity of *Anogeissus leiocarpus*, traditionally used in Burkina Faso, for the treatment of infected burn wounds. **Methods:** Investigations were carried out on methanol extract from *A. leiocarpus* stem bark. The reporter strains *Chromobacterium violaceum* CV026 and *P. aeruginosa* PAO1 derivatives were used to evidence any interference with the bacterial quorum sensing and expression of related genes. *P. aeruginosa* PAO1 was used to measure the impact on pyocyanin production. **Results:** At a sub-inhibitory concentration (100 μg/mL), *A. leiocarpus* methanol extract quenched the quorum sensing mechanism of *P. aeruginosa* PAO1 by down-streaming the *rhlR* gene, with a subsequent reduction of pyocyanin production. Moreover, the antioxidant polyphenols evidenced are able to reduce the oxidative stress induced by pyocyanin. **Conclusion:** The antioxidant and anti-quorum sensing activities of *A. leiocarpus* stem bark could justify its traditional use in the treatment of infected burn wounds.

Keywords: *Anogeissus leiocarpus*; *Chromobacterium violaceum* CV026; *Pseudomonas aeruginosa* PAO1; pyocyanin; quorum sensing

1. Introduction

Pseudomonas aeruginosa infections are common following burn injuries [1] and often present as wound infections [2]. Due to its extensive arsenal of virulence factors and inherent resistance to several antibiotics, approximately 80% of burn patients infected with *P. aeruginosa* die of septicaemia [3]. Production of virulence factors by *P. aeruginosa* is under the control of a cell-to-cell communication system termed quorum sensing (QS), which is a mechanism used by many bacteria to detect their critical cell numbers through the release and perception of small diffusible signal molecules called auto inducers, in order to coordinate a common behavior [4–6].

In *P. aeruginosa*, two QS systems (lasI/lasR and rhlI/RhlR) drive the production (by the synthetases LasI and RhlI) and the perception (by the transcription factors LasR and RhlR) of the auto inducers acyl homoserine lactones (AHL)—*N*-(3-oxododecanoyl)-L-homoserine lactone (3-oxo-C12-HSL) and *N*-butanoyl-L-homoserine lactone (C4-HSL), respectively [4,5,7,8]. A third

QS system, based on quinolone signals, links and interacts in an intricate way with the lasI/lasR and rhlI/RhlR quorum-sensing systems [9–12].

Following injuries, inflammation process (representing a non-specific immune response to chemical or biological aggression) takes place in order to pathogen elimination and tissue injury reparation [13–15].

Inflammatory reactions start with the release of inflammatory mediators (e.g., cytokines, endotoxins, prostaglandins, leukotrienes, and histamine) as well as reactive oxygen species (ROS) by injured cells.

In non-pathogenic conditions, cells are normally able to defend themselves against ROS damage through the use of endogen enzymatic and non-enzymatic antioxidants agents. Since *P. aeruginosa* infection during a burn wound dramatically boosts the level of ROS, antioxidant defense systems of cells are overpassed, resulting in oxidative stress with significant damage to cell structures [16,17].

In the ongoing struggle against bacterial infection, antibiotics are commonly used to kill pathogenic bacteria. However, bacteria increasingly exhibit resistance against available antimicrobial drugs [18,19]. To cope with these limitations, the alternative approach consisting in attenuating the expression of bacterial virulence factor without affecting their viability by using anti-QS agents has become a rational preventive strategy [20,21].

In Burkina Faso, more than 80% of the population relies on traditional practices and medicinal plants to treat various diseases [22]. Some medicinal plants have been reported to present anti-inflammatory activity and wound healing effects without any antibacterial activity [22,23], which suggests a non-antimicrobial modulation of virulence factors.

In this study, *Anogeissus leiocarpus* (DC) Guill. & Perr. (Combretaceae), which is traditionally involved in Burkina Faso for the treatment of infected burn wounds [22], was investigated for its ability to reduce the production of pyocyanin, one of the QS-controlled virulence factors produced by *P. aeruginosa*, and to interfere with the bacterial QS system. Total polyphenol and flavonoid content as well as the antioxidant potentiality of this medicinal plant were also assessed.

2. Materials and Methods

2.1. Bacterial Strains, Plasmids, and Culture Conditions

Chromobacterium violaceum CV026, *Pseudomonas aeruginosa* PAO1, and its derivatives (Table S1) harboring plasmids pPCS1001 (P_{lasR}-*lacZ* transcriptional fusion), pβ03 (P_{lasI}-*lacZ* transcriptional fusion), pPCS1002 (P_{rhlR}-*lacZ* transcriptional fusion), pLPR1 (P_{rhlI}-*lacZ* transcriptional fusion), pTB4124 (P_{acAe}-*lacZ* transcriptional fusion) and pβ02 (P_{rhlA}-*lacZ* transcriptional fusion) were provided from the Laboratoire de Biotechnologie Vegetale (Université Libre de Bruxelles, Gosselies, Belgium). *P. aeruginosa* PAO1 (37 °C, agitation 175 rpm) and *C. violaceum* CV026 (30 °C, agitation 175 rpm) were grown in LB broth. *P. aeruginosa* PAO1 derivatives strains were grown (37 °C, agitation 175 rpm) in LB-MOPS broth (50 mM, pH 7) supplemented with carbenicillin (300 μg/mL).

2.2. Plant Material Collection and Extraction

Stem bark of *Anogeissus leiocarpus* (DC) Guill. et Perr. (Combretaceae) was collected in August 2014 at Gampela (25 km, east of Ouagadougou, Burkina Faso). Botanical identity was assessed by Dr. Amade Ouedraogo from the Laboratoire de Biologie et Ecologie Vegetale (Université Ouaga 1 Pr. Joseph Ki-Zerbo, Ouagadougou, Burkina Faso) where a voucher specimen (ID: 16883) was deposited. Plant material was dried at room temperature, ground into fine powder, and stored in an airtight bag until use.

Powdered plant material (100 g) was defatted with petroleum ether (500 mL) in a soxhlet extractor (Wheaton industries Inc., Millvile, NJ, USA) and soaked (24 h, 25 °C, continuous stirring) in methanol. Extract was filtrated, concentrated in a vacuum evaporator (Büchi Labortechnik AG, Postfach, Flawil, Switzerland) and dried to obtain 14.4 g of plant extract. Plant extract (100 mg/mL) was dissolve either in methanol for phytochemical purpose or in dimethyl sulfoxide (DMSO) for testing on bacterial strains. Test samples were stored at 4 °C until use.

2.3. Total Polyphenol and Flavonoid Content Determination

Total polyphenol was determined according to the colorimetric method of Folin–Ciocalteu [24]. Plant extract (25 μL, 100 μg/mL in methanol) was mixed with Folin–Ciocalteu Reagent (125 μL, 0.2 N) and, 5 min later, with sodium bicarbonate (100 μL, 75 g/L). After incubation (1 h, room temperature), absorbance was measured at 760 nm against a methanol blank. Gallic acid (0–100 mg/L) was used to generate a standard calibration curve ($Y = 0.005X + 0.00968$; $R^2 = 0.99$), and total polyphenol content was expressed as mg gallic acid equivalent to 100 mg of plant extract (mg GAE/100 mg).

Total flavonoid was estimated according to the Dowd method [24]. Plant extract (75 μL, 100 μg/mL in methanol) was mixed with aluminium trichloride (75 μL, 2% in methanol). Absorbance was subsequently read at 415 nm after incubation (10 min, room temperature) against a methanol blank. Quercetin (0–100 mg/L) was used to plot a standard calibration curve ($Y = 0.02891X + 0.0036$; $R^2 = 0.99$), and total flavonoid content was expressed as mg of quercetin equivalent to 100 mg of plant extract (mg QE/100 mg).

2.4. Antioxidant Assays

Antioxidant activity was measured through 2,2-diphenyl-1-picrylhydrazyl (DPPH) and ferric reducing antioxidant power (FRAP) assays as previously described [24].

For the DPPH assay, freshly prepared DPPH solution (200 μL, 0.02 mg/mL in methanol) was mixed with plant extract (100 μL, 100 to 0.39 μg/mL in methanol). The mixture was subsequently shacked and incubated (15 min in darkness, room temperature), and absorbance was measured at 517 nm against a methanol blank. DPPH radical scavenging activities were plotted against sample concentrations, and the result was expressed as a sample concentration scavenging 50% of DPPH radicals (IC50). Quercetin was used as positive controls.

For FRAP testing, plant extract (100 μL, 100 μg/mL in methanol) was mixed with a phosphate buffer (250 μL, 0.2 M, pH 6.6) and a potassium hexacyanoferrate solution (250 μL, 1% in water). After incubation (30 min, 50 °C), trichloroacetic acid (250, 10% in water) was added, and the mixture centrifuged (2000× *g* for 10 min). The supernatant (125 μL) was mixed with water (125 μL) and a fresh $FeCl_3$ solution (25 μL, 0.1% in water) to read absorbance at 700 nm. Ascorbic acid was used to plot a calibration curve ($R^2 = 0.99$). Reducing power was expressed as μM ascorbic acid equivalent per gram of plant extract (μM AAE/g). Quercetin was used as positive controls.

2.5. Determination of MIC and MBC

MIC (minimum inhibitory concentration) values on *P. aeruginosa* PAO1 and *C. violaceum* CV026 were determined according to the micro dilution method, using *p*-iodonitrotetrazolium (INT) as an indicator of bacterial growth [25]. In brief, an overnight bacterial culture was diluted with LB broth to obtain a starting inoculum (109 CFU/mL). Inoculum (180 μL) was added to serial dilutions of test extract (20 μL; 50 to 0.39 mg/mL in DMSO 10%) to obtain a final concentration range of 5 mg/mL to 0.039 mg/mL. Mixtures were incubated for 18 h (37 °C, 175 rpm agitation). After 18 h of incubation, 50 μL of INT (0.2 mg/mL) was added to each well, and the microplate was further incubated (37 °C, 30 min). Bacterial growth was indicated by a red color within the microplate wells (Greiner Bio-One GmbH, Frieckenhausen, Germany).

To determine the MBC, aliquots of 20 μL from all dilutions not showing any bacterial growth were spread onto LB agar plates and incubated (37 °C, 24 h). The minimum concentration for which there is no visible growth on agar plate was recorded as MBC [26].

2.6. *Quantitative Analysis of Pyocyanin Production in P. aeruginosa PAO1*

Inhibition of pyocyanin production was assessed according to previously described procedures [27]. *P. aeruginosa* PAO1 was grown (18 h in LB broth, 37 °C, 175 rpm agitation), and cells were washed twice in fresh LB medium. In 18 culture tubes, appropriately diluted PAO1 cell suspension (250 μL) was added to the LB medium (4.7 mL, starting OD600nm ranged between 0.02 and 0.03) and supplemented with plant extract (50 μL, 10 mg/mL in DMSO) or DMSO. At periodic time intervals (3 h), tubes ($n = 3$) were sampled to assess bacterial growth (ufc/mL) and pyocyanin content.

From each tube, 100 μL of bacterial culture were removed and diluted in LB broth to be plated onto LB agar and incubated (24 h, 37 °C) for colony counting, while 200 μL of bacterial culture was used to determine optical density at 600 nm. Remaining bacterial culture was centrifuged (7000 rpm, 10 min, 24 °C) to obtain culture supernatant. Pyocyanin was extracted from the supernatant (4 mL) with chloroform (2 mL) and re-extracted from chloroform with 0.2 M HCl (1 mL). Optical density reading at 380 nm allows pyocyanin determination.

2.7. *Quantitative Analysis of Violacein Production in C. violaceum CV026*

Inhibition of violacein production in *C. violaceum* CV026 was tested according to [27]. Violacein production was induced in *C. violaceum* CV026 by adding exogenous *N*-hexanoyl-L-homoserine lactone (HHL; Sigma-Aldrich Chemie GmbH, Darmstadt, Germany).

An appropriately diluted overnight culture of *C. violaceum* CV026 (200 μL) was incubated (30 °C, 48 h, 175 rpm agitation) in 18 culture tubes containing LB broth (4.7 mL) supplemented with HHL (50 μL, 10 mM in DMSO) and plant extract (50 μL, 10 mg/mL in DMSO) or DMSO. At periodic time intervals (6 h), tubes ($n = 3$) were sampled to assess bacterial growth (ufc/mL and OD600 nm) and pyocyanin content, while violacein was quantified after 48 h growth.

From each tube, bacterial culture (1 mL) was centrifuged (7000 rpm, 10 min) and DMSO (1 mL) was added to the pellet. The solution was vortexed to dissolve violacein, and cell debris was discarded by centrifugation (7000 rpm, 10 min). Violacein content in supernatant was measured by the absorbance at 585 nm.

2.8. *β-Galactosidase Assay*

β-Galactosidase measurements were performed as previously described [27]. After growth in liquid LB-MOPS-Carbenicillin (37 °C with 175 rpm agitation) for 18 h, PAO1 reporter strains harboring plasmids (Table S1) were washed twice in fresh LB medium and resuspended in fresh liquid LB-MOPS-Carbenicillin. PAO1 reporter strains inoculums (50 μL) were incubated (37 °C with 175 rpm agitation) for 8 or 18 h in 1 mL of LB-MOPS-Carbenicillin (initial OD600 nm of culture comprised between 0.020 and 0.025) supplemented with 10 μL of plant extracts (100 μg/mL final concentration) or 10 μL of DMSO. After incubation, bacterial density was assessed by spectrophotometry (OD600 nm), and the sample used for cell growth assessment was used to perform the β-galactosidase assay with O-nitrophenyl-β-D-galactopyranoside as described elsewhere [28].

2.9. *Statistical Analysis*

All experiments were performed in triplicate (independent assays), and data were expressed as mean ± SD. Data analysis was performed via analysis of variance (one-way ANOVA or two-way ANOVA) followed by a Tukey or Bonferonni test, using GraphPad Prism software (version 5.00 for window, GraphPad Software, San Diego, CA, USA) p value ≤ 0.05 was considered significant.

3. Results

3.1. Antioxidant Activity, Total Polyphenol, and Flavovoid Content

Total polyphenol and total flavonoid were quantified from methanol extract of *A. leiocarpus* stem bark together with its antioxidant capacity through radicals DPPH scavenging activity and ferric reducing power, and each antioxidant assay involved a different antioxidant mechanism. The amount of total polyphenol was particularly high (82.62 ± 3.16 mg GAE/100 mg) in addition to a low content of total flavonoid (15.14 ± 0. 39 mg QE/100 mg). As shown, an interesting antioxidant potential was found. *A. leiocarpus* exhibits the same DPPH radical scavenging activity (1.82 ± 0.07 µg/mL) as quercetin (1.40 ± 0.15 µg/mL), while its ferric-reducing power (4.29 ± 0.19 µM AAE/g) was only two-fold lower than that of our antioxidant reference (7.66 ± 0.39 µM AAE/g).

3.2. Inhibition of Pyocianin Production

The MIC (1.25 mg/mL) and MBC (>5.00 mg/mL) values evaluated allow for the selection of a sub-inhibitory concentration for the bioassay on *P. aeruginosa* PAO1. Methanol extract from *A. leiocarpus* stem bark (100 µg/mL) was incubated for 18 h in *P. aeruginosa* PAO1 culture to access its capacity to interfere with the production of pyocyanin, a QS-dependent extracellular virulence factor of the bacteria. As shown, methanol extract from *A. leiocarpus* (100 µg/mL final concentration) significantly impact ($p < 0.05$) in a kinetic way the production of pyocyanin (Figure 1a) without any effect on bacterial kinetic growth (Figure 1b). Hence, the reduction of pyocyanin production recorded within 18 h was not the consequence of any bactericidal or bacteriostatic effect but probably the effect of some interference with the QS mechanism of *P. aeruginosa* PAO1, controlling the production of pyocyanin.

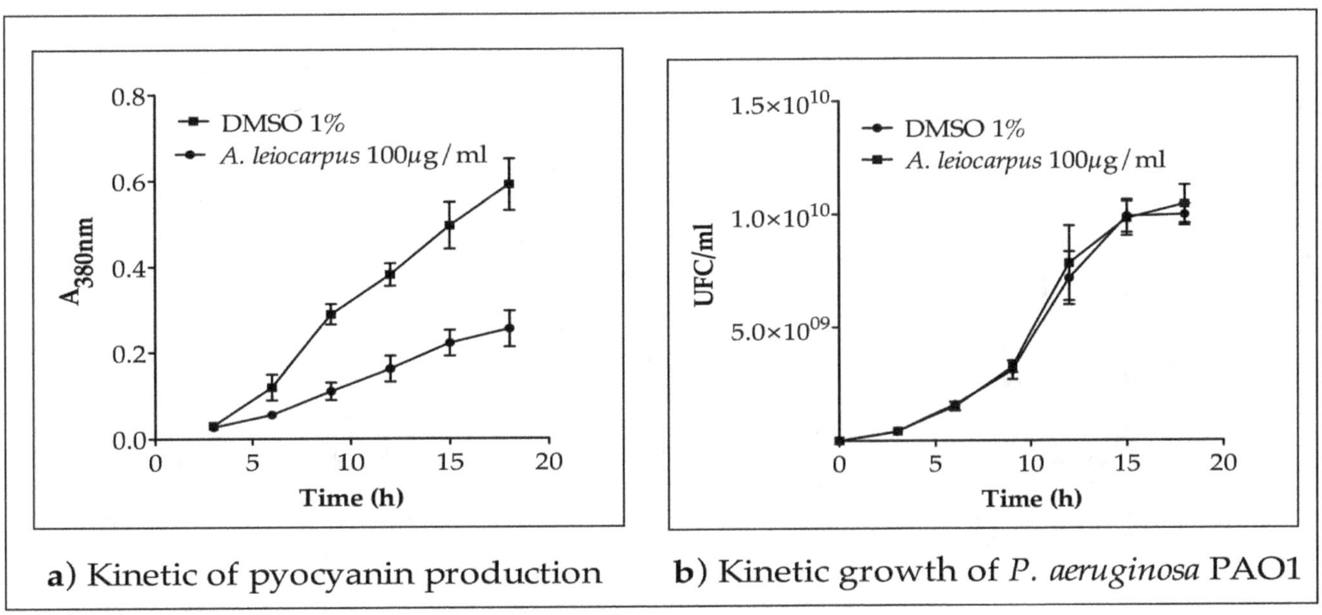

Figure 1. Methanol extract from *A. leiocarpus* reduce pyocyanin production in *P. aeruginosa* PAO1. (**a**) *A. leiocarpus* extract (100 µg/mL) significantly reduced ($p > 0.05$) pyocyanin production within 18 h compared to DMSO used as control; (**b**) *A. leiocarpus* extract (100 µg/mL) did not exhibit a significant effect on *P. aeruginosa* PAO1 kinetic growth within 18 h. Dimethyl sulfoxide (DMSO) was used as negative control. *P. aeruginosa* PAO1 was grown (37 °C, 175 rpm agitation) in the LB broth. Mean values ± SD of triplicate independent experiments are shown.

3.3. Anti-Quorum Sensing Activity

To assess the ability of the methanol extract from *A leiocarpus* stem bark to interfere with the quorum sensing mechanism, the reporter strain *C. violaceum* CV026, deficient in the homoserine-lactone synthase gene *cviI*, was used. This strain is unable to produce quorum sensing auto inducers (homoserine-lactones) by itself, nor therefore the QS-related violacein, without an external supply of homoserine-lactone. The MIC (0.62 mg/mL) and MBC (2.50 mg/mL) values evaluated allow for the selection of a sub-inhibitory concentration for the bioassay on *C. violaceum* CV026. Methanol extract from *A. leiocarpus* (100 μg/mL final concentration) reduced violacein production by up to 50% (Figure 2a) without any effect on bacterial kinetic growth (Figure 2b). Therefore, the reduction of violacein production observed was not due to any bactericidal or bacteriostatic effect, but to a quenching of the QS system of the bacteria. When extract was added to *C. violaceum* CV026 growth medium without a HHL supply, violacein was not produced, indicating that *A. leiocarpus* extract do not contain mimic HHL compound (data not shown).

In order to evidence any interference with the expression of quorum sensing (QS) genes of *P. aeruginosa* PAO1, we focused on the transcriptional level after 18 h of incubation. Therefore, the expression of the HHL synthetases genes (*lasI* and *rhlI*), the QS regulator genes (*lasR* and *rhlR*), and the virulence factor QS-controlled genes (*lasB* and *rhlA*) were evaluated. As shown (Figure 3), methanol extract of *A. leiocarpus* stem bark did not significantly affect ($p < 0.05$) the transcription level of the quorum sensing *lasI*, *lasR*, and *rhlI* genes, while expression of *rhlR* was significantly ($p < 0.05$) downstreamed.

To determine whether the drop in β-galactosidase activity recorded was not due to an effect on the transcription/translation mechanisms, nor to an inhibition of the enzyme (β-galactosidase), a *P. aeruginosa* PAO1 strain harboring the aceA-lacZ fusion (*aceA* gene encoding for isocitrate lyase) was tested. As shown, *A. leiocarpus* extract had no effect on the transcription of the *aceA* gene, demonstrating that it affects the expression of QS-related genes without interfering with the entire transcription machinery of *P. aeruginosa* PAO1. Hence, *A. leiocarpus* methanol extract clearly exhibited anti-QS activity on *P. aeruginosa* PAO1.

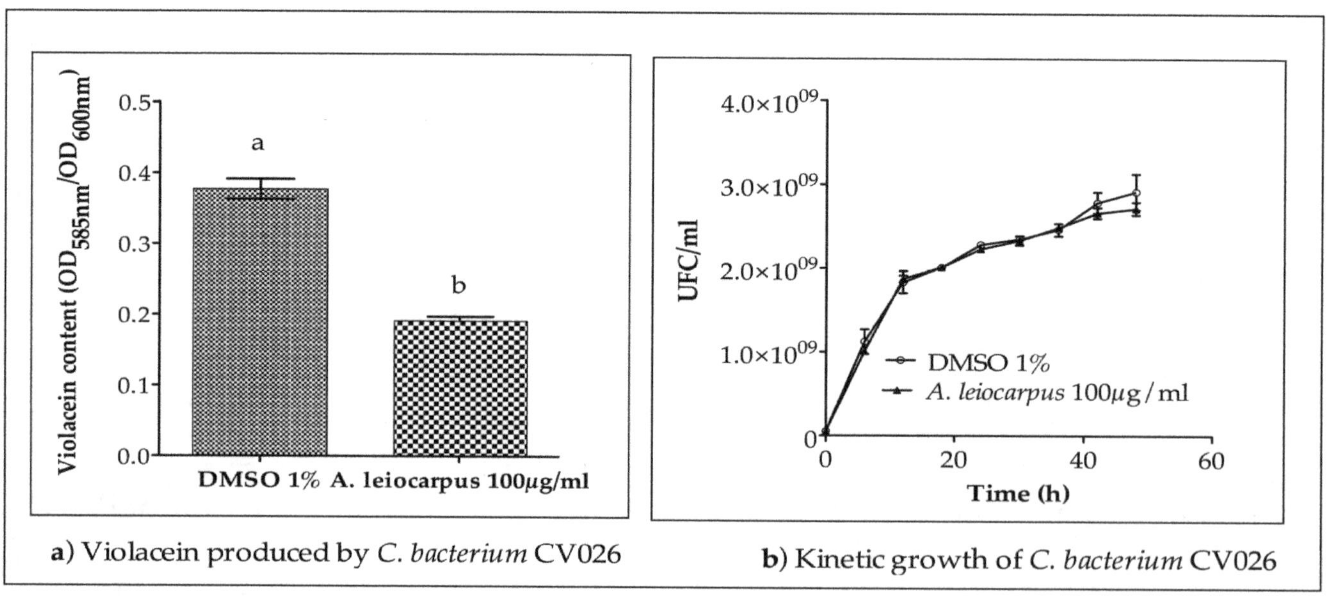

Figure 2. Anti-quorum sensing (QS) activity of methanol extract from *A. leiocarpus*. (**a**) *A. leiocarpus* extract (100 μg/mL) significantly reduces ($p > 0.05$) violacein production by *C. violaceum* CV026 within 48 h (**b**) *A. leiocarpus* extract (100 μg/mL) did not exhibit a significant effect of on *C. violaceum* CV026 kinetic growth within 48 h. Dimethyl sulfoxide (DMSO) was used as a negative control. *C. violaceum* CV026 was grown (30 °C, 175 rpm agitation) in LB broth supplemented with HHL (10 μM in DMSO). Mean values of triplicate independent experiments and SD are shown. Data with different letters in superscript are significantly different ($p > 0.05$).

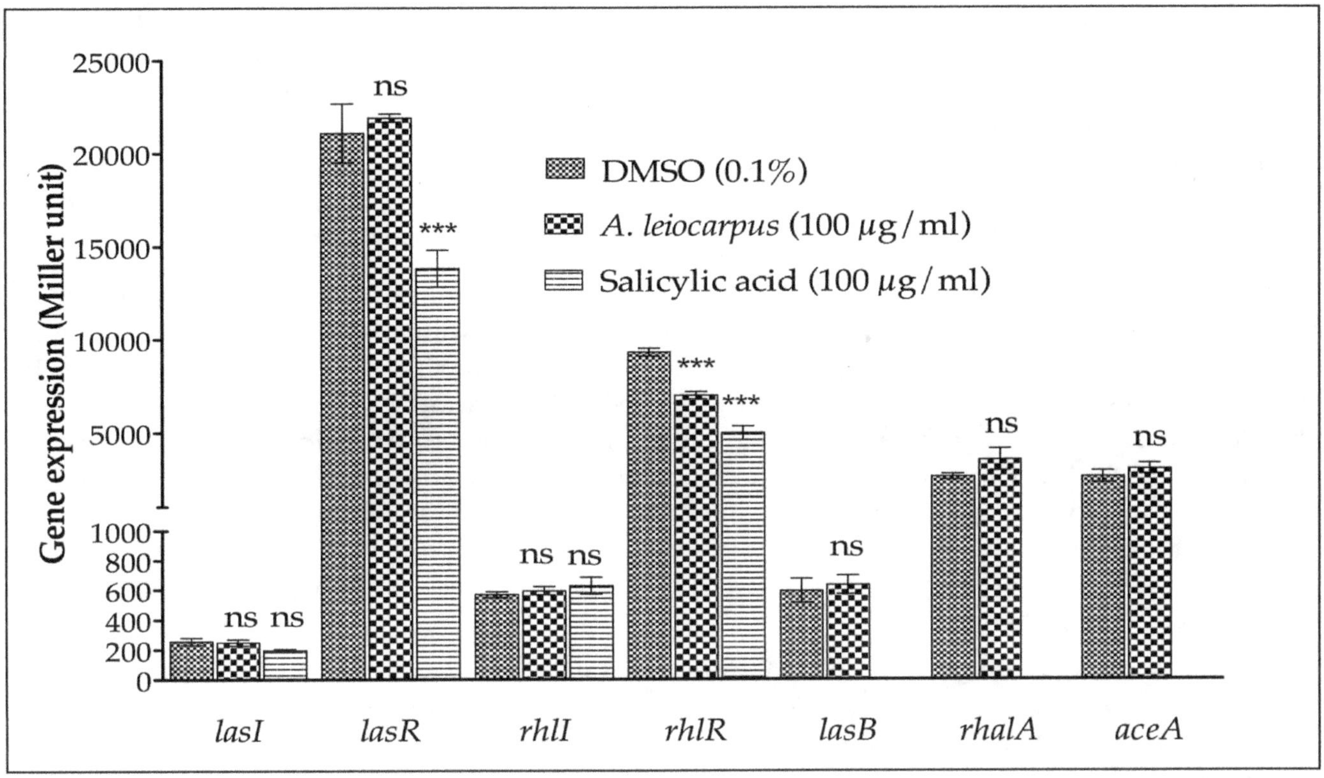

Figure 3. Effect of *A. leiocarpus* extract on the transcription level of *lasRI* and *rhlRI* QS genes. Data are expressed as mean ± SD of 3 independent essays. Dimethyl sulfoxide (DMSO) was used as negative control. Salicylic acid was used as positive control. *** Significantly different compared with DMSO treatment ($p < 0.05$). ns: not significantly different compared to DMSO treatment. Gene expression was measured as the β-galactosidase activity of the *lacZ* gene fusions and expressed in Miller units. Expression of the *aceA* gene is used as a quorum-sensing independent control. *P. aeruginosa* PAO1 strains were grown.

4. Discussion

Our in vitro investigations show that methanol extract from *A. leiocarpus* stem bark exhibits promising antioxidant capacity along with anti-QS activity with a subsequent reduction of pyocyanin production. Since *phz*, the biosynthesis genes of pyocyanin, is under the control of *las* and *rhl* QS systems [29,30], the observed decrease in pyocyanin production is related to the downstreaming of the QS regulator gene *rhlR*.

P. aeruginosa PAO1 QS systems *las* and *rhl* seems to be important for a successful infection in burn wounds, as the virulence of PAO1 mutants defective in either *lasI*, *lasR*, or *rhlI* is reduced [31]. Consistent with this, the inability of QS-deficient strains to induce a successful infection was proposed to be linked with a decreased production of virulence factors such as pyocyanin among other virulence factors, and the most significant virulence reduction was detected with the mutant defective in both *lasI* and *rhlI* [31]. Hence, the anti-QS demonstrated might explain the traditional usage of *A. leiocarpus* stem bark to treat infected burn wounds.

Within the Combretaceae family, to which belongs *A. leiocarpus*, anti-QS medicinal plants have been previously reported. *Bucida buceras*, *Combretum albiflorum*, and *Conocarpus erectus* quench the QS mechanism of *P. aeruginosa* PAO1 with a subsequent inhibition of the bacteria virulence factors [27,32]. Polyphenols and flavonoids are also known for their anti-QS potentiality. The flavonoids catechin, isolated from *Combretum albiflorum* and naringenin have been reported to inhibit QS-regulated virulence factors expression in *P. aeruginosa* and thought to possibly interfere with the perception of the native AHL by LasR and RhlR [27,33]. Epigallocatechin gallate, tannic acid, and ellagic acid also demonstrated their anti-QS potential against *Pseudomonas putida* [34]. Vescalagin and castalagin, two ellagitannins isolated from *Conocarpus erectus*, decrease AHL production, QS gene expression and elastases production [35]. The anti-QS activity and related reduction of pyocyanin production observed within our study might be due to castalagin, since it has been previously isolated from the stem bark of *A. leiocarpus* [36]. Furthermore, 3,3′,4′-tri-*O*-methylflavellagic acid, 3,3′-di-*O*-methylellagic acid, and 3,4,3′-tri-*O*-methylflavellagic acid-4′-β-D-glucoside, three ellagic acid derivatives isolated from *A. leiocarpus* stem bark [37], might contribute to the anti-QS bioactivity we demonstrated.

Among several virulence factors produced by *P. aeruginosa*, pyocyanin is known to be involved in cell host degradation and the production of ROS [38,39]. Pyocyanin alters the redox cycle involved in cellular respiration and increases the oxidative stress on host cells [1]. The mechanism by which pyocyanin causes cell cycle arrest is related to its redox (oxidation–reduction) properties, and its ability to reduce molecular oxygen into reactive oxygen species induces low-level, yet persistent, oxidative stress [40,41]. Thus, pyocyanin is able to delay cicatrization and might also lead to chronic inflammation in wound and burn injuries infected by *P. aeruginosa*. Polyphenols and flavonoids responsible for the antioxidant activity of *A. leiocarpus* could therefore contribute to the reduction of the oxidative stress caused by pyocyanin and thus reduce inflammatory intensity independently of pyocyanin reduction, a benefit for wound healing.

Taken together, anti-QS and antioxidant activities of *A. leiocarpus* could contribute to an explanation of its wound-healing benefit. The antioxidant activities could represent a preventive action to minimize ROS due to inflammation but also counterbalance the high level production of ROS when burn injuries are infected by opportunistic pathogens. Additionally, the anti-QS activity also preserves a minimal ROS level as it reduces virulence factor production such as pyocyanin, and more importantly reduce the abilities of pathogens to degrade host tissue and to resist host immune responses that can maintain inflammation and delay the healing process.

5. Conclusions

Our study demonstrated the antioxidant and anti-QS activities of the methanol extract from *A. leiocarpus* stem bark. Based on bibliographic reports, catalagin and ellagic acid derivatives might be responsible for the anti-QS property demonstrated. These results contribute to the establishment of the traditional use of *A. leiocarpus* stem bark in the management of infected burn wounds on a rational basis. By reducing the production of pyocyanin and related oxidative stress within infected tissues in a QS manner, *A. leiocarpus* stem bark benefits to the healing process of septic injuries.

In future investigations, we will focus on the interference of the anti-QS molecules from *A. leiocarpus* either with the mechanisms of perception or production of homoserine lactones (lasI/lasR, rhlI/rhlR QS systems) or with the quinolone signal (the third QS system) within *P. aeruginosa*.

Acknowledgments: The authors are grateful to Prof Mondher EL JAZIRI from the Laboratoire de Biotechnologie Vegetale, Univerté Libre de Bruxelles, Belgium, for providing the bacterial strains used in this study. This research was funded by The World Academy of Science (TWAS) under the research grant 12-044/RG/BIO/AF/AC-G-UNESCO FR: 3240271326.

Author Contributions: M.K. conceived and designed the experiments; V.O. performed the experiments; M.K. and V.O. analyzed the data and wrote the paper; M.K. provided reagents and material through a research grant awarded to him.

References

1. Liu, G.Y.; Nizet, V. Color me bad: Microbial pigments as virulence factors. *Trends Microbiol.* **2009**, *17*, 406–413. [CrossRef] [PubMed]

2. Rumbaugh, K.P.; Griswold, J.A.; Hamood, A.N. The role of quorum sensing in the in vivo virulence of *Pseudomonas aeruginosa*. *Microbes Infect.* **2000**, *2*, 1721–1731. [CrossRef]
3. Richard, P.; le Floch, R.; Chamoux, C.; Pannier, M.; Espaze, E.; Richet, H. *Pseudomonas aeruginosa* outbreak in a burn unit: Role of antimicrobials in the emergence of multiply resistant strains. *J. Infect. Dis.* **1994**, *170*, 377–383. [CrossRef] [PubMed]
4. Greenberg, E.P. Acyl-homosérine lactone quorum sensing in bacteria. *J. Microbiol.* **2000**, *38*, 117–121.
5. Jimenez, P.N.; Koch, G.; Thompson, J.A.; Xavier, K.B.; Cool, R.H.; Quax, W.J. The multiple signaling systems regulating virulence in *Pseudomonas aeruginosa*. *Microbiol. Mol. Biol. Rev.* **2012**, *76*, 46–65. [CrossRef] [PubMed]
6. Parsek, M.R.; Greenberg, E.P. Sociomicrobiology: The connections between quorum sensing and biofilms. *Trends Microbiol.* **2005**, *13*, 27–33. [CrossRef] [PubMed]
7. Pesci, E.C.; Pearson, J.P.; Seed, P.C.; Iglewski, B.H. Regulation of *las* and *rhl* quorum sensing in *Pseudomonas aeruginosa*. *J. Bacteriol.* **1997**, *179*, 3127–3132. [PubMed]
8. Venturi, V. Regulation of quorum sensing in *Pseudomonas*. *FEMS Microbiol. Rev.* **2006**, *30*, 274–291. [CrossRef] [PubMed]
9. Diggle, S.P.; Winzer, K.; Chhabra, S.R.; Worrall, K.E.; Cámara, M.; Williams, P. The *Pseudomonas aeruginosa* quinolone signal molecule overcomes the cell density-dependency of the quorum sensing hierarchy, regulates *rhl*-dependent genes at the onset of stationary phase and can be produced in the absence of LasR. *Mol. Microbiol.* **2003**, *50*, 29–43. [CrossRef] [PubMed]
10. McKnight, S.L.; Iglewski, B.H.; Pesci, E.C. The *Pseudomonas* quinolone signal regulates *rhl* quorum sensing in *Pseudomonas aeruginosa*. *J. Bacteriol.* **2000**, *182*, 2702–2708. [CrossRef] [PubMed]
11. Pesci, E.C.; Milbank, J.B.; Pearson, J.P.; McKnight, S.; Kende, A.S.; Greenberg, E.P.; Iglewski, B.H. Quinolone signaling in the cell-to-cell communication system of *Pseudomonas aeruginosa*. *Proc. Natl. Acad. Sci. USA* **1999**, *96*, 11229–11234. [CrossRef] [PubMed]
12. Wade, D.S.; Calfee, M.W.; Rocha, E.R.; Ling, E.A.; Engstrom, E.; Coleman, J.P.; Pesci, E.C. Regulation of *Pseudomonas* quinolone signal synthesis in *Pseudomonas aeruginosa*. *J. Bacteriol.* **2005**, *187*, 4372–4380. [CrossRef] [PubMed]
13. Gibran, N.S.; Heimbach, D.M. Current status of burn wound pathophysiology. *Clin. Plast. Surg.* **2000**, *27*, 11–22. [PubMed]
14. Farina, J.A., Jr.; Rosique, M.J.; Rosique, R.G. Curbing inflammation in burn patients. *Int. J. Inflamm.* **2013**. [CrossRef] [PubMed]
15. Ward, P.A.; Lentsch, A.B. The acute inflammatory response and its regulation. *Arch. Surg.* **1999**, *134*, 666–669. [CrossRef] [PubMed]
16. Rahman, I.; MacNee, W. Regulation of redox glutathione levels and gene transcription in lung inflammation: Therapeutic approaches. *Free Radic. Biol. Med.* **2000**, *28*, 1405–1420. [CrossRef]
17. Wang, J.; Blanchard, T.G.; Ernst, P.B. *Host Inflammatory Response to Infection in Helicobacter pylori: Physiology and Genetics*; Mobley, H.L.T., Mendz, G.L., Hazell, S.L., Eds.; ASM Press: Washington, DC, USA, 2001.
18. Epps, L.C.; Walker, P.D. Fluoroquinolone consumption and emerging resistance. *US Pharm.* **2006**, *10*, 47–54.
19. English, B.K.; Gaur, A.H. The use and abuse of antibiotics and the development of antibiotic resistance. *Adv. Exp. Med. Biol.* **2010**, *659*, 73–82. [PubMed]
20. Bjarnsholt, T.; Givskov, M. The role of quorum sensing in the pathogenicity of the cunning aggressor *Pseudomonas aeruginosa*. *Anal. Bioanal. Chem.* **2007**, *387*, 409–414. [CrossRef] [PubMed]
21. Hentzer, M.; Givskov, M. Pharmacological inhibition of quorum sensing for the treatment of chronic bacterial infections. *J. Clin. Investig.* **2003**, *112*, 1300–1307. [CrossRef] [PubMed]
22. Nacoulma, O.G. *Plantes Médicinales et Pratiques Médicinales Traditionnelles au Burkina*; Université de Ouagadougou: Ouagadougou, Burkina Faso, 1996. (In French)
23. Agyare, C.; Asase, A.; Lechtenberg, M.; Niehues, M.; Deters, A.; Hensel, A. An ethnopharmacological survey and in vitro confirmation of ethnopharmacological use of medicinal plants used for wound healing in Bosomtwi-Atwima-Kwanwoma area, Ghana. *J. Ethnopharmacol.* **2009**, *125*, 393–403. [CrossRef] [PubMed]
24. Lamien-Meda, A.; Lamien, C.E.; Compaoré, M.M.Y.; Meda, N.T.R.; Kiendrebeogo, M.; Zeba, B.; Millogo, J.F.; Nacoulma, O.G. Polyphenol content and antioxidant activity of fourteen wild edible fruits from Burkina Faso. *Molecules* **2008**, *13*, 581–594. [CrossRef] [PubMed]

25. Eloff, J.N. A sensitive and quick microplate method to determine the minimal inhibitory concentration of plant extracts for bacteria. *Planta Med.* **1998**, *64*, 711–713. [CrossRef] [PubMed]
26. Escalona-Arranz, J.C.; Péres-Roses, R.; Urdaneta-Laffita, I.; Camacho-Pozo, M.I.; Rodríguez-Amado, J.; Licea-Jiménez, I. Antimicrobial activity of extracts from *Tamarindus indica* L. leaves. *Pharmacogn. Mag.* **2010**, *6*, 242–247. [CrossRef] [PubMed]
27. Vandeputte, O.M.; Kiendrebeogo, M.; Rajaonson, S.; Diallo, B.; Mol, A.; El Jaziri, M.; Baucher, M. Identification of catechin as one of the flavonoids from *Combretum albiflorum* bark extract that reduces the production of quorum-sensing-controlled virulence factors in *Pseudomonas aeruginosa* PAO1. *Appl. Environ. Microbiol.* **2010**, *76*, 243–253. [CrossRef] [PubMed]
28. Zhang, X.; Bremer, H. Control of the *Escherichia coli* rrnB P1 promoter strength by ppGpp. *J. Biol. Chem.* **1995**, *270*, 11181–11189. [CrossRef] [PubMed]
29. Pearson, J.P.; Pesci, E.C.; Iglewski, B.H. Roles of *Pseudomonas aeruginosa las* and *rhl* quorum-sensing systems in control of elastase and rhamnolipid biosynthesis genes. *J. Bacteriol.* **1997**, *179*, 5756–5767. [PubMed]
30. Brint, J.; Ohman, D.E. Synthesis of multiple exoproducts in *Pseudomonas aeruginosa* is under the control of RhlR-RhlI, another set of regulators in strain PAO1 with homology to the autoinducer-responsive LuxR-LuxI family. *J. Bacteriol.* **1995**, *177*, 7155–7163. [PubMed]
31. Rumbaugh, K.P.; Griswold, J.A.; Iglewski, B.H.; Hamood, A.N. Contribution of quorum sensing to the virulence of *Pseudomonas aeruginosa* in burn wound infections. *Infect. Immun.* **1999**, *67*, 5854–5862. [PubMed]
32. Adonizio, A.; Kong, K.; Mathee, K. Inhibition of quorum sensing-controlled virulence factor production in *Pseudomonas aeruginosa* by south Florida plant extracts. *Antimicrob. Agents Chemother.* **2008**, *52*, 198–203. [CrossRef] [PubMed]
33. Vandeputte, O.M.; Kiendrebeogo, M.; Rasamiravaka, T.; Stévigny, C.; Duez, P.; Rajaonson, S.; Diallo, B.; Mol, A.; Baucher, M.; El Jaziri, M. The flavanone naringenin reduces the production of quorum sensing-controlled virulence factors in *Pseudomonas aeruginosa* PAO1. *Microbiology* **2011**, *157*, 2120–2132. [CrossRef] [PubMed]
34. Huber, B.; Eberl, L.; Feucht, W.; Polster, J. Influence of polyphenols on bacterial biofilm formation and quorum-sensing. *Z. Naturforsch. C* **2003**, *58*, 879–884. [CrossRef] [PubMed]
35. Adonizio, A.L. *Anti-Quorum Sensing Agents from South Florida Medicinal Plants and Their Attenuation of Pseudomonas aeruginosa Pathogenicity*; Florida International University: Miami, FL, USA, 2008.
36. Shuaibu, M.N.; Pandey, K.; Wuyep, P.A.; Yanagi, T.; Hirayama, K.; Ichinose, A.; Tanaka, T.; Kouno, I. Castalagin from *Anogeissus leiocarpus* mediates the killing of *Leishmania* in vitro. *Parasitol. Res.* **2008**, *103*, 1333–1338. [CrossRef] [PubMed]
37. Chaabi, M.; Benayache, S.; Benayache, F.; N'Gom, S.; Koné, M.; Anton, R.; Weniger, B.; Lobstein, A. Triterpenes and polyphenols from *Anogeissus leiocarpus* (Combretaceae). *Biochem. Syst. Ecol.* **2007**, *36*, 59–62. [CrossRef]
38. Gloyne, L.S.; Grant, G.D.; Perkins, A.V.; Powell, K.L.; McDermott, C.M.; Johnson, P.V.; Anderson, G.J.; Kiefel, M.; Anoopkumar-Dukie, S. Pyocyanin-induced toxicity in A549 respiratory cells is causally linked to oxidative stress. *Toxicol. In Vitro* **2011**, *25*, 1353–1358. [CrossRef] [PubMed]
39. Tamura, Y.; Suzuki, S.; Kijima, M.; Takahashi, T.; Nakamura, M. Effect of proteolytic enzyme on experimental infection of mice with *Pseudomonas aeruginosa*. *J. Vet. Med. Sci.* **1992**, *54*, 597–599. [CrossRef] [PubMed]
40. Muller, M. Premature cellular senescence induced by pyocyanin, a redox-active *Pseudomonas aeruginosa* toxin. *Free Radic. Biol. Med.* **2006**, *41*, 1670–1677. [CrossRef] [PubMed]
41. Muller, M.; Li, Z.; Maitz, P.K. *Pseudomonas* pyocyanin inhibits wound repair by inducing premature cellular senescence: Role for p38 mitogen-activated protein kinase. *Burns* **2009**, *35*, 500–508. [CrossRef] [PubMed]

10

Terpenoids from Octocorals of the Genus *Pachyclavularia*

Yu-Chia Chang [1,2,3,4], Jyh-Horng Sheu [4,*], Yang-Chang Wu [5,6,7,*] and Ping-Jyun Sung [1,4,5,8,9,*]

1 National Museum of Marine Biology and Aquarium, Pingtung 944, Taiwan; jay0404@gmail.com
2 Greenhouse Systems Technology Center, Central Region Campus, Industrial Technology Research Institute, Nantou 540, Taiwan
3 Forcean Marine International Corporation, Kaohsiung 800, Taiwan
4 Department of Marine Biotechnology and Resources, National Sun Yat-sen University, Kaohsiung 804, Taiwan
5 Graduate Institute of Natural Products, Kaohsiung Medical University, Kaohsiung 807, Taiwan
6 Research Center for Natural Products and Drug Development, Kaohsiung Medical University, Kaohsiung 807, Taiwan
7 Department of Medical Research, Kaohsiung Medical University Hospital, Kaohsiung 807, Taiwan
8 Graduate Institute of Marine Biology, National Dong Hwa University, Pingtung 944, Taiwan
9 Chinese Medicine Research and Development Center, China Medical University Hospital, Taichung 404, Taiwan
* Correspondence: sheu@mail.nsysu.edu.tw (J.-H.S.); yachwu@kmu.edu.tw (Y.-C.W.); pjsung@nmmba.gov.tw (P.-J.S.)

Abstract: In this paper, we reviewed natural compounds isolated from octocorals belonging to the genus *Pachyclavularia*, including 20 cembrane-, 39 briarane-, and eight briarellin-related diterpenoids, and one secosterol. The chemical constituents of these 68 secondary metabolites, and their names, structures, and bioactivities, along with studies of their biological activities, are summarized in this review. Based on the literature, many of these compounds possess bioactivities, including anti-inflammation properties, cytotoxicity, and ichthyotoxicity, suggesting that they may have the potential to be developed into biomedical agents for treatment.

Keywords: *Pachyclavularia*; octocoral; cembrane; briarane; briarellin; secosterol; bioactivity

1. Introduction

Octocorals of the genus *Pachyclavularia* (phylum Cnidaria, class Anthozoa, order Alcyonacea, family Briareidae) [1], which originally belonged to the family Tubiporidae [2], distributed in the subtropical and tropical waters of the Indo-Pacific Ocean, have been investigated. Since the initial study in 1979 discovered a cembranoid diterpene, pachyclavulariadiol (**1**), from the Australian octocoral *P. violacea* [3], subsequent studies over the past few decades have yielded a series of interesting secondary metabolites, particularly diterpenoids originally synthesized from cyclized cembranoids, including briarane- and briarellin-related analogues (Scheme 1) [4]. In this article, we have listed the different types of compounds isolated from two Indo-Pacific octocorals, *Pachyclavularia violacea* (Scheme 1) and *Pachyclavularia* sp., and summarized their chemical constituents and research into the biological activities of these metabolites.

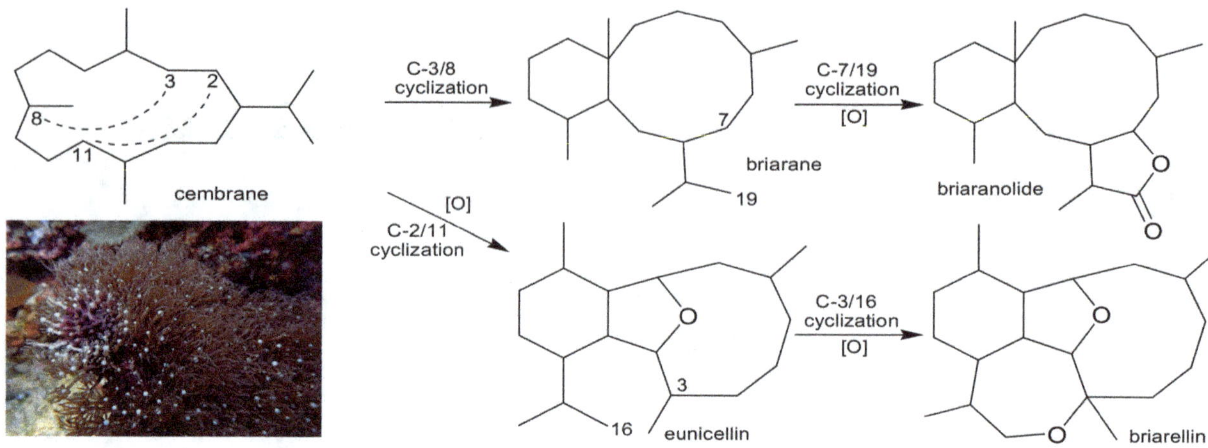

Scheme 1. Octocoral *P. violacea* and the proposed biosynthetic pathways of the cembrane, briarane, and briarellin carbon skeletons [4].

2. Cembranoids from *Pachyclavularia violacea* (Quoy and Gaimard, 1833) (=*Clavularia violacea, Briareum violaceum*)

The *Pachyclavularia* genus includes one very common species, *Pachyclavularia violacea* [2,3]. Bowden and colleagues [3] isolated several compounds, including three new cembrane-type diterpenes, pachyclavulariadiol (**1**), and its naturally-derived mono- and di-acetylated derivatives (**2** and **3**), from octocoral *P. violacea* collected in Australia (Figure 1). The study also established the structures, including the relative configurations, of new furanocembranoids **1–3** and determined the configuration of **1** by spectroscopic/chemical methods and X-ray diffraction, respectively.

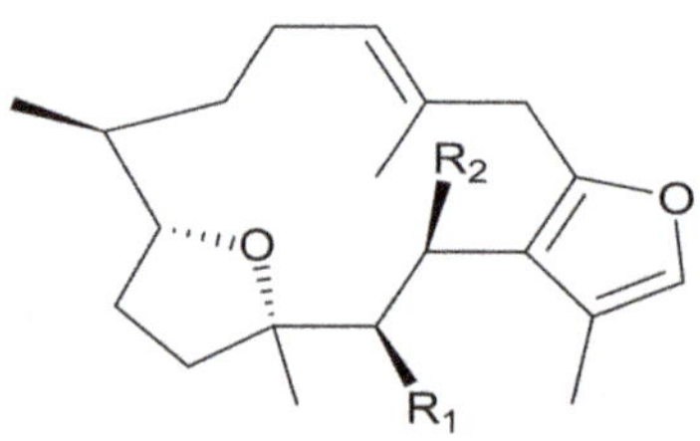

1: $R_1 = R_2 = OH$
2: $R_1 = OH$, $R_2 = OAc$
3: $R_1 = R_2 = OAc$

Figure 1. Structures of pachyclavulariadiol (**1**) and its natural mono- and di-acetylated derivatives **2** and **3**.

In 1989, Inman and Crews [5] reported the isolation of a new cembranolide from *P. violacea* collected from Vanuatu waters, and named the compound pachyclavularolide (**4**) (Figure 2). Later, the structure of **4**, including the relative configuration, was determined using spectroscopic methods and molecular mechanics calculations, and further confirmed by single-crystal X-ray analyses in a study by Sheu et al. [6]. The former study was the first to present a detailed conformational analysis of a 14-membered cembrane ring [5].

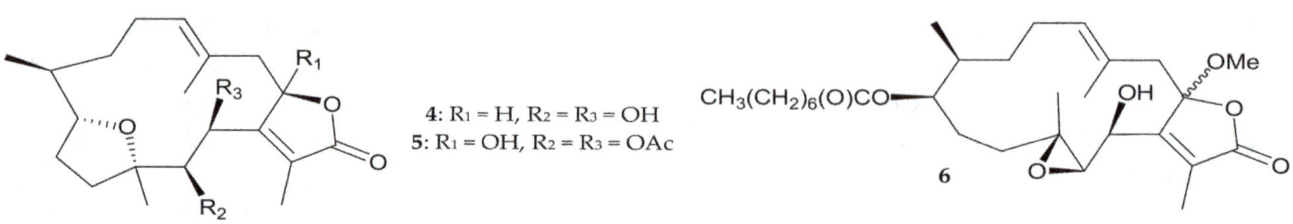

4: $R_1 = H$, $R_2 = R_3 = OH$
5: $R_1 = OH$, $R_2 = R_3 = OAc$

Figure 2. Structures of pachyclavularolide (**4**) and pachyclavulariolides E (**5**) and F (**6**).

Two new cembranes, pachyclavulariolides E (**5**) and F (**6**) (Figure 2), were isolated from *P. violacea* samples collected from waters off Madang in Papua New Guinea in 2000 [7]. The structures of **5** and **6**, including the relative configurations, which were elucidated from spectroscopic data [7], and the structure, including the relative configuration of **5**, was further confirmed from single-crystal X-ray analysis by Sheu et al. [6]. A cytotoxic assay showed that compound **6** had an IC_{50} value of 1.0 μg/mL in the treatment of murine leukemia P388 cells [7], though this compound was claimed to be an artifact due to methanol used in the extraction procedure [7].

Twelve new cembranolides, pachyclavulariolides G–R (**7–18**) (Figure 3), and two known analogues, pachyclavulariolide (**4**) and pachyclavulariolide E (**5**) [5,7] (Figure 2), were obtained from *P. violacea* specimens collected from Kenting Coast, Taiwan [6,8]. The structures, including the relative configurations, of cembranolides **7–18** were established by spectroscopic/chemical methods [6,8], and the structures of **4**, **5**, **7**, and **8** were also verified by single-crystal analyses [6]. However, the hydroxy group at C-2 in briarane **11** was still unconfirmed at that stage [6], and information regarding the reasonable biosynthetic pathway suggested that briarane **12** could be the precursor of briarane **16** [8]. Cytotoxic assays revealed that pachyclavulariolide K (**11**) had ED_{50} values of 2.8, 3.3, 6.7, and 7.6 μg/mL against P388 (mouse lymphoma), HT-29 (human colorectal adenocarcinoma), A549 (human epithelial carcinoma), and KB cells (human nasopharynx carcinoma), respectvively, while pachyclavulariolides E (**5**), I (**9**), J (**10**), and M (**13**) had ED_{50} values against P388 cells of 4.0, 1.3, 2.5, and 3.2 μg/mL, respectively [6,8].

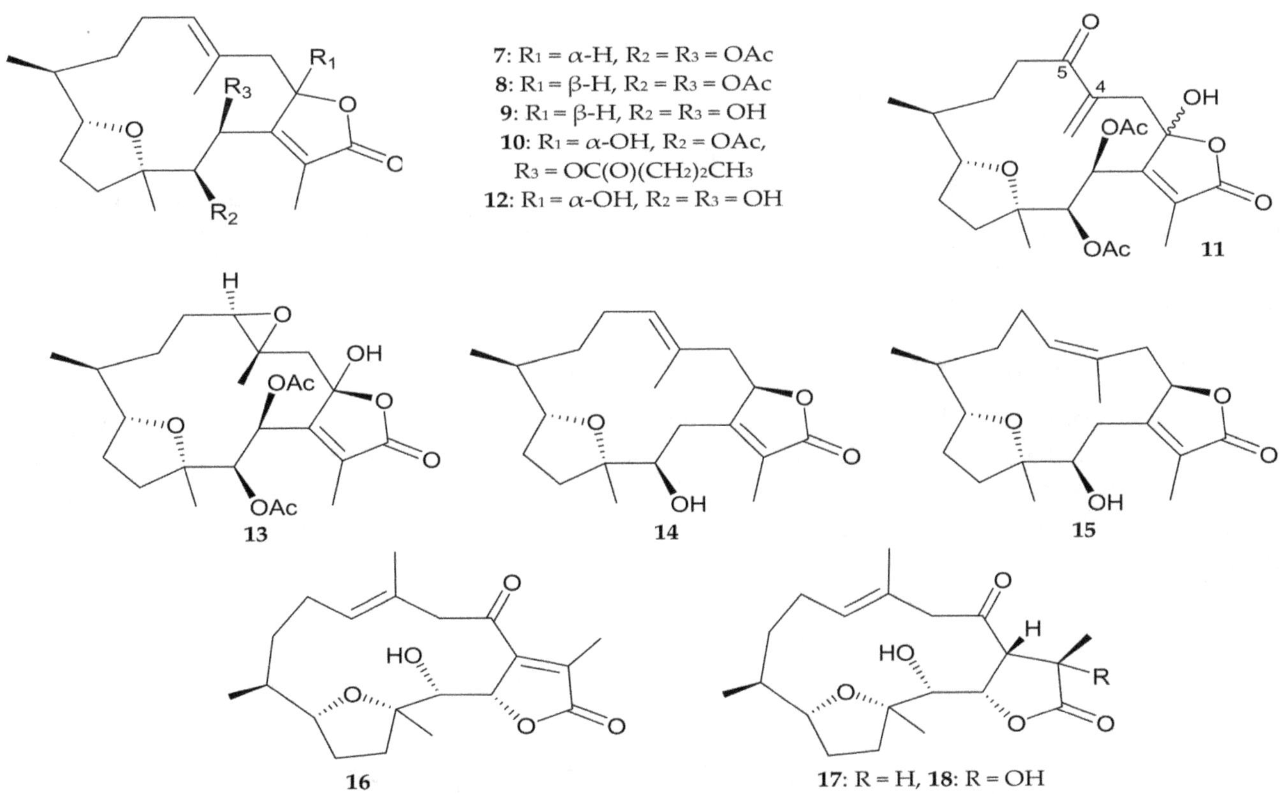

Figure 3. Structures of pachyclavulariolides G–R (**7–18**).

A new cytotoxic cembranoid, claviolide (**19**) (Figure 4), was isolated from the dichloromethane extract of *Clavularia violacea*, collected at a depth of 5–6 m off Green Island, Taiwan. The structure, including the relative configuration, of **19** was established using a spectroscopic approach, and this compound was found to exhibit significant cytotoxicity towards P388 and HT-29 tumor cells, with ED_{50} values of 0.84 and 0.38 μg/mL, respectively [9].

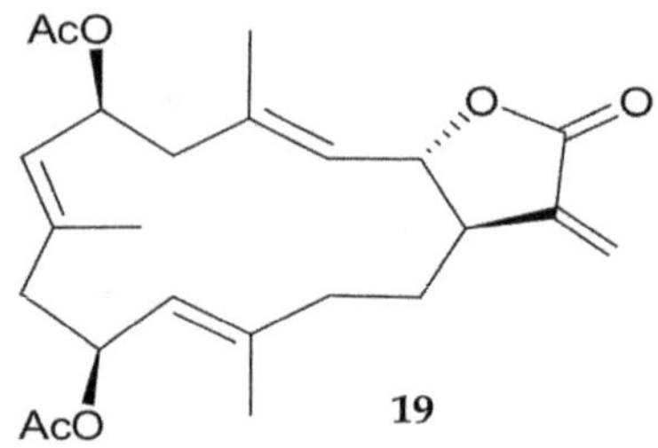

19

Figure 4. Structure of claviolide (**19**).

Chang and coworkers isolated a new cembranoid, briaviodiol A (**20**) (Figure 5), from the organic extract of *Briareum violaceum* [2] collected off Pingtung Coast, Southern Taiwan, and confirmed its structure, including the relative configuration, by single-crystal X-ray diffraction analysis [10].

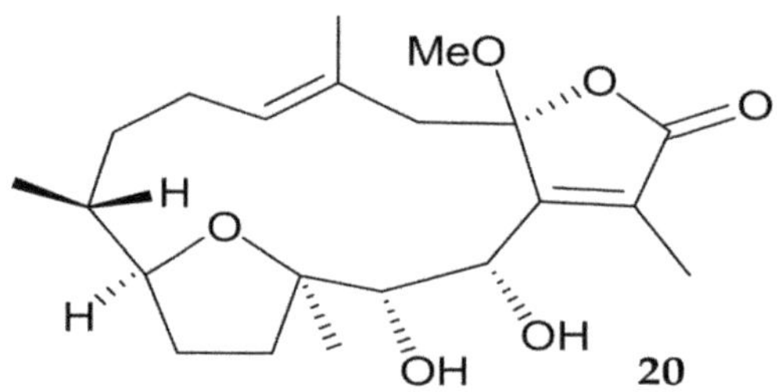

20

Figure 5. Structure of briaviodiol A (**20**).

Interestingly, with the exception of cembranoids **6** (pachyclavulariolide F) and **19** (claviolide), cembranoids (18/20) from *P. violacea* have been found to possess a tetrahydrofuran moiety, and these furanocembranoids are likely to be chemical markers of cembranoids obtained from *P. violacea*. Among the furanocembranoids, the α,β-unsaturated ketone moiety in pachyclavulariolide K (**11**) seems to enhance cytotoxicity toward various tumor cells.

3. Briaranes from *Pachyclavularia* sp. and *Pachyclavularia violacea*

Uchio and colleagues [11] identified three new unnamed briaranes, **21–23** (Figure 6), from specimens of the octocoral *Pachyclavularia* sp. collected off the Great Barrier Reef, Australia. The authors established the structures of **21–23**, including the relative configurations, using a spectroscopic approach, and also found that briarane **21** exhibited ichthyotoxicity towards the mosquito fish *Gambusia affinis*.

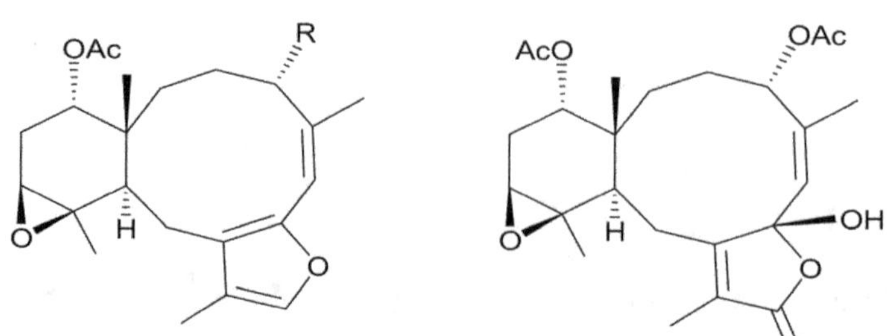

21: R = OAc, **22**: R = H **23**

Figure 6. Structures of briaranes **21–23**.

Five briarane diterpenoids, including three new metabolites 2β-acetoxy-2-(debutyryloxy)-stecholide E (**24**), 9-deacetylstylatulide lactone (**25**), and 4β-acetoxy-9-deacetylstylatulide lactone (**26**), along with two known metabolites, brianthein W (**27**) [12] and 9-deacetylbriareolide H (**28**) [13,14]

(Figure 7), were isolated from a Taiwanese soft coral *Briareum* sp., which was originally identified as *Pachyclavularia violacea* collected off the coast of Kenting, Taiwan [15]. The structures of new briaranes **24–26**, including the relative configurations, were established by chemical/spectroscopic methods. Cytotoxic assays were performed on briaranes **24–28** to assess their toxicity against P388, HT-29, KB, and A549 tumor cells, and the results showed that all briaranes except **26** exhibited cytotoxicity against P388 cells, with ED_{50} values of 0.61, 1.12, 0.76 and 0.28 μg/mL, respectively [15], indicating that the acetoxy group at C-4 in **26** redeuce the cytotoxicity. Briaranes **25** and **28** showed cytotoxicity towards HT-29 and KB cells, with ED_{50} values of 1.79 and 0.27 μg/mL, respectively [15]. The cytotoxicities of 9-hydroxybriaranes **24**, **25**, and **28** were not significantly different to their corresponding 9-acetyl derivatives, 2β-acetoxy-2-(debutyryloxy)-stecholide E acetate, stylatulide lactone [16], and briareolide H [13], respectively [15].

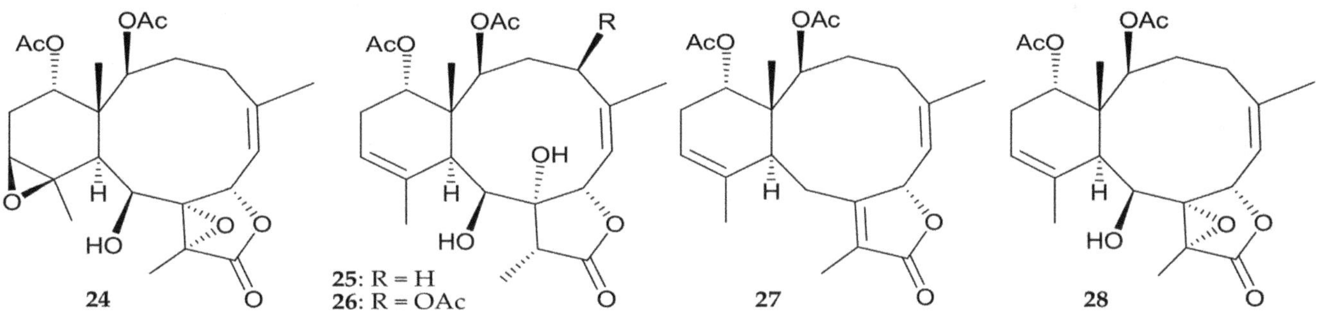

Figure 7. Structures of 2β-acetoxy-2-(debutyryloxy)stecholide E (**24**), 9-deacetylstylatulide lactone (**25**), 4β-acetoxy-9-deacetylstylatulide lactone (**26**), brianthein W (**27**), and 9-deacetylbriareolide H (**28**).

In 2000, Xu et al. [7] isolated four new briarane derivatives, pachyclavulariolides A–D (**29–32**) (Figure 8), from *P. violacea* specimens collected from reefs off Madang, Papua New Guinea. The authors used a spectroscopic approach to determine the structures, including the relative configurations, of **29–32**, and further employed single-crystal X-ray diffraction analysis to identify the structure, including the relative configuration, of briarane **30** (pachyclavulariolide B). They also found that briaranes **29–32** were the first briaranes of this type to possess an 11,14-ether bridge that resulted in an oxanorbornane structure.

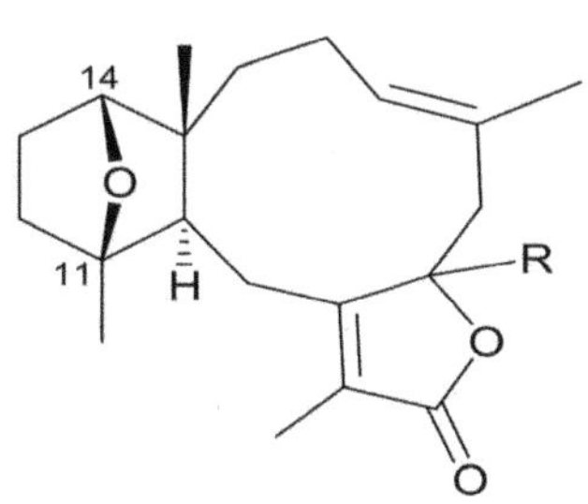

29: R = α-H
30: R = α-OH
31: R = α-OMe
32: R = β-OMe

Figure 8. Structures of pachyclavulariolides A–D (**29–32**).

Research by a group in Japan identified nine new briaranes, pachyclavulides A–I (**33–41**) (Figure 9), from *P. violacea* collected off Okinawa, and determined their structures, including the relative configurations, using spectroscopic methods [17,18]. The absolute configuration of pachyclavulide A (**33**) was determined by single-crystal X-ray diffraction analysis of its *p*-bromobenzoyl ester [17]. Pachyclavulides B (**34**) and E (**37**) were found to show cytotoxicity against human central neural system (CNS) SNB-75 and A549 (human alveolar epithelial carcinoma) tumor cells, with GI_{50} values of 5.2 and 5.1 μM, respectively [18] and pachyclavulide C (**35**) was not cytotoxic toward SNB-75 cells. It seems that the hydroxy group at C-16 in briarane **34** will enhance the cytotoxity. Enantioselective preparation of the six-membered ring of pachyclavulide B (**34**) was also achieved [19].

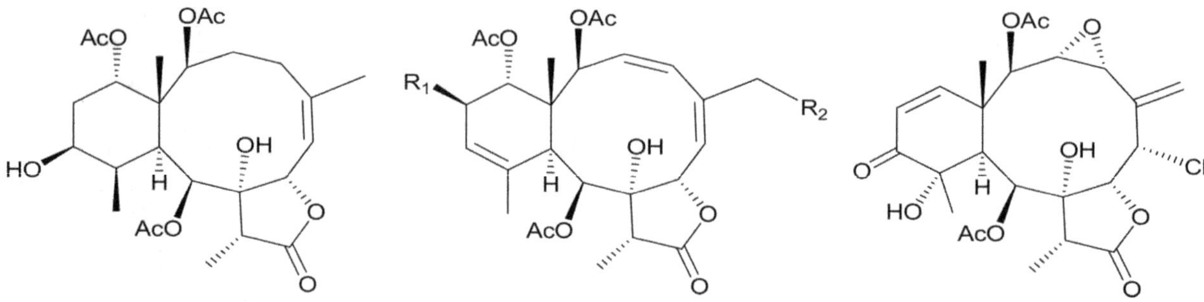

33 **34**: R_1 = H, R_2 = OH, **35**: R_1 = H, R_2 = OAc, **41**: R_1 = OH, R_2 = OMe **36**

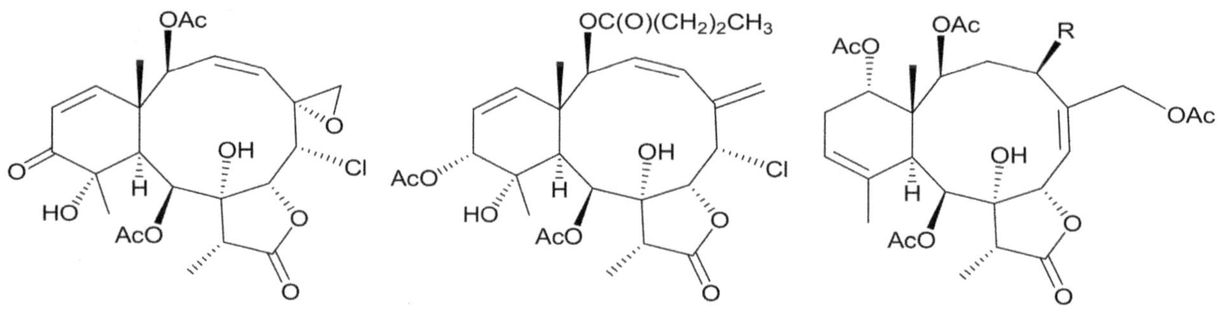

37 **38** **39**: R = OH, **40**: R = H

Figure 9. Structures of pachyclavulides A–I (**33**–**41**).

In addition, another group of researchers isolated four new briaranes, brianodins A–D (**42**–**45**), from soft coral identified as *Pachyclavularia* sp. from Okinawa, Japan [20]. They established the structures, including the relative configurations, of briaranes **42**–**45** by interpretation of spectroscopic data, and determined the absolute configurations of brianodins C (**44**) and D (**45**) by the modified Mosher's method (Figure 10). The 1,2-diol moiety at C-8 and C-17 in **43**–**45** is rarely found in briarane analogues [21–26].

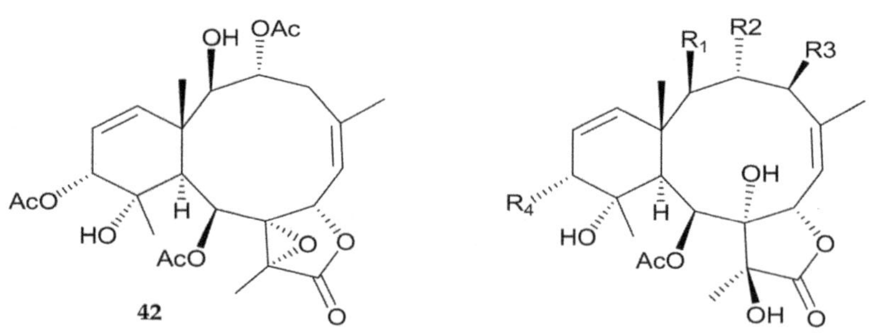

42

43: R_1 = R_3 = R_4 = OAc, R_2 = OH
44: R_1 = R_3 = OAc, R_2 = R_4 = OH
45: R_1 = R_4 = OH, R_2 = OAc, R_3 = H

Figure 10. Structures of brianodins A–D (**42**–**45**).

Sixteen briarane analogues, including ten new metabolites briaviolides A–J (**46**–**55**), along with six known briaranes, solenolides A (**56**) and D (**57**) [27], excavatolide A (**58**) [28], briaexcavatolide I (**59**) [29] (Figure 11), 4β-acetoxy-9-deacetylstulatulide lactone (**26**) and 9-deacetylstylatulide lactone (**25**) [15] (Figure 7), were isolated from *Briareum violaceum* [2] collected in the waters of Taiwan [30]. Using spectroscopic/chemical methods, the structures, including the relative configurations, of new briaranes **46**–**55** were determined, and the absolute configuration of briaviolide A (**46**) was further confirmed by X-ray crystallographic analysis [30]. In anti-inflammatory activity assays, briaviolides E (**50**) and I (**54**) were found to possess inhibitory effects against the production of superoxide anions by human neutrophils in vitro (inhibition rates = 34.17% and 28.66%, respectively), and inhibited the release of elastase (inhibition rates = 26.03% and 28.81%, respectively) at a concentration of 10 μg/mL; while the monobenzoyl derivative of 46 was found to possess selective activity to inhibit elastase release (inhibition rate = 28.60%) at a concentration of 10 μg/mL [30]. By comparison of the structure-activity relationships between briaranes **53** (briaviolide H) and **54** (briaviolide I), indicating that the hydroperoxy group at C-12 in **54** enhance the activity to inhibit the elastase release and the generation of superoxide anions.

A study performed by Cheng et al. revised the structure of solenolide D (**57**) [31], and this compound was later found to be a potent anti-inflammatory agent with an efficacy comparable to that of indomethacin [27]. Potency in excess of a 70% reduction of edema was observed at a concentration of approximately 15 μg/per ear (mouse ear assay) [27].

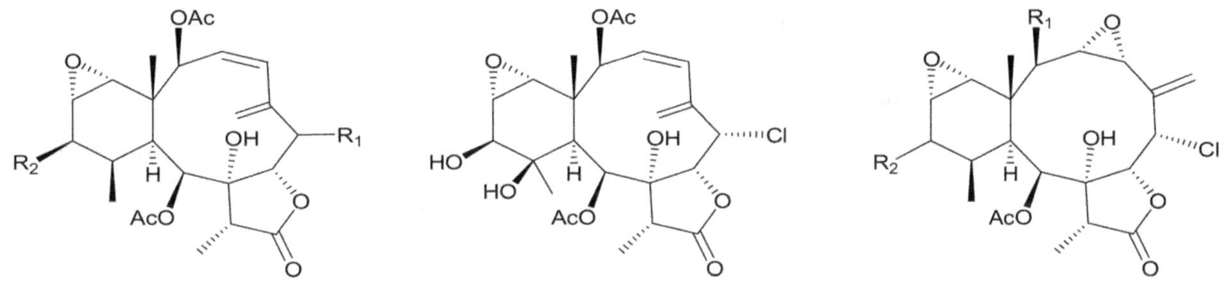

46: R_1 = α-Cl, R_2 = OH
47: R_1 = α-Cl, R_2 = $OC(O)CH_2CH_3$
48: R_1 = β-OAc, R_2 = OAc
59: R_1 = α-Cl, R_2 = OAc

49

50: R_1 = OAc, R_2 = β-$OC(O)CH_2CH(CH_3)_2$
51: R_1 = OH, R_2 = α-$OC(O)(CH_2)_4CH_3$
52: R_1 = OAc, R_2 = α-OAc
57: R_1 = OAc, R_2 = β-OAc

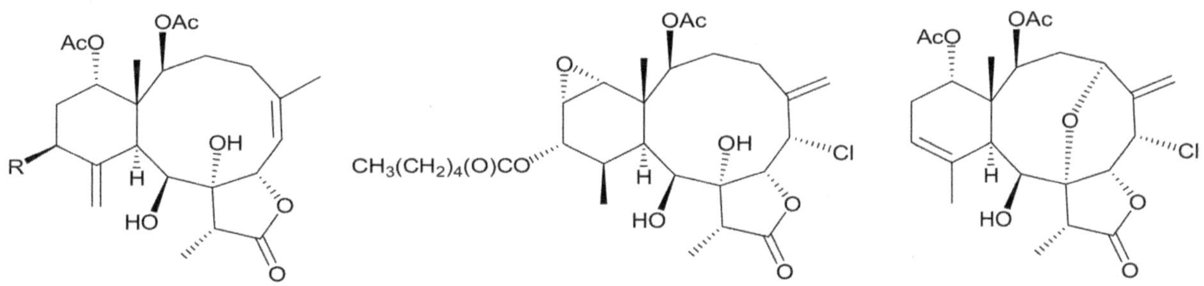

53: R = OH, **54**: R = OOH, **55**: R = OAc

56

58

Figure 11. Structures of briaviolides A–J (**46–55**), solenolides A (**56**) and D (**57**), excavatolide A (**58**), and briaexcavatolide I (**59**).

4. Briarellins from *Pachyclavularia violacea*

Eight novel briarellins, including pachyclavulariaenones A–G (**60–66**) [32,33] and secopachyclavulariaenone A (**67**) [6] (Figure 12), were isolated from *P. violacea* collected off Kenting Coast, Taiwan. Pachyclavulariaenone B (**61**) was also isolated from *P. violacea* specimens collected in the Togian Islands near Sulawesi Island, Indonesia [34]. The structures, including the relative configurations, of briarellins **60–67** were established by spectroscopic methods, and the structures, including the relative configurations, of briarellins **62** (pachyclavulariaenone C) [32] and **65** (pachyclavulariaenone F) [33] were further confirmed by single-crystal X-ray diffraction analyses. Briarellins **60–67** were found to be unprecedented examples of this type of compound, as they possess a six-membered carbocyclic ring *cis*-fused to both the ten-membered carbocyclic ring and seven-membered ether ring, making three ring-junction protons *cis* to each other [6,32,33]. Cytotoxic assays revealed that pachyclavulariaenone G (**66**) exhibited cytotoxicity towards P388 and HT-29 tumor cells, with ED_{50} values of 0.2 and 3.2 μg/mL, respectively [33]. It is obvious to note that the hydroxy groups at C-4 and C-6 in 66 caused this compound to be more cytotoxic than its analogues **62, 64**, and **65**.

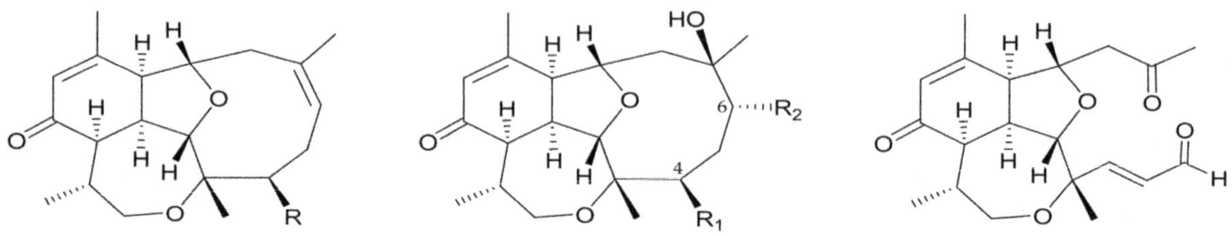

60: R = $OC(O)(CH_2)_2CH_3$
61: R = OAc
63: R = OH

62: R_1 = OAc, R_2 = OH
64: R_1 = R_2 = OAc
65: R_1 = OH, R_2 = OAc
66: R_1 = R_2 = OH

67

Figure 12. Structures of pachyclavulariaenones A–G (**60–66**) and secopachyclavulariaenone A (**67**).

5. Secosterol from *Pachyclavularia violacea*

A new 9,11-secosterol, (24*S**)-3β,11-dihydroxy-5β,6β-epoxy-24-methyl-9,11-secocholestan-9-one (**68**) (Figure 13), was isolated from *P. violacea* specimens collected off the Togian Islands, Indonesia, and its structure, including the relative configurations, was elucidated on the basis of spectroscopic data [34].

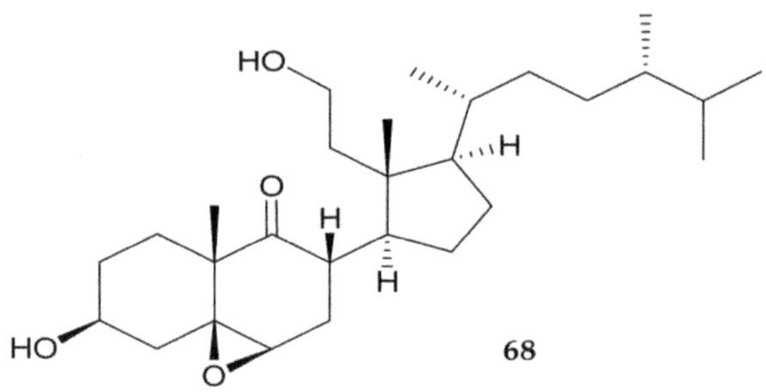

68

Figure 13. Structure of secosterol **68**.

6. Conclusions

Ever since pachyclavulariadiol (**1**) was obtained from a specimen of the octocoral *P. violacea* collected in Australia [4], 68 interesting secondary metabolites, including 20 cembranes (29.41%), 39 briaranes (57.35%), eight briarellins (11.76%), and one secosterol (1.47%), have been isolated from octocorals belonging to the genus *Pachyclavularia*. Many studies have reported that compounds obtained from *Pachyclavularia* spp. possess various biologic activities, such as cytotoxicity (seven cembranes, six briaranes, and one briarellin), anti-inflammatory activity (three briaranes), and ichthyotoxicity (one briarane). It is interesting to note that all compounds from *Pachyclavularia* spp. reported as having been isolated between 1979 and 2014 were collected from octocorals distributed in the Indo-Pacific Ocean. The briarane-type natural products act as a chemical marker of octocorals belonging to the family Briareidae. Up to date, 379 briaranes [35–40], 13 eunicellins, 34 asbestinane, one cembrane, and one pyranone [4], have been isolated from the octocorals belonging to the family Briareidae, including the genera *Briareum* and *Erythropodium*. As more than 50% of the compounds obtained from the *Pachyclavularia* genus are briarane-type diterpenoids, we support that the taxonomic position of the *Pachyclavularia* genus should be readjusted and placed under the family Briareidae. Based on above findings, these results suggest that continuing investigation of new terpenoid analogues with the potential bioactivities from this marine organism are worthwhile for further development. The octocoral *Pachyclavularia violacea* had been transplanted to culturing tanks located in the National Museum of Marine Biology and Aquarium, Taiwan, for extraction of additional natural products to establish a stable supply of bioactive material.

Acknowledgments: This research was supported by grants from the National Museum of Marine Biology and Aquarium; the National Dong Hwa University; the National Sun Yat-sen University; and the Ministry of Science and Technology (grant nos. MOST 106-2320-B-291-001-MY3 and 104-2320-B-291-001-MY3), Taiwan, awarded to Ping-Jyun Sung.

Author Contributions: Yu-Chia Chang contributed in terms of writing the manuscript. Jyh-Horng Sheu, Yang-Chang Wu, and Ping-Jyun Sung conceived and designed the format of the manuscript. All the authors contributed in terms of critical reading and discussion of the manuscript.

References

1. Samimi-Namin, K.; van Ofwegen, L.P. Overview of the genus *Briareum* (Cnidaria, Octocorallia, Briareidae) in the Indo-Pacific, with the description of a new species. *ZooKeys* **2016**, *557*, 1–44. [CrossRef] [PubMed]
2. Bayer, F.M. Key to the genera of octocorallia exclusive of Pennatulacea (Coelenterata: Anthozoa), with diagnoses of new taxa. *Proc. Biol. Soc. Wash.* **1981**, *94*, 902–947.
3. Bowden, B.F.; Coll, J.C.; Mitchell, S.J.; Raston, C.L.; Stokie, G.J.; White, A.H. Studies of Australian soft corals. XV. The structure of pachyclavulariadiol, a novel furano-diterpene from *Pachyclavularia violacea*. *Aust. J. Chem.* **1979**, *32*, 2265–2274. [CrossRef]
4. Sung, P.-J.; Chen, M.-C. The heterocyclic natural products of gorgonian corals of genus *Briareum* exclusive of briarane-type diterpenoids. *Heterocycles* **2002**, *57*, 1705–1715. [CrossRef]
5. Inman, W.; Crews, P. The structure and conformational properties of a cembranolide diterpene from *Clavularia violacea*. *J. Org. Chem.* **1989**, *54*, 2526–2529. [CrossRef]
6. Sheu, J.-H.; Wang, G.-H.; Sung, P.-J.; Duh, C.-Y.; Chiang, M.Y. Pachyclavulariolides G–L and secopachyclavulariaenone A, seven novel diterpenoids from the soft coral *Pachyclavularia violacea*. *Tetrahedron* **2001**, *57*, 7639–7648. [CrossRef]
7. Xu, L.; Patrick, B.O.; Roberge, M.; Allen, T.; van Ofwegen, L.; Andersen, R.J. New diterpenoids from the octocoral *Pachyclavularia violacea* collected in Papua New Guinea. *Tetrahedron* **2000**, *56*, 9031–9037. [CrossRef]
8. Sheu, J.-H.; Wang, G.-H.; Duh, C.-Y.; Soong, K. Pachyclavulariolides M–R, six novel diterpenoids from a Taiwanese soft coral *Pachyclavularia violacea*. *J. Nat. Prod.* **2003**, *66*, 662–666. [CrossRef] [PubMed]
9. Duh, C.-Y.; El-Gamal, A.A.H.; Chu, C.-J.; Wang, S.-K.; Dai, C.-F. New cytotoxic constituents from the Formosan soft corals *Clavularia viridis* and *Clavularia violacea*. *J. Nat. Prod.* **2002**, *65*, 1535–1539. [CrossRef] [PubMed]
10. Chang, Y.-C.; Huang, I.-C.; Chiang, M.Y.-N.; Hwang, T.-L.; Kung, T.-H.; Lin, C.-S.; Sheu, J.-H.; Sung, P.-J. Briaviodiol A, a new cembranoid from a soft coral *Briareum violacea*. *Chem. Pharm. Bull.* **2010**, *58*, 1666–1668. [CrossRef] [PubMed]
11. Uchio, Y.; Fukazawa, Y.; Bowden, B.F.; Coll, J.C. New diterpenes from an Australian *Pachyclavularia* species (Coelenterata, Anthozoa, Octocorallia). *Tennen Yuki Kagobutsu Toronkai Koen Yoshishu* **1989**, *31*, 548–553.
12. Cardellina, J.H., II; James, T.R., Jr.; Chen, M.H.M.; Clardy, J. Structure of brianthein W, from the soft coral *Briareum polyanthes*. *J. Org. Chem.* **1984**, *49*, 3398–3399. [CrossRef]
13. Pordesimo, E.O.; Schmitz, F.J.; Ciereszko, L.S.; Hossain, M.B.; van der Helm, D. New briarein diterpenes from the Caribbean gorgonians *Erythropodium caribaeorum* and *Briareum* sp. *J. Org. Chem.* **1991**, *56*, 2344–2357. [CrossRef]
14. Bowden, B.F.; Coll, J.C.; König, G.M. Studies of Australian soft corals. XLVIII. New briaran diterpenoids from the gorgonian coral *Junceella gemmacea*. *Aust. J. Chem.* **1990**, *43*, 151–159. [CrossRef]
15. Sheu, J.-H.; Sung, P.-J.; Huang, L.-H.; Lee, S.-F.; Wu, T.; Chang, B.-Y.; Duh, C.-Y.; Fang, L.-S.; Soong, K.; Lee, T.-J. New cytotoxic briaran diterpenes from the Formosan gorgonian *Briareum* sp. *J. Nat. Prod.* **1996**, *59*, 935–938. [CrossRef] [PubMed]
16. Wratten, S.J.; Faulkner, D.J. Some diterpenes from the sea pen *Stylatula* sp. *Tetrahedron* **1979**, *35*, 1907–1912. [CrossRef]
17. Iwasaki, J.; Ito, H.; Aoyagi, M.; Sato, Y.; Iguchi, K. Briarane-type diterpenoids from the Okinawan soft coral *Pachyclavularia violacea*. *J. Nat. Prod.* **2006**, *69*, 2–6. [CrossRef] [PubMed]
18. Ito, H.; Iwasaki, J.; Sato, Y.; Aoyagi, M.; Iguchi, K.; Yamori, T. Marine diterpenoids with a briarane skeleton from the Okinawan soft coral *Pachyclavularia violacea*. *Chem. Pharm. Bull.* **2007**, *55*, 1671–1676. [CrossRef] [PubMed]

19. Iwasaki, J.; Ito, H.; Nakamura, M.; Iguchi, K. A synthetic study of briarane-type marine diterpenoid, pachyclavulide B. *Tetrahedron Lett.* **2006**, *47*, 1483–1486. [CrossRef]
20. Ishiyama, H.; Okubo, T.; Yasuda, T.; Takahashi, Y.; Iguchi, K.; Kobayashi, J. Brianodins A–D, briarane-type diterpenoids from soft coral *Pachyclavularia* sp. *J. Nat. Prod.* **2008**, *71*, 633–636. [CrossRef] [PubMed]
21. Iwagawa, T.; Takayama, K.; Okamura, H.; Nakatani, M.; Doe, M.; Takemura, K.; Shiro, M. Cytotoxic briarane diterpenes from a gorgonacean *Briareum* sp. *Heterocycles* **1999**, *51*, 2619–2625. [CrossRef]
22. Iwagawa, T.; Hirose, T.; Takayama, K.; Okamura, H.; Nakatani, M.; Doe, M.; Takemura, K. Violides N–P, new briarane diterpenes from a gorgonacean *Briareum* sp. *Heterocycles* **2000**, *53*, 1789–1792. [CrossRef]
23. Sung, P.-J.; Su, J.-H.; Duh, C.-Y.; Chiang, M.Y.; Sheu, J.-H. Briaexcavatolides K–N, new briarane diterpenes from the gorgonian *Briareum excavatum*. *J. Nat. Prod.* **2001**, *64*, 318–323. [CrossRef] [PubMed]
24. Sung, P.-J.; Hu, W.-P.; Wu, S.-L.; Su, J.-H.; Fang, L.-S.; Wang, J.-J.; Sheu, J.-H. Briaexcavatolides X–Z, three new briarane-related derivatives from the gorgonian coral *Briareum excavatum*. *Tetrahedron* **2004**, *60*, 8975–8979. [CrossRef]
25. Iwagawa, T.; Babazono, K.; Nakatani, M.; Doe, M.; Morimoto, Y.; Takemura, K. Briarane diterpenes from a gorgonian *Briareum* sp. *Heterocycles* **2005**, *65*, 607–617. [CrossRef]
26. Sung, P.-J.; Su, Y.-D.; Li, G.-Y.; Chiang, M.Y.; Lin, M.-R.; Huang, I.-C.; Li, J.-J.; Fang, L.-S.; Wang, W.-H. Excavatoids A–D, new polyoxygenated briaranes from the octocoral *Briareum excavatum*. *Tetrahedron* **2009**, *65*, 6918–6924. [CrossRef]
27. Groweiss, A.; Look, S.A.; Fenical, W. Solenolides, new antiinflammatory and antiviral diterpenoids from a marine octocoral of the genus *Solenopodium*. *J. Org. Chem.* **1988**, *53*, 2401–2406. [CrossRef]
28. Sheu, J.-H.; Sung, P.-J.; Cheng, M.-C.; Liu, H.-Y.; Fang, L.-S.; Duh, C.-Y.; Chiang, M.Y. Novel cytotoxic diterpenes, excavatolides A–E, isolated from the Formosan gorgonian *Briareum excavatum*. *J. Nat. Prod.* **1998**, *61*, 602–608. [CrossRef] [PubMed]
29. Sheu, J.-H.; Sung, P.-J.; Su, J.-H.; Liu, H.-Y.; Duh, C.-Y.; Chiang, M.Y. Briaexcavatolides A–J, new diterpenes from the gorgonian *Briareum excavatum*. *Tetrahedron* **1999**, *55*, 14555–14564. [CrossRef]
30. Liaw, C.-C.; Cheng, Y.-B.; Lin, Y.-S.; Kuo, Y.-H.; Hwang, T.-L.; Shen, Y.-C. New briarane diterpenoids from Taiwanese soft coral *Briareum violacea*. *Mar. Drugs* **2014**, *12*, 4677–4692. [CrossRef] [PubMed]
31. Cheng, J.-F.; Yamamura, S.; Terada, Y. Stereochemistry of the brianolide acetate (=solenolide D) by the molecular mechanics calculations. *Tetrahedron Lett.* **1992**, *33*, 101–104. [CrossRef]
32. Wang, G.-H.; Sheu, J.-H.; Chiang, M.Y.; Lee, T.-J. Pachyclavulariaenones A–C, three novel diterpenoids from the soft coral *Pachyclavularia violacea*. *Tetrahedron Lett.* **2001**, *42*, 2333–2336. [CrossRef]
33. Wang, G.-H.; Sheu, J.-H.; Duh, C.-Y.; Chiang, M.Y. Pachyclavulariaenones D–G, new diterpenoids from the soft coral *Pachyclavularia violacea*. *J. Nat. Prod.* **2002**, *65*, 1475–1478. [CrossRef] [PubMed]
34. Anta, C.; González, N.; Rodríguez, J.; Jiménez, C. A new secosterol from the Indonesian octocoral *Pachyclavularia violacea*. *J. Nat. Prod.* **2002**, *65*, 1357–1359. [CrossRef] [PubMed]
35. Sung, P.-J.; Sheu, J.-H.; Xu, J.-P. Survey of briarane-type diterpenoids of marine origin. *Heterocycles* **2002**, *57*, 535–579. [CrossRef]
36. Sung, P.-J.; Chang, P.-J.; Fang, L.-S.; Sheu, J.-H.; Chen, W.-C.; Chen, Y.-P.; Lin, M.-R. Survey of briarane-type diterpenoids-Part II. *Heterocycles* **2005**, *65*, 195–204. [CrossRef]
37. Sung, P.-J.; Sheu, J.-H.; Wang, W.-H.; Fang, L.-S.; Chung, H.-M.; Pai, C.-H.; Su, Y.-D.; Tsai, W.-T.; Chen, B.-Y.; Lin, M.-R.; et al. Survey of briarane-type diterpenoids-Part III. *Heterocycles* **2008**, *75*, 2627–2648. [CrossRef]
38. Sung, P.-J.; Su, J.-H.; Wang, W.-H.; Sheu, J.-H.; Fang, L.-S.; Wu, Y.-C.; Chen, Y.-H.; Chung, H.-M.; Su, Y.-D.; Chang, Y.-C. Survey of briarane-type diterpenoids-Part IV. *Heterocycles* **2011**, *83*, 1241–1258. [CrossRef]
39. Sheu, J.-H.; Chen, Y.-H.; Chen, Y.-H.; Su, Y.-D.; Chang, Y.-C.; Su, J.-H.; Weng, C.-F.; Lee, C.-H.; Fang, L.-S.; Wang, W.-H.; et al. Briarane diterpenoids isolated from gorgonian corals between 2011 and 2013. *Mar. Drugs* **2014**, *12*, 2164–2181. [CrossRef] [PubMed]
40. Su, Y.-D.; Su, J.-H.; Hwang, T.-L.; Wen, Z.-H.; Sheu, J.-H.; Wu, Y.-C.; Sung, P.-J. Briarane diterpenoids isolated from octocorals between 2014 and 2016. *Mar. Drugs* **2017**, *15*, 44. [CrossRef] [PubMed]

11

Chemical Composition, Cytotoxic, Apoptotic and Antioxidant Activities of Main Commercial Essential Oils in Palestine

Mohammad A. Al-Tamimi [1,*], Bob Rastall [2] and Ibrahim M. Abu-Reidah [1,3]

1 Deptartment of Nutrition and Food Technology, An-Najah National University, PO Box 7, Nablus 415, Palestine
2 Department of Food and Nutritional Sciences, The University of Reading, Whiteknights, Reading RG6 6AP, UK; r.a.rastall@reading.ac.uk
3 Deptartment of Chemistry, An-Najah National University, PO Box 7, Nablus 415, Palestine; iabureidah@gmail.com or iabureidah@najah.edu
* Correspondence: m.altamimi@najah.edu

Academic Editor: James D. Adams

Abstract: Background: Essential oils (EOs) are complex mixtures of several components gifted with a wide array of biological activities. The present research was designed to evaluate whether commercial essential oils could be effective by examining their in vitro antioxidant, cytotoxic, and apoptotic properties of nine commercially available EOs in Palestine, namely, African rue, basil, chamomile, fennel, fenugreek, ginger, spearmint, sage, and thyme, and to assure their effective use. **Methods:** The cytotoxic activity was determined using HT29-19(A) non-muco secreting and HT29-muco secreting (MS) cell lines. MTT, and trypan blue tests, and DPPH radical scavenging have also been assayed on the studied EOs. **Results:** In this work chamomile oil showed the lowest IC_{50} at the content of 60 µL/mL, while all other EOs reached such a decrease when 70–80 µL/mL was used on HT-29 (MS) cell lines. In HT-29 19(A) cells, 50% of viability was obtained when 80 µL/mL of ginger and African rue was used, while all other EOs needed more than 80 µL/mL to reach such a decline in viability. Otherwise, an MTT assay on HT-29 (MS) displayed ginger EO with the lowest IC_{50}, followed by African rue and sage, with 40, 48 and 53 µL/mL, respectively. Otherwise, for the rest of the EOs, the IC_{50} was obtained by assaying around 80 µL/mL. Ginger showed the lowest IC_{50} with 60 µL/mL and thyme was the highest with 77 µL/mL when HT-29 19(A) cells were used. **Conclusion:** The most active EOs were found to be ginger, chamomile oil, and African rue. In general, the results demonstrate that most commercial EOs tested in this work possess low, or no biological activities; this may be due to processing, storage conditions, and handling or other reasons, which may cause losses in the biological and pharmacological properties that endemically exist in the Eos; hence, more investigation is still required on commercial EOs before they are recommended to the public.

Keywords: essential oils (EOs); cytotoxicity; apoptosis; antioxidants; cell lines; anti-cancer activity

---

1. Introduction

Aromatic plants (APs) have been used since antiquity as a potential source of drug discovery and development of disease chemoprevention, in folk medicine, and as preservatives in foods [1]. The best known aromatic plants: viz, chamomile, fennel, ginger, thyme, basil, and sage, originate from the Mediterranean area. The Middle East in general and Palestine in particular, are areas with many endemic plants whose compounds could be used in medicine [2,3]. Many APs are used for different industrial purposes such as food, drugs, and perfumery manufacturing.

APs contain many biologically active compounds, mainly phenolics and EOs, which have been found to possess antioxidant, antiparasitic, antimicrobial, anti-carcinogenic, and anti-inflammatory properties, among others [4]. Essential oils (EOs) are also used for the management of chronic diseases like cardiovascular, diabetes, Alzheimer's, cancer, and others [5].

EOs are natural, concentrated, volatile aromatic compounds isolated from plants which have long been used in medicine, pharmaceutical, perfumery, cosmetic, and in many food applications. Initially, EOs have been utilized in medicine, but in the last decades their use as fragrance and essence ingredients has improved to become the major employment. Up to now, about 3000 EOs are well-known, of which, around 10% is engaged commercially in the flavor and aroma markets [6].

It is well-known that EOs are found in lots of APs, which possess a wide array of biological and pharmacological activities, which are associated with traditional and complementary medicine [4].

EOs are highly complex mixtures involving several tens to hundreds of different types of individual volatile compounds such as terpenoid, oxygenated terpenes, sesquiterpenes, and hydrocarbons, which are responsible for their characteristic aroma. EOs are hydrophobic liquids with a particular odor and taste aroma which are often poorly soluble in water. EOs have been widely used for their virucidal, bactericidal, fungicidal, anticancer, antioxidant, antidiabetic activities [7,8]. They are usually prepared by fragrance extraction techniques such as distillation (hydro or steam distillation), cold pressing, extraction (maceration), or by using of supercritical carbon dioxide extraction [9,10]. The biological activity of EOs is strictly linked to their chemical composition.

Table 1 presents a list of common EOs commercially available in Palestine and their sources.

Commercial EOs are of great interest for consumers with people being prescribed them as traditional remedies. Doses of 5 to 20 mL of EOs can be prescribed to people to relieve pains, headaches, joint arthritis and problems in the digestive system (personal observation).

Indeed, there is a relationship between the production of reactive oxygen species (ROS) to the origin of oxidation and inflammation that can lead to cancer [11]. Oxidative stress is a major contributor to the pathogenesis of a number of chronic diseases, that is why antioxidant behavior is one of the most commonly determined biological activities in extracts of plants such as EOs [12]. It has been reported that more than half of most cancer cases and their consequent deaths worldwide are potentially preventable [13]. Therefore, modification in dietary habits by increasing consumption of functional foods rich in antioxidants such as EOs is greatly supported [14].

The anticancer activity of EOs has been described in more than five hundred scientific reports; those first published dated to the 1960s [15].

So far, the effects of EOs have been investigated on glioblastoma, melanoma, leukemia and oral cancers, as well as on bone, breast, cervix, colon, lung, prostate, and uterus cancers [16]. Among the anticancer medications, 70% of drugs approved between 1940 and 2002 are either natural products or developed based on knowledge gained from natural products [17]. Most researchers who experimented on the anti-proliferation properties of natural compounds have examined the apoptosis process of certain cancer cells [18].

In spite of all the information available on several EOs, the investigation dealing with this kind of commercial product has been inadequate. Moreover, to the best of our knowledge, there are no reports available about in vitro cytotoxicity of these studied commercial EOs against HT29-19A non-muco secreting and HT29-muco secreting cell line types. Therefore, the aim of the present work has been to study and compare the antioxidant, cytotoxic, and apoptotic activities of nine commercially available EOs together with their in vitro anticancer activity assayed by methyl thiazol tetrazolium (MTT) and trypan blue tests, in order to evaluate their significance for traditional use.

Table 1. A list of the main popular commercial EOs in Palestine.

Essential Oil	Plant Family	Traditional Use and Activity	Reference
African rue (*Peganum harmala* L.)	Nitrariaceae (Zygophyllaceae)	Coughs, hypertension, diabetes, asthma, jaundice, lumbago, and many other human ailments, skin and subcutaneous tumors, skin diseases, wounds and lice.	[10,19]
Basil (*Ocimum basilicum* L.)	Lamiaceae	Antifungal, physicochemical and insect-repelling activity, antiseptic (postpartum infections) depression, migraine, stomach and intestinal ache.	[11]
Chamomile (*Matricaria chamomilla* L.)	Asteraceae	Abscesses, allergies, arthritis, boils, colic, cuts, cystitis, dermatitis, dysmenorrhea, earache, flatulence, hair, headache, inflamed skin, insect bites, insomnia, nausea, neuralgia, PMS, rheumatism, sores, sprains, strains, stress, wounds.	[12]
Fennel (*Foeniculum vulgare* Mill.)	Apiaceae (Umbelliferae)	Fennel essential oil is used as flavoring agents in food products also used as a constituent in cosmetic and pharmaceutical products. Herbal drugs and essential oil of fennel have antispasmodic, diuretic, anti-inflammatory, analgesic and antioxidant effects are active for dyspeptic complaints, flatulence and bloating. The volatile oil showed antimicrobial and hepatoprotective activity.	[13]
Fenugreek (*Trigonellafoenum-graecum* L.)	Fabaceae	Diabetes, sexual weakness, stomach and intestinal pain. The oil in the seeds is used as a skin softener and emollient. Fenugreek essential oil is rich in terpenenes.	[14,15]
Ginger (*Zingiber officinale* R.)	Zingiberaceae	wide application in flavor and perfumery industries, anti-emetic effect or control of nausea and vomiting, prevention of coronary artery disease, healing and prevention of both arthritic conditions and stomach ulcers.	[16]
Spearmint (*Mentha spicata* L.)	Lamiaceae	Food, cosmetic, confectionary, chewing gum, toothpaste and pharmaceutical industries. strong insecticidal and mutagenic activity.	[17]
Sage (*Salvia fruticosa* Mill.)	Lamiaceae	Antibacterial, cytostatic, antiviral and antioxidant activities. Moreover, they are frequently used in traditional medicine to treat diarrhea, eye diseases, gonorrhea; they possess antiseptic and antispasmodic activities. Also, the essential oils of Salvia species are used as cosmetics and as flavoring agents in perfumery.	[18]
Thyme (*Thymus vulgaris* L.)	Lamiaceae	Natural antimutagen	[20]

2. Materials and Methods

2.1. Essential Oils

The following commercial EOs were purchased from a local market in the city of Tulkarm, Palestine in May 2015, which was the end of the season for most aromatic plants grown locally, without knowing the conditions of production of these EOs. They are: African rue, basil, chamomile, fennel, fenugreek, ginger, mint, sage, and thyme, which are widely used in Palestine. All oils were micro-filtered using 0.2 μM disc (Sartorius Stedim Biotech, Goettingen, Germany) in order to eliminate any impurity present in the EO, then EOs were kept at 4 °C in dark containers till they were used for the experiment.

2.2. Gas Chromatography-Mass Spectrometry (GC-MS)

The analysis of the commercial EOs was performed on a GC-MS HP model 5975B inert MSD (Agilent Technologies, J&W Scientific Products, Palo Alto, CA, USA), equipped with an Agilent Technologies capillary DB-5MS column (30 m length; 0.25 mm i.d.; 0.25 mm film thickness), and coupled to a mass selective detector (MSD5975B, ionization voltage 70 eV; all Agilent, Santa Clara, CA, USA). The carrier gas (He) was used at a 1 mL min^{-1} flow rate. The oven temperature program was as follows: 1 min at 100 °C ramped from 100 to 260 °C at 4 °C min^{-1} and 10 min at 260 °C. The component concentration was obtained by semi-quantification by peak area integration from GC peaks.

2.3. Cell Culture Maintenance and Preparation

Mucus-secreting HT29-MS and non-mucus-secreting HT29-A (19) cells were obtained from the cells and culture collection at the University of Reading, UK. All cells were cultured in Dulbecco's modified Eagle medium (DMEM)-high glucose, contains sodium pyruvate (Life Technologies, Paisley, UK), supplemented with 10% defibrinated fetal bovine serum, 5% GlutaMAX™ (Life Technologies, Paisley, UK) and 1% antibacterial/antimycotic solution (Sigma-Aldrich, Pool, UK). All cells were grown in T-75 cm^2 flask and incubated at 37 °C with 5% CO_2 and 95% relative humidity. Media were changed every other day.

After reaching 70%–80% confluence, cells were split as follows; media were aspirated and cells were washed twice with 5 mL pre-warmed Phosphate buffered saline (Sigma-Aldrich, Pool, UK), then 5 mL trypsin-EDTA (0.5 g/L, Sigma-Aldrich, Pool, UK) was added and cells were re-incubated for a further 10 min. Trypsin was deactivated by adding 5 mL fresh medium and the suspension was centrifuged at 1800 rpm for 5 min. Supernatant was aspirated, then pelleted cells were reconstituted with 1 mL fresh medium. Cell count was conducted using a hemocytometer and microscopy and 105 cells/mL were recultured in a sterile flask. Flasks were monitored daily and checked microscopically for any contamination.

For the experiment, cells were cultured as above for 21 days and 15 days for HT29-(MS) and HT29-19 (A), respectively, so they reach maturation then they were used for viability, cytotoxicity and apoptosis tests.

2.4. Trypan Blue Exclusion Assay

To determine the effect of the EOs on the viability of cells, approximately, 105 mature cells/mL were transferred in a 12-well tissue culture plate and left for 48 h to establish adherence to plate before different concentrations of EOs were mixed with DMEM media and 500 μL/mL of such mixture were pipetted into each well. Some wells with media containing no EOs were used as control. After 24 h the media were aspirated and cells were trypsinized, collected and resuspended in an equivolume of 0.4% Trypan blue (Sigma-Aldrich, Pool, UK). This experiment was done in triplicates and repeated three times. The percentages of viable cells were counted using an inverted microscope and the percent of viability was determined in comparison with the control. Photos for cells under the microscope at different time intervals were taken using a Nikon™ Coolpix, 5400 digital camera (Nikon Inc., Melville, NY, USA).

2.5. MTT Cytotoxicity Assay

The in vitro cytotoxic activity of the EOs on HT29-19 (A) and HT29-(MS) was determined using the MTT (3-[4,5-dimethylthiazol-2-yl]-2,5-diphenyl tetrazolium bromide) assay as follows. Briefly, 200 μL/mL of medium containing cells at a density of 2 × 105 mature cells/mL were seeded in each well of a flat-bottom 96-well plate. Cells were permitted to adhere to the plate for 48 h. Then media were replaced with 180 μL/mL of various concentrations of the EOs (0%–100% of original EOs mixed with DMEM media) and incubated for 24 h. After that, MTT solution (0.5 mg/mL, Sigma-Aldrich) 20 μL/mL was added. Plates were incubated at 37 °C for another 4 h after which cultures were removed from incubator and the resulting formazan crystals were dissolve by adding an amount of MTT solubilizing solution (10% Triton X-100 with 0.1 N HCl in anhydrous isopropanol) equal to the original culture medium volume. All tests and analyses were run in triplicate. Pipetting up and down was required to completely dissolve the MTT formazan crystals. DMSO was used as the positive control and wells were left with no cells for the negative control. The absorbance of each well was determined by a spectrophotometer at dual wavelengths of 570 and 690 nm for the background on a multi-well plate reader with software (Tecan Group Ltd., Mannedorf, Switzerland). The viability percentage was calculated by the following formula: the concentration providing 50% inhibition (IC_{50}) was calculated from a graph plotting inhibition percentage against different EOs concentration.

Each experimental condition was analyzed in triplicate, with three experiments for each EO. Growth inhibition was calculated as follows:

$$\% \text{ Viability} = (OD_{sample} - OD_{blank}/OD_{control} - OD_{blank}) \times 100$$

2.6. DPPH Radical Scavenging Assay

DPPH (2,2-Diphenyl-1-picrylhydrazyl, Sigma-Aldrich, Pool, UK) radical scavenging activity was measured as described by Molyneux [21] with some modifications. Briefly, 0.5 mL of EO (8 mg/mL in methanol) was added to 1 mL of DPPH solution (20 mg/mL in methanol) freshly prepared. After shaking, the mixture was incubated for 15 min in darkness at room temperature and then absorbance was measured at 517 nm against a control (mixture without EO). Quercetin (Sigma-Aldrich, Pool, UK) was used as positive control. The inhibition percentage of free DPPH radicals (I%) was calculated following the formula:

$$\text{Percentage of radical scavenging} = (Abs_{control} - (Abs_{sample}/Abs_{control})) \times 100$$

where $Abs_{control}$ is the absorbance of the control reaction (blank with methanol and DPPH) and Abs_{sample} is the absorbance of the sample reaction (essential oil diluted in methanol and DPPH). The sample concentration (in 1 mL reaction mixture) providing 50% inhibition was estimated by plotting the percentages of inhibition against essential oil concentrations (Table 2). All determinations were performed in triplicate.

Table 2. DPPH Scavenging activity of the tested EOs.

Commercial EOs	African Rue	Basil	Chamomile	Fennel	Fenugreek	Ginger	Mint	Sage	Thyme
Quercetin equivalent (μg/mL)	20	20	20	20	<20	<20	<20	<20	<20

Five hundred µL of EO (8 mg/mL in methanol) was added to 1 mL of DPPH solution (20 mg/mL in methanol) freshly prepared. After shaking, the mixture was incubated for 15 min in darkness at room temperature and then absorbance was measured at 517 nm against a control. Quercetin was used for comparison.

2.7. Apoptosis Assay

Depending on cytotoxicity results, ginger oil was selected for examining apoptosis property which was measured using caspase-3 activity kit (Abcam, Cambridge, UK) according to the instructions of the manufacturer. Briefly, apoptosis was induced in cells by adding ginger oil, and the cells were incubated for 2 h. In addition, a control culture without induction was concurrently incubated. Cells were pelleted and counted almost 1×10^6 cells. Cells were also re-suspended in 50 µL of chilled cell lysis buffer and incubated on ice for 10 min. Finally, they were centrifuged for 1 min in a micro-centrifuge ($10{,}000\times g$).

3. Results

3.1. EOs Composition

For the used commercial oils, the supplier provided no data about their contents or chemical analysis, which is presumed to be the company's copyright. However, a simple chemical analysis was performed in order to have a gross estimate of the components of the employed essential oils as % composition (Table 3).

Table 3. Main chemical components of the investigated EOs using GC-MS.

Components of EOs	A. Rue (%)	Basil (%)	Chamomile (%)	Fennel (%)	Fenugreek (%)	Ginger (%)	Mint (%)	Sage (%)	Thyme (%)
(E)-Anethol	13								
Eugenol	20								
Cicloysosativene	5								
3-Decanone	1								
α-Isomethyl-(E)-ionol	7								
Carvone	2						80		
Carvacrol	6								8
Dihydrocarvenyl acetate							1		
Caryophyllene	3	1			15		1		
Neral (cis-citral)					17	9			
Methyl chavicol		76							
Limonene	1						9		15
Linalool		15							
Thymol	7								25
ρ-Cymene									14
α-Pinene				1	2		0.5		12
β-Pinene					15				
Anethole				75					
Fenchone				13					
Cis-thujone								30	
Camphor	3				17			22	
1,8-Cineole								8	
α-Selinene					4.5				
Geranial					5	10			
2,5-Dimethylpyrazine					7				
α-Bisabolol oxide A			24						
Chamazulene			10						
α-Bisabolone oxide A			19						
α-Bisabolol oxide B			30						
Spathulenol			4						
α-Zingiberene						17.4			
Camphene						8			
α-Farnesene						6			
β-Sesquiphellandrene						6.6			
Total identified chemicals	66%	92%	87%	89%	82.5%	57%	91.5%	60%	74%

3.2. Viability Test by Trypan Blue

Viability test of both cell lines by trypan blue is shown in Figure 1a,b. HT-29 (MS) cell line viability decreased by 50% when 60 μL/mL of chamomile were used while all other EOs reached such a decrease when 70–80 μL/mL were used. In HT-29 19(A), 50% of viability was obtained when using 80 μL/mL of ginger and African rue, while all other EOs needed more than 80 μL/mL to reach such a decline in viability. However, apart from mint, all EOs produced 0% to 10% viability when concentrations were increased to 100 μL/mL.

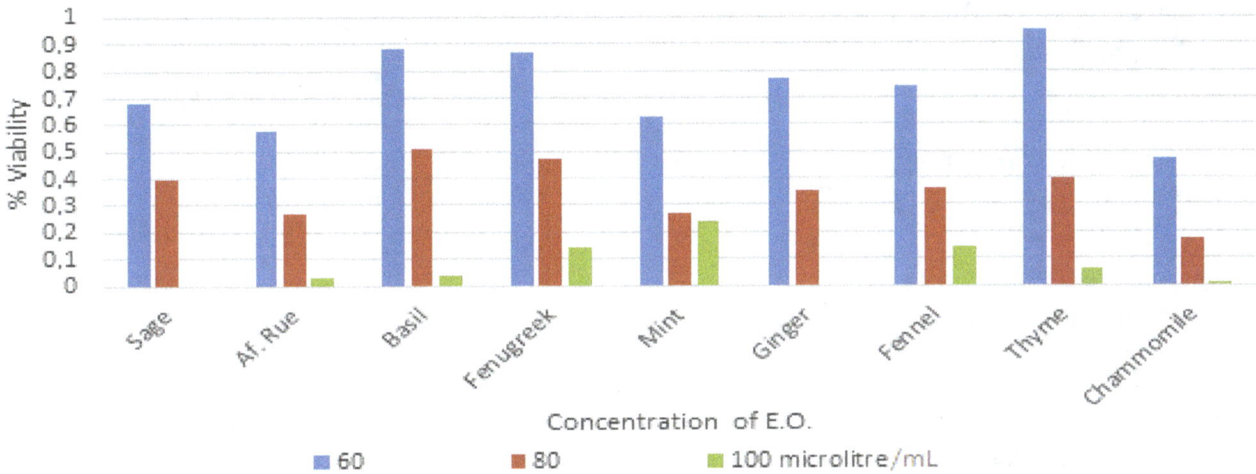

(a) Viability test of by trypan blue on HT-29 (MS) cell lines

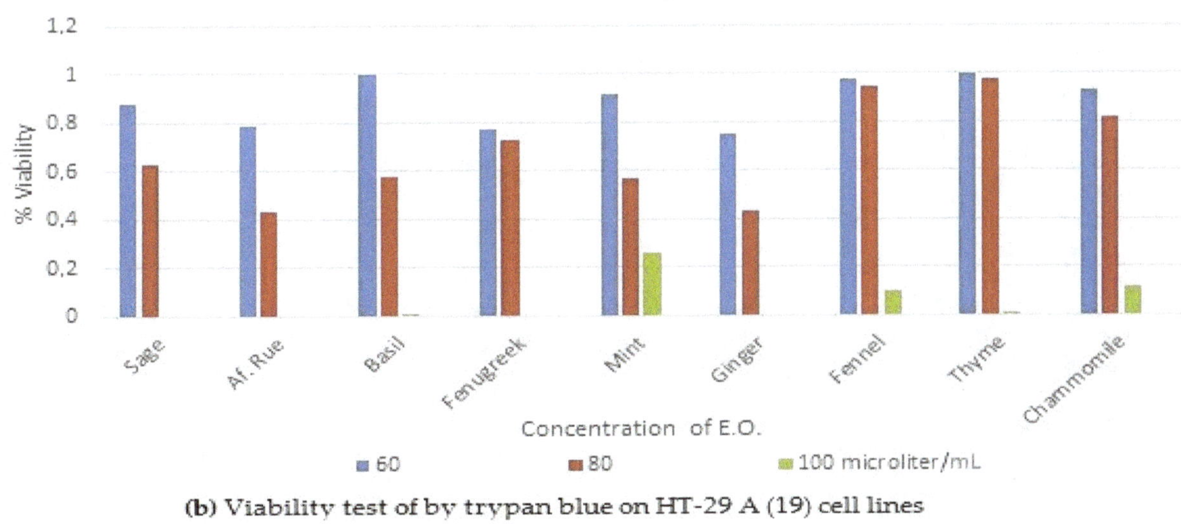

(b) Viability test of by trypan blue on HT-29 A (19) cell lines

Figure 1. Viability percentages of: (**a**) HT29-19(A) non-muco secreting and (**b**) HT29-muco secreting (MS) cell lines treated for 48 h with EOs.

Photos of ginger oil effect on cells at different time intervals are shown in Figure 2a–c.

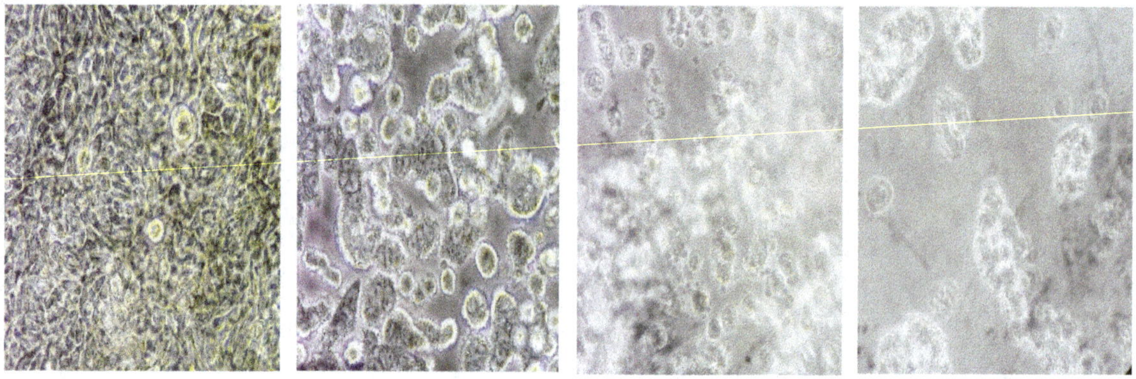

(a) (b) (c) (d)

Figure 2. Effect of ginger oil on the HT-29 (MS) cell line as observed under the microscope. × 400 (**a**), represents cells at time 0 min; (**b–d**) cell at 30 min intervals after ginger oil addition.

3.3. MTT Assay

The MTT cytotoxicity test for both cell lines is shown in Figure 3a,b. IC_{50} for EOs using HT-29 (MS) has revealed that ginger was the lowest in concentration to achieve IC_{50} followed by African rue and sage, with 40, 48 and 53 μL/mL respectively. Whereas, the rest of EOs showed IC_{50} at contents around 80 μL/mL. In the HT-29 19(A) cells, the same trend was obtained, in which ginger got the lowest concentration (60 μL/mL) then thyme was the highest with 77 μL/mL.

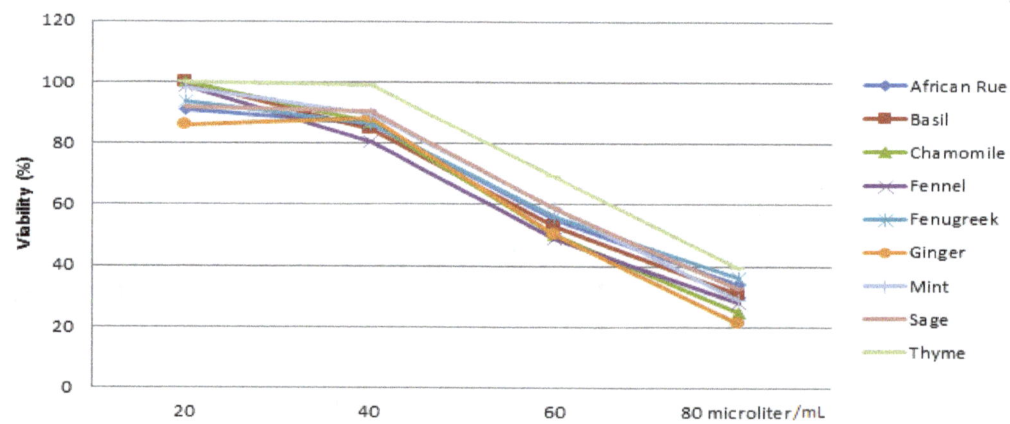

(a)IC_{50} for EOs using HT-29 19(A)

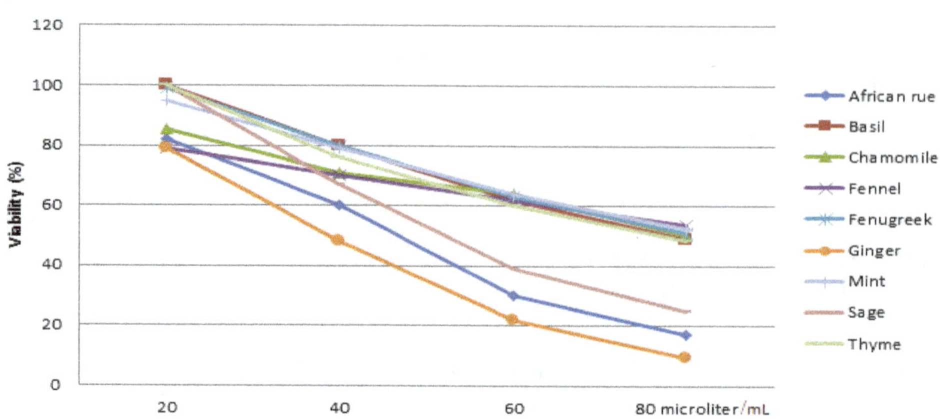

(b) IC_{50} for EOs using HT-29 (MS)

Figure 3. MTT assay using cell lines treated with EOs for 48 h: (**a**) IC_{50} on HT-29 19(A); (**b**) IC_{50} on HT-29 (MS).

3.4. DPPH Radical Scavenging

The reduction ability of DPPH radicals' formation was determined by the decrease in the absorbance at 517 nm induced by antioxidants. DPPH is a stable free radical and accepts an electron (hydrogen radical) to become a stable diamagnetic molecule. A DPPH assay revealed that all commercial EOs assayed in this study have got a very weak or no scavenging capacity compared with the control. These results may be a result of the low quality control of the production or the handling of these EOs products.

Scavenging activity was equivalent to ≤20 μg/mL quercetin, which was the lowest concentration used in the experiment.

3.5. Apoptosis

Ginger oil failed to show an ability to induce apoptosis within the time frame of this experiment. On the other side, caspase-3 activity has not been detected. The same was found for the rest of the EOs. This may be justified by the change in quality of the EOs composition due to many factors including the oxidation, adulteration, or aging [20,21]. As for the S-1 sample, the total amount was determined.

4. Discussion

As it can be noticed from the trypan blue experiment results, most of the EOs have been shown to have a similar trend to inhibit 50% growth (IC_{50}) at the content of 80 μL/mL. Indeed, chamomile was very effective when used on HT-29 (MS), whereas, ginger and African rue showed superior effect in comparison with other EOs on HT-29 19(A) cells.

From the latest studies, ginger constituents were reported to have a vital effect in the control of tumor development through up-regulation of the tumor suppressor gene, induction of apoptosis and inactivation of VEGF pathways. For instance, 6-gingerol was found to have a role in the suppression of the hyper-proliferation, transformation, and inflammatory routes that take part in numerous steps of carcinogenesis, angiogenesis and metastasis; in addition, it acts in the initiation of apoptosis in the prostate cancer cell line via inhibition of cell invasion reduction of matrix metalloproteinase-9 expression. Also, 6-gingerol stimulates apoptosis through up-regulation of NAG-1 and G1 cell cycle arrest through down-regulation of cyclin D1 [22]. Besides, other abundant terpenoids also have been found to be present in the ginger like, neral, geranial, zingerberene, camphene, and other oxygenated monoterpenes [23] which may exert a synergistic anticancer activity.

Otherwise, *Peganum harmala* is traditionally used to treat many diseases including cancer. Recent studies show that the alkaloids of *Peganum harmala* are cytotoxic to several tumor cell lines in vitro and have an antitumor effect in a tumor model in vivo. Harmine, a major identified indole alkaloid in the African rue and vasicinone, were the most potent components in inhibiting cell growth and as an antiproliferating agent [24,25]. The active principle at a dose of 50 mg/kg given orally to mice for 40 days was found to have significant anti-tumoral activity [26].

The only difference between both cell lines was the ability of cells to secrete mucus. The negative effect of chamomile, in the case of HT-29 19 (A) cells, is not clear. Mucus in the gut plays a major role in protecting the gut linen from foreign (bio)chemicals. In vitro, a lack of secreting mucus may induce other protective mechanisms that enabled HT-29 19(A) to withstand the impact of higher concentration of EOs. However, as soon as this mechanism was damaged, the viability dramatically declined. On the other side, protection, by mucus, from the effect of the EOs in HT-29 (MS) has gradually decreased as the concentrations of the EOs were increasing.

Scavenging ability of antioxidants decreases by several factors, such as direct light exposure, storage temperature and processing (time needed in open air and temperature) [20]. Commercial EOs are treated and stored in a way in which they can lose their antioxidant and other biological properties. Indeed, there are inevitable factors due to oxidation in the extraction process and in the storage bulk scale of essential oil [20]. Moreover, in Palestine, some EOs are displayed on the shelves in transparent containers, and the temperature may exceed 35 °C in summer time. However, the compositional change in the EOs may be unavoidable even at 5 °C. Such bad preservation conditions may prevent the products from retaining their ability as free radical scavengers.

In fact, EOs which possess high levels of unsaturation might be generally unstable due to many factors such as heat, light, hydration and oxidation.

5. Conclusions

From the EOs tested in this study, we noticed that some had potential activities against the cancer cell tested. Interestingly, in this work, chamomile oil showed the lowest IC_{50} at a content of 60 μL/mL in HT-29 (MS) cell lines. In HT-29 19(A) cells, 50% of the viability was obtained when 80 μL/mL of ginger and African rue EOs were used. An MTT assay on HT-29 (MS) cells showed that ginger IC_{50} was the lowest, followed by African rue and sage, with 40, 48 and 53 μL/mL, respectively. On the other hand, ginger had the lowest IC_{50} with 60 μL/mL whilst thyme was the highest with 77 μL/mL in HT-29 19(A) cells. However, the used commercial EOs did not show any biological activities in the antioxidant and caspase-3 assays.

Factors such as processing, handling, and storage conditions may be responsible for the faintness in the biological and pharmacological properties of the commercial EOs, which originally possess significant biological activities, suggesting that more investigation on commercial Eos is required before recommending their use to the public.

Acknowledgments: The authors acknowledge the help of Zamalah and Cooperative Bank, Palestine for funding through research project.

Author Contributions: The list authors contributed to this work as follows: M.A.A.-T. and B.R. conceived and designed the experiments; M.A.A.-T. and I.M.A.-R. performed research and analyzed the data and wrote the paper. B.R., I.M.A.-R. polished the paper. All authors read and approved the final manuscript.

References

1. Lis-Balchin, M. Essential oils and 'aromatherapy': Their modern role in healing. *J. R. Soc. Promot. Health* **1997**, *117*, 324–329. [CrossRef]
2. Alzeer, B.J.; Vummidi, R.; Arafeh, R.; Rimawi, W.; Saleem, H.; Luedtke, N.W. The influence of extraction solvents on the anticancer activities of Palestinian medicinal plants. *J. Med. Plants Res.* **2014**, *8*, 408–415.
3. Christaki, E.; Bonos, E.; Giannenas, I.; Florou-Paneri, P. Aromatic Plants as a Source of Bioactive Compounds. *Agriculture* **2012**, *2*, 228–243. [CrossRef]
4. Bruneton, J. *Pharmacognosy, Phytochemistry, Medicinal Plants*; Technique & Documentation; Lavoisier: Andover, France, 1999.
5. Turek, C.; Stintzing, F.C. Stability of Essential Oils: A Review. *Compr. Rev. Food Sci. Food Saf.* **2013**, *12*, 40–53. [CrossRef]
6. Baser, K.H.C.; Buchbauer, G. *Handbook of Essential Oils: Science, Technology, and Applications*; CRC Press: Boca Raton, FL, USA, 2009.
7. Calo, J.R.; Crandall, P.G.; O'Bryan, C.A.; Ricke, S.C. Essential oils as antimicrobials in food systems—Review. *Food Control* **2015**, *54*, 111–119. [CrossRef]
8. Hyldgaard, M.; Mygind, T.; Meyer, R.L. Essential Oils in Food Preservation: Mode of Action, Synergies, and Interactions with Food Matrix Components. *Front. Microbiol.* **2012**, *3*. [CrossRef] [PubMed]
9. Li, Y.; Fabiano-Tixier, A.S.; Chémat, F. *Essential Oils as Reagents in Green Chemistry*; Springer: Avignon, France, 2014.
10. Lubbe, A.; Verpoorte, R. Cultivation of medicinal and aromatic plants for specialty industrial materials. *Ind. Crops Prod.* **2011**, *34*, 785–801. [CrossRef]
11. Reuter, S.; Gupta, S.C.; Chaturvedi, M.M.; Aggarwal, B.B. Oxidative stress, inflammation, and cancer: How are they linked? *Free Radic. Biol. Med.* **2010**, *49*, 1603–1616. [CrossRef] [PubMed]

12. Moylan, J.S.; Reid, M.B. Oxidative stress, chronic disease, and muscle wasting. *Muscle Nerve* **2007**, *35*, 411–429. [CrossRef] [PubMed]
13. Tantamango-Bartley, Y.; Jaceldo-Siegl, K.; Fan, J.; Fraser, G. Vegetarian Diets and the Incidence of Cancer in a Low-risk Population. *Cancer Epidemiol. Biomark. Prev.* **2013**, *22*, 286–294. [CrossRef] [PubMed]
14. Namvar, F.; Rahman, H.S.; Mohamad, R.; Baharara, J.; Mahdavi, M.; Amini, E.; Chartrand, M.S.; Yeap, S.K. Cytotoxic effect of magnetic iron oxide nanoparticles synthesized via seaweed aqueous extract. *Int. J. Nanomed.* **2014**, *9*, 2479–2488. [CrossRef] [PubMed]
15. Bayala, B.; Bassole, I.H.; Scifo, R.; Gnoula, C.; Morel, L.; Lobaccaro, J.-M.A.; Simpore, J. Anticancer activity of essential oils and their chemical components—A review. *Am. J. Cancer Res.* **2014**, *4*, 591–607. [PubMed]
16. Bayala, B.; Bassole, I.H.; Gnoula, C.; Nebie, R.; Yonli, A.; Morel, L.; Figueredo, G.; Nikiema, J.B.; Lobaccaro, J.M.; Simpore, J. Chemical Composition, Antioxidant, Anti-Inflammatory and Anti-Proliferative Activities of Essential Oils of Plants from Burkina Faso. *PLoS ONE* **2014**, *9*. [CrossRef] [PubMed]
17. Sak, K. Cytotoxicity of dietary flavonoids on different human cancer types. *Int. J. Pharmacogn.* **2014**, *8*, 122–146. [CrossRef] [PubMed]
18. Gordaliza, M. Natural products as leads to anticancer drugs. *Clin. Transl. Oncol.* **2007**, *9*, 767–776. [CrossRef] [PubMed]
19. Nóbrega de Almeida, R.; Agra, M.D.F.; Souto Maior, F.N.; Pergentino de Sousa, D. Essential oils and their constituents: Anticonvulsant activity. *Molecules* **2011**, *16*, 2726–2742. [CrossRef] [PubMed]
20. Sawamura, M.; Son, U.-S.; Choi, H.-S.; Kim, M.-S.L.; Fears, M.; Phi, N.T.L.; Kumagai, C. Compositional changes in commercial lemon essential oil for aromatherapy. *Int. J. Aromather.* **2004**, *14*, 27–36. [CrossRef]
21. Wabner, D. The peroxide value—A new tool for the quality control of essential oils. *Int. J. Aromather.* **2002**, *12*, 216–218. [CrossRef]
22. Molyneux, P. The use of the stable free radical diphenylpicrylhydrazyl (DPPH) for estimating antioxidant activity. *Songklanakarin J. Sci. Technol.* **2004**, *26*, 211–219.
23. Chagonda, L.S.; Chalchat, J.-C. Essential oil Composition of *Zingiber officinale* Roscoe from Eastern Zimbabwe. *J. Essent. Oil Bear. Plants* **2016**, *19*, 510–515. [CrossRef]
24. Lamchouri, F.; Zemzami, M.; Jossang, A.; Abdellatif, A.; Israili, Z.H.; Lyoussi, B. Cytotoxicity of alkaloids isolated from Peganum harmala seeds. *Pak. J. Pharm. Sci.* **2013**, *26*, 699–706. [PubMed]
25. Aihetasham, A.; Umer, M.; Akhtar, M.S.; Din, M.I.; Rasib, K.Z. Bioactivity of medicinal plants *Mentha arvensis* and *Peganum harmala* extracts against *Heterotermes indicola* (Wasmann) (Isoptera). *Int. J. Biosci.* **2015**, *7*, 116–126.
26. Lamchouri, F.; Settaf, A.; Cherrah, Y.; Zemzami, M.; Lyoussi, B.; Zaid, A.; Atif, N.; Hassar, M. Antitumour principles from *Peganum harmala* seeds. *Therapie* **1999**, *54*, 753–758. [PubMed]

12

Antidermatophytic Activity of the Fruticose Lichen *Usnea orientalis*

Ashutosh Pathak [1], Dalip Kumar Upreti [2] and Anupam Dikshit [1,*]

1 Biological Product Lab, Department of Botany, University of Allahabad, Allahabad 211002, India; ashupathaks@rediffmail.com
2 Lichenology Laboratory, CSIR-National Botanical Research Institute, Rana Pratap Marg, Lucknow 226001, India; upretidknbri@gmail.com
* Correspondence: anupambplau@rediffmail.com

Academic Editor: James D. Adams

Abstract: In the present study, the new biological sources in the form of lichen *Usnea orientalis* Motyka was screened for its antidermatophytic potential. Six species of dermatophytes were chosen on the basis of their prevalence for antidermatophytic assays, and the Clinical Laboratory Standard Institute (CLSI)-recommended broth microdilution procedure was used to detect the efficacy of extract against dermatophytes. Thin layer chromatography of lichen extracts reveals the presence of two secondary metabolites viz. salazinic acid and usnic acid. *U. orientalis* extract exhibited promising antidermatophytic activity against all tested pathogens. Amongst all tested pathogens, *Epidermophyton floccosum* exhibited most susceptibility towards extract, whereas *Trichophyton mentagrophytes* exhibited the least susceptibility. Topical application of *U. orientalis* extract might be helpful in the cure of dermal infections.

Keywords: antidermatophytic; dermatophytes; DPPH; Lichen

---

1. Introduction

Lichen thallus (a composite organism) is mainly composed of mycobiont and photobiont in a mutualistic relationship [1]. Lichens are known for their secondary metabolites, which are quite unique to them and have several properties such as photoprotection, allelopathy, and antioxidant, antimicrobial, and antiviral activities [2]. The genus *Usnea* is well known for the worldwide distribution and for the role of secondary metabolite, i.e., usnic acid, in medicines. More than 300 species of genus *Usnea* were reported throughout the world, of which 57 are from India [3]. *Usnea orientalis* Motyka (fruticose and corticolous lichen) was used ethno-medicinally in urinary tract problems, swelling, and edema [4]. Cutaneous infections caused by fungi generally produce boggy nodular swelling called kerion [5]. Cutaneous mycoses (skin infection) caused by filamentous keratinophilic fungi known as dermatophytes, composed of the three genera *Trichophyton*, *Microsporum*, and *Epidermophyton* [6]. In humans, about 30 species of dermatophytes have been identified as pathogens [7]. Dermatophytes are cosmopolitan in distribution. Several reports from different parts of the world have reported the occurrence of dermatophytes. A study involving 16 European countries showed that 35%–40% of the analyzed individuals had infection of the foot (tinea pedis) caused by dermatophytes [8]. A study in the US revealed that between 22% and 55% had hair scalp infection of dermatophytes [9]. Another study conducted in Brazil showed that *Trichophyton rubrum*, *Microsporum canis*, and *Epidermophyton floccosum* were the most prevalent species infecting humans in developing countries [10]. The World Health Organization estimated that dermatophytes affect about 25% of the world population [6]. Apart from wide prevalence, the dermatophytes have exhibited resistance against griseofulvin, terbinafine, and fluconazole [6,11–14]. Although the prevalence of drug resistance in dermatophytes is rare, recurrence in patients is common with 60%–80% [5]. Based on the aforementioned literature, the new biological source in the form of *U. orientalis* was screened for its antidermatophytic property.

2. Material and Methods

2.1. Preparation and Percent Yield of Extract

Lichen thalli were collected from Koti, Chakrata district, Uttarakhand, India and identified with the help of relevant keys [15]. The voucher specimen was deposited in the Botanical Survey of India, Allahabad, India: *U. orientalis* (Accession No. BSA-8760). Two grams of air-dried thallus (vegetative as well as fruiting) was washed thoroughly using tap water followed by distilled water and pat-dried. Then, thalli were subjected to cold extraction of secondary metabolites in 50 mL of acetone. Subsequently, the solvent was filtered by Whatman No. 1 filter paper after 48 h.

The weight of crude extract obtained was 0.16 g after vacuum drying the filtrate via rotary evaporator. Percent yield of crude extract was calculated according to the equation below:

$$\text{Percent yield } (\%) = (\text{Dry weight of extract/Dry weight of sample}) \times 100.$$

Stock solution (50 mg/mL) of crude extract was prepared in dimethyl sulphoxide (DMSO) for the evaluation of antidermatophytic and free radical scavenging activity.

2.2. Thin Layer Chromatography of Extract

Solvent A (Toluene (180 mL) 1,4 dioxane (45 mL): Acetic acid (5 mL)) and Solvent C (Toluene (170 mL): Acetic acid (30 mL)) was used as mobile phase, whereas silica-coated aluminum plate (TLC Silica gel 60 F254, Merck KGaA, Darmstadt, Germany) was used as stationary phase and Usnic acid (Chemical Industry Co., Ltd., Tokyo, Japan) was taken as standard [16].

2.3. Test Pathogens and Inocula Preparation

Fungal cultures of *Epidermophyton floccosum* (MTCC No. 7880), *Microsporum canis* (MTCC No. 3270), *M. fulvum* (MTCC No. 7684), *M. gypseum* (MTCC No. 2867), *Trichophyton rubrum* (MTCC No. 296), and *T. mentagrophytes* (MTCC No. 7687) were procured from Microbial Type Culture Collection and Gene Bank (MTCC), Chandigarh, India, and were subcultured on Sabouraud Dextrose Agar (SDA) medium under laminar flow cabinet (Laminar flow ultra clean air unit, Micro-Filt, Pune, India). Inocula were prepared in saline media and then adjusted to a 0.5 McFarland standard, corresponding to ca 0.5×10^6 CFU/mL, and transmittance of inocula prepared were 70%–72% at 520 nm for each pathogen [17].

2.4. Antifungal Assay for Opportunistic Filamentous Fungi

2.4.1. Determination of Fungistatic Concentration

Antifungal susceptibility test was performed according to the Clinical Laboratory Standard Institute (CLSI)-recommended broth microdilution method in RPMI-1640 medium HEPES modification (Sigma Aldrich, St. Louis, MO, USA) supplemented with MOPS buffer (3-morphollinopropane-1-sulfonic acid) (Qualigens Fine Chemicals, Mumbai, India) [18]. Brief steps involved per plate were as follows: Inocula prepared was diluted 1:50 times in testing media, i.e., RPMI 1640; the test was performed in 96-well flat bottom microtiter plates; Column 1 was named as negative control consisting of 100 µL of RPMI-1640 broth media and 100 µL of inocula prepared in formaldehyde (less than 0.5%); Column 2 was named as broth control consisting of 200 µL of media; Columns 3 and 4, 6 and 7, and 9 and 10 were vertically diluted with extract having a final concentration of 1.25 to 0.009 mg/mL and named as treated; Column 5, 8, and 11 were taken as positive controls and contained only 100 µL of inocula and 100 µL of RPMI-1640 broth media, respectively; Column 12 was named as extract control and contained vertically diluted extract in the aforementioned concentrations. To nullify the effect of extract color, optical density (O.D.) of the extract control was subtracted from treated columns corresponding to extract treated [19]. Percent inhibition was calculated using following equation:

$$\text{Per cent Inhibition (\%)} = ((\text{O.D. positive control} - \text{O.D. extract-treated}) / (\text{O.D. positive control})) \times 100.$$

Minimum inhibition concentrations (MICs) was calculated based on optical density recorded with a spectrophotometer (SpectraMax Plus^{384}, Molecular Devices Corporation, Orleans Drive, Sunnyvale, CA, USA) at 530 nm after 96 h of incubation at 30 ± 2 °C (Figure 1).

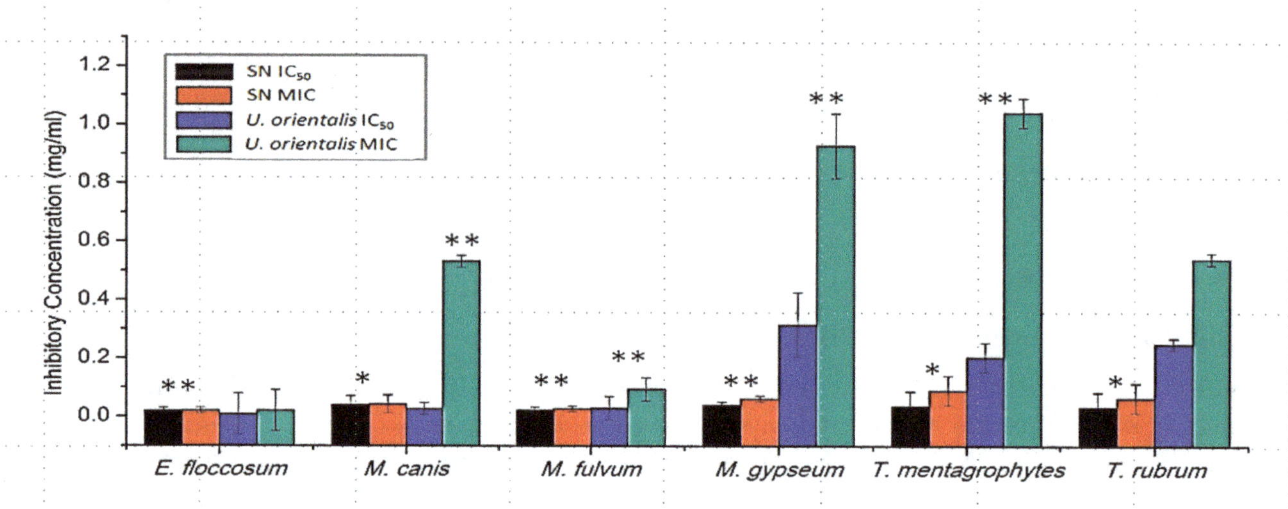

Figure 1. Antidermatophytic activity *U. orientalis* extract compared with Sertaconazole nitrate. Error bars show the standard error mean. ** Level of significance ≤ 0.01. * Level of significance ≤ 0.05.

The antifungal activity of the chemical drug Sertaconazole nitrateBP (SN) (Glenmark Pharmaceuticals, Nasik, India) was taken as the reference standard. An amount of 50 mg/mL of stock solution of SN was prepared and tested at the same concentrations as the *U. orientalis* extract.

2.4.2. Determination of Fungicidal Concentration

A portion of 20 µL of *U. orientalis*-treated columns from the above MIC wells were transferred into 7-mL tubes of a fresh RPMI 1640 medium. Tubes were incubated at 30 ± 2 °C for 4 weeks and checked for the turbidity. The aforementioned procedure was performed with SN, and the concentration at which no turbidity has been achieved was defined as the minimum fungicidal concentration (MFC) [20,21].

2.5. Statistical Analysis

An independent sample *t*-test was performed between the positive control and sertacoazole-treated dermatophytes; and between the positive control and extract-treated dermatophytes for the measure of Levene's test for equality of variances and *t*-test for equality of means via SPSS v20.

3. Results and Discussion

3.1. Percent Yield of Extract

Percent yield of extract obtained from *U. orientalis* thallus was 8%.

3.2. Thin Layer Chromatography

A light yellow turning into a green-colored spot was observed and confirmed as usnic acid in *U. orientalis* extract and the other compound was salazinic acid. The chromatographic study confirmed the presence of two compounds viz. usnic acid and salazinic acid in the *U. orientalis* extract.

3.3. Antifungal Test for Opportunistic Filamentous Fungi

U. orientalis, fruticose lichen, contains usnic and salazinic acid and is used ethno-medicinally in swelling. The *U. orientalis* extract was tested for its efficacy against six dermatophytic species and compared with sertaconazole nitrate. Sertaconazole nitrate is a highly active chemical drug having low fungistatic and fungicidal activities, but it causes inflammation and itching in patients [22]. Due to the side effects of SN and the development of resistance in dermatophytes against first-line clinical drugs, there is a need for new antidermatophytic compounds. The antidermatophytic activity of SN and *U. orientalis* were represented graphically in the form of IC_{50} (50% inhibitory concentration) and MIC (minimum inhibitory concentration) values were represented graphically in Figure 1.

E. floccosum exhibited equal susceptibility towards SN and *U. orientalis* extract with an MIC value equivalent to 0.021 mg/mL and an MFC value equivalent to 0.039 mg/mL. The IC_{50} value for *E. floccosum* was achieved at 0.009 mg/mL against *U. orientalis* and 0.020 mg/mL against SN. *M. gypseum* was found least susceptible among *Microsporum* spp. with IC_{50} = 0.040 mg/mL; MIC = 0.062 mg/mL; MFC = 0.078 mg/mL against SN and IC_{50} = 0.316 mg/mL; MIC = 0.927 mg/mL; MFC = 1.250 mg/mL against *U. orientalis*. *M. fulvum* was found most susceptible among *Microsporum* spp. with IC_{50} = 0.022 mg/mL; MIC = 0.027 mg/mL; MFC = 0.039 mg/mL against SN and IC_{50} = 0.029 mg/mL; MIC = 0.094 mg/mL; MFC = 0.156 mg/mL against *U. orientalis*. The IC_{50}, MIC, and MFC for *M. canis* were obtained at 0.040 mg/mL, 0.043 mg/mL, and 0.078 mg/mL for SN and 0.027 mg/mL, 0.531 mg/mL, and 0.625 mg/mL for *U. orientalis* extract.

The IC_{50}, MIC, and MFC for *T. rubrum* were achieved at 0.033 mg/mL, 0.064 mg/mL, and 0.078 mg/mL against SN and 0.249 mg/mL, 0.54 mg/mL, and 0.625 mg/mL against *U. orientalis* extract. *T. mentagrophytes* was found least susceptible amongst all tested pathogens with IC_{50} = 0.037 mg/mL, MIC = 0.09 mg/mL, and MFC = 0.156 mg/mL against SN and IC_{50} = 0.204 mg/mL, MIC = 1.04 mg/mL, and MFC = 1.25 mg/mL against *U. orientalis* extract. The efficacy of *U. orientalis* extract is equivalent to sertaconazole nitrate against *E. floccosum*, but was found to be less effective against all other dermatophytes.

In another study, extracts of *U. florida* exhibited an MIC between 0.050 and 0.100 mg/mL against *M. gypseum*, *T. mentagrophytes*, and *T. rubrum* [23]. In the present study *U. orientalis* exhibited a MIC between 0.531 and 1.04 mg/mL and was found to be less active than *U. florida*. The ethno-medicinal use of *U. orientalis* extract in swelling caused by dermatophyte infection might be cured, but in vivo efficacy and potency of the lichen extract needs to be investigated.

3.4. Statistical Analysis

The level of significance was calculated in terms of *p*-value. Results obtained were statistically significant except between *U. orientalis* treatments and control *T. rubrum* (p-value = 0.19) and *U. orientalis* treatments and control *E. floccosum* (p-value = 0.19); *p*-values calculated for SN-treated *E. floccosum*, *M. fulvum*, and *M. gypseum* were less than 0.01, whereas, for *M. canis*, *T. mentagrophytes*, and *T. rubrum*, *p*-values were less than 0.05. *p*-value calculated for *U. orientalis* treated all pathogens except *T. rubrum*, *which* showed a level of significance less than 0.01 (Figure 1).

4. Conclusions

U. orientalis extract exhibited broad-range antidermatophytic activity against all three genera of dermatophytes, and usnic acid (a well-known antifungal compound) was present in the lichen extract. Topical application of lichen extract might be helpful in the cure of cutaneous infections.

Acknowledgments: Gopal Prasad Sinha, Head of Office, Central Regional Centre, Botanical Survey of India, Allahabad for accepting the voucher specimens of Lichens, and University Grant Commission (UGC) New Delhi, India, for financial assistance.

Author Contributions: Dalip Kumar Upreti identified the lichen; Ashutosh Pathak, Dalip Kumar Upreti and Anupam Dikshit designed the experiments, analyzed the results and proof reading of the manuscript; Ashutosh Pathak collected the lichen thallus, performed the experiments and wrote the manuscript.

References

1. Hawksworth, D.L. Freshwater and marine lichen-forming. In *Aquatic Mycology across the Millennium*; Hyde, K.D., Ho, W.H., Pointing, S.B., Eds.; Fungal Diversity: Hong Kong, China, 2000; Volume 5.
2. Molnar, K.; Farkas, E. Current results on Biological Activities of Lichen Secondary Metabolites: A Review. *Z. Naturforschung C* **2010**, *65*, 157–173. [CrossRef]
3. Shukla, P.; Upreti, D.K.; Tewari, L.M. Secondary metabolite variability in genus *Usnea* in India: A potential source for bioprospection. *J. Environ. Sci. Technol.* **2015**, *2*, 44–55.
4. Wang, L.S.; Qian, Z.G. *Pictorial Handbook to Medicinal Lichens in Chin*; Yunnan Provincial Science and Technology Publishers: Kunming, China, 2013.
5. Dias, M.F.R.G.; Quaresma-Santos, M.V.P.; Bernardes-Filho, F.; Amorim, A.G.F.; Schechtman, R.C.; Azulay, D.R. Update on therapy for superficial mycoses: Review article part 1. *An. Bras. Dermatol.* **2013**, *88*, 764–774. [CrossRef] [PubMed]
6. Peres, N.T.A.; Maranhão, F.C.A.; Rossi, A.; Martinez-Rossi, N.M. Dermatophytes: Host-pathogen interaction and antifungal resistance. *An. Bras. Dermatol.* **2010**, *85*, 657–667. [CrossRef] [PubMed]
7. White, T.C.; Oliver, B.G.; Graser, Y.; Henn, M.R. Generating and testing molecular hypotheses in the dermatophytes. *Eukaryot. Cell* **2008**, *7*, 1238–1245. [CrossRef] [PubMed]
8. Burzykowski, T.; Molenberghs, G.; Abeck, D.; Haneke, E.; Hay, R.; Katsambas, A.; Roseeuw, D.; van de Kerkhof, P.; van Aelst, R.; Marynissen, G. High prevalence of foot diseases in Europe: Results of the Achilles Project. *Mycoses* **2003**, *46*, 496–505. [CrossRef] [PubMed]
9. Abdel-Rahman, S.M.; Simon, S.; Wright, K.J.; Ndjountche, L.; Gaedigk, A. Tracking *Trichophyton tonsurans* through a large urban child care center: Defining infection prevalence and transmission patterns by molecular strain typing. *Pediatrics* **2006**, *118*, 2365–2373. [CrossRef] [PubMed]
10. Heidrich, D.; Garcia, M.R.; Stopiglia, C.D.O.; Magagnin, C.M.; Daboit, T.C.; Vetoratto, G.; Schwartz, J.; Amaro, T.G.; Scroferneker, M.L. Dermatophytosis: A 16-year retrospective study in a metropolitan area in southern Brazil. *J. Infect. Dev. Ctries.* **2015**, *9*, 865–871. [CrossRef] [PubMed]
11. Stephenson, J. Investigators seeking new ways to stem rising tide of resistant fungi. *J. Am. Med. Assoc.* **1997**, *277*, 5–6. [CrossRef]
12. Wingfield, A.B.; Fernandez-Obregon, A.C.; Wignall, F.S.; Greer, D.L. Treatment of tinea imbricata: A randomized clinical trial using griseofulvin, terbinafine, itraconazole and fluconazole. *Br. J. Dermatol.* **2004**, *150*, 119–126. [CrossRef] [PubMed]
13. Smith, K.J.; Warnock, D.W.; Kennedy, C.T.; Johnson, E.M.; Hopwood, V.; van Cutsem, J.; Vanden Bossche, H. Azole resistance in *Candida albicans*. *Med. Mycol.* **1986**, *24*, 133–144. [CrossRef]
14. Orozco, A.; Higginbotham, L.; Hitchcock, C.; Parkinson, T.; Falconer, D.; Ibrahim, A.; Ghannoum, M.A.; Filler, S.G. Mechanism of fluconazole resistance in *Candida krusei*. *Antimicrob. Agents Chemother.* **1998**, *42*, 2645–2649. [PubMed]
15. Awasthi, D.D. *A compendium of the Macrolichens from India, Nepal and Sri Lanka*; Bishen Singh Mahendra Pal Singh: Dehradun, India, 2007.
16. Orange, A.; James, P.W.; White, F.J. *Microchemical Methods for Identification of Lichens*; British Lichen Society: London, UK, 2001.
17. Santos, D.A.; Barros, M.E.S.; Hamdan, J.S. Establishing a method of inoculum preparation for susceptibility testing of *Trichophyton rubrum* and *Trichophyton mentagrophytes*. *J. Clin. Microbial.* **2006**, *44*, 98–101. [CrossRef] [PubMed]
18. Rex, J.H.; Alexander, B.D.; Andes, D.; Arthington-Skaggs, B.; Brown, S.D.; Chaturveli, V.; Espinel-Ingroff, A.; Ghannoum, M.A.; Knapp, C.C.; Motyl, M.R.; et al. *Reference Method for Broth Dilution Antifungal Susceptibility*

Testing of Filamentous Fungi, Approved Standard, 2nd ed.; M38A2 28(16); Clinical and Laboratory Standard Institute (CLSI): Wayne, PA, USA, 2008.

19. Pathak, A.; Shukla, S.K.; Pandey, A.; Mishra, R.K.; Kumar, R.; Dikshit, A. In vitro antibacterial activity of ethno medicinally used lichens against three wound infecting genera of Enterobacteriaceae. *Proc. Natl. Acad. Sci. India Sect. B Biol. Sci.* **2015**. [CrossRef]
20. Veinovic, G.; Cerar, T.; Strle, F.; Lotric-Furlan, S.; Maraspin, V.; Cimperman, J.; Ruzic-Sabjic, E. In vitro susceptibility of European human *Borrelia burgdorferi* sensu stricto strains to antimicrobial agents. *Int. J. Antimicrob. Agents* **2013**, *41*, 288–291. [CrossRef] [PubMed]
21. Pathak, A.; Mishra, R.K.; Shukla, S.K.; Kumar, R.; Pandey, M.; Pandey, M.; Qidwai, A. In vitro evaluation of antidermatophytic activity of five lichens. *Cogent Biol.* **2016**. [CrossRef]
22. Liebel, F.; Lyte, P.; Garay, M.; Babad, J.; Southall, M.D. Anti-inflammatory and anti-itch activity of sertaconazole nitrate. *Arch. Dermatol. Res.* **2006**, *298*, 191–199. [CrossRef] [PubMed]
23. Schmeda-Hirschmann, G.; Tapia, A.; Lima, B.; Pertino, M.; Sortino, M.; Zacchino, S.; Arias, A.R.; Feresin, G.E. A new antifungal and antiprotozoal depside from the Andean lichen *Protousnea poeppigii*. *Phytother. Res.* **2008**, *22*, 349–355. [CrossRef] [PubMed]

13

The Bioactive Extract of *Pinnigorgia* sp. Induces Apoptosis of Hepatic Stellate Cells via ROS-ERK/JNK-Caspase-3 Signaling

Liang-Mou Kuo [1,2,†], Po-Jen Chen [3,4,†], Ping-Jyun Sung [5,6,7,8,9], Yu-Chia Chang [6,10], Chun-Ting Ho [3], Yi-Hsiu Wu [3] and Tsong-Long Hwang [3,4,11,12,*]

1 Graduate Institute of Clinical Medical Sciences, College of Medicine, Chang Gung University, Taoyuan 333, Taiwan; kuo33410@yahoo.com.tw
2 Department of General Surgery, Chang Gung Memorial Hospital, Chiayi 613, Taiwan
3 Graduate Institute of Natural Products, College of Medicine, Chang Gung University, Taoyuan 333, Taiwan; litlep@hotmail.com (P.-J.C.); Tsudanyer@hotmail.com (C.-T.H.); modemtw@gmail.com (Y.-H.W.)
4 Chinese Herbal Medicine Research Team, Healthy Aging Research Center, Chang Gung University, Taoyuan 333, Taiwan
5 Graduate Institute of Marine Biology, National Dong Hwa University, Pingtung 944, Taiwan; pjsung@nmmba.gov.tw
6 National Museum of Marine Biology and Aquarium, Pingtung 944, Taiwan; jay0404@gmail.com
7 Chinese Medicine Research and Development Center, China Medical University Hospital, Taichung 404, Taiwan
8 Graduate Institute of Natural Products, Kaohsiung Medical University, Kaohsiung 807, Taiwan
9 Department of Marine Biotechnology and Resources, National Sun Yat-sen University, Kaohsiung 804, Taiwan
10 Doctoral Degree Program in Marine Biotechnology, National Sun Yat-sen University & Academia Sinica, Kaohsiung 804, Taiwan
11 Research Center for Chinese Herbal Medicine, Research Center for Food and Cosmetic Safety, Graduate Institute of Health Industry Technology, College of Human Ecology, Chang Gung University of Science and Technology, Taoyuan 333, Taiwan
12 Department of Anaesthesiology, Chang Gung Memorial Hospital, Taoyuan 333, Taiwan
* Correspondence: htl@mail.cgu.edu.tw
† These authors contributed equally to this work.

Abstract: The activation of hepatic stellate cells (HSCs) is a significant phenomenon during the pathogenesis of liver disorders, including liver cirrhosis and fibrosis. Here, we identified that the extract from a gorgonian coral *Pinnigorgia* sp. (Pin) induced apoptosis of HSC-T6 cells. Pin inhibited the viability of HSC-T6 cells and increased their subG1 population, DNA fragmentation, caspase-3 activation, and reactive oxygen species (ROS) production in a concentration-dependent manner. The Pin-induced ROS generation and apoptotic effects were significantly reversed by a thiol antioxidant, *N*-acetylcysteine (NAC). Additionally, Pin induced ERK/JNK phosphorylation and pharmacological inhibition of ERK/JNK rescued the Pin-induced cell death. Pin-activated ERK/JNK were significantly reduced after the administration of NAC; however, the inhibition of ERK/JNK failed to change the Pin-induced ROS production. Similarly, pinnigorgiol A, a pure compound isolated from Pin, elicited ROS production and apoptosis in HSC-T6 cells. The pinnigorgiol A-induced apoptosis was retrained by NAC. Together, it appears that Pin leads to apoptosis in HSC-T6 cells through ROS-mediated ERK/JNK signaling and caspase-3 activation. Pinnigorgiol A serves as a bioactive compound of Pin and may exhibit therapeutic potential by clearance of HSCs.

Keywords: hepatic stellate cells; *Pinnigorgia* sp.; ROS; apoptosis; caspase-3; MAPK

1. Introduction

Hepatic fibrosis is an early significant lesion in chronic liver diseases such as liver cirrhosis and hepatocellular carcinoma. The excessive activation and proliferation of hepatic stellate cells (HSCs) gives rise to pro-inflammatory growth factors and extracellular matrix proteins during the pathogenesis of hepatic fibrosis, initiating matrix deposition in the liver [1–3]. Emerging evidences reveal that the restriction of activated HSCs is a potential strategy for hepatic fibrosis therapy via repressing proliferation or inducing apoptosis of HSCs [4–7]. So far, natural products derived from marine organisms display various potential pharmacological activities, including those applicable in liver disorder [8–10]. It is desirable to develop novel and useful marine natural products as better remedial strategies for hepatic disease through reversing the activated HSCs back to their quiescent status.

The *Pinnigorgia* sp. (Figure 1A) was first isolated and identified as in Taiwan [11]. Taxonomically, gorgonian coral *Pinnigorgia* sp. belongs to the animal kingdom (Kingdom Animalia), Cnidaria (Phylum Cnidaria), Anthozoa (Class Anthozoa), Octocorals subclass (Subclass Octocorallia), Gorgonian head (Order Gorgonacea), Holaxonia suborder, Family Gorgoniidae. Recently, various natural compounds from a gorgonian coral *Pinnigorgia* sp. have been shown to exhibit anti-inflammatory potential in human neutrophils [11–15]. In addition, the coralline extract from *Pinnigorgia* sp. (Pin) reduces the survival rate of HSCs [11,16], although the underlying mechanisms are still elusive. Therefore, it can be suggested that Pin may possess potential application to attenuate liver fibrosis via retraining the HSCs activation.

The aim of this study was to uncover the pharmacological mechanism of Pin-inhibited cell viability in a rat HSC cell line, HSC-T6 cells. During proliferation and activation of HSCs, intracellular redox homeostasis tightly controls the cell viability. Intracellular glutathione (GSH) level is an important factor to modulate redox balance [17]. GSH depletion induces reactive oxygen species (ROS) accumulation, leading to caspase-3-dependent apoptosis in HSCs [18–20]. Moreover, mitogen-activated protein kinases (MAPKs) signaling is also involved in redox homeostasis and apoptosis in HSCs [20–23].

In the present study, we found that the Pin-repressed cell viability in HSCs was dependent on caspase-3-, ROS-, and ERK/JNK-mediated apoptosis. Pin-induced ERK/JNK activation occurred through ROS production. The caspase-3 inhibitor, thiol antioxidants, and ERK/JNK inhibitors significantly abolished the Pin-induced cell death in HSCs. Moreover, pinnigorgiol A served as a bioactive compound of Pin that triggered the apoptosis and ROS production in HSCs. Our findings suggest that marine natural products from gorgonian coral including Pin and pinnigorgiol A exhibit therapeutic potentials by clearance of HSCs.

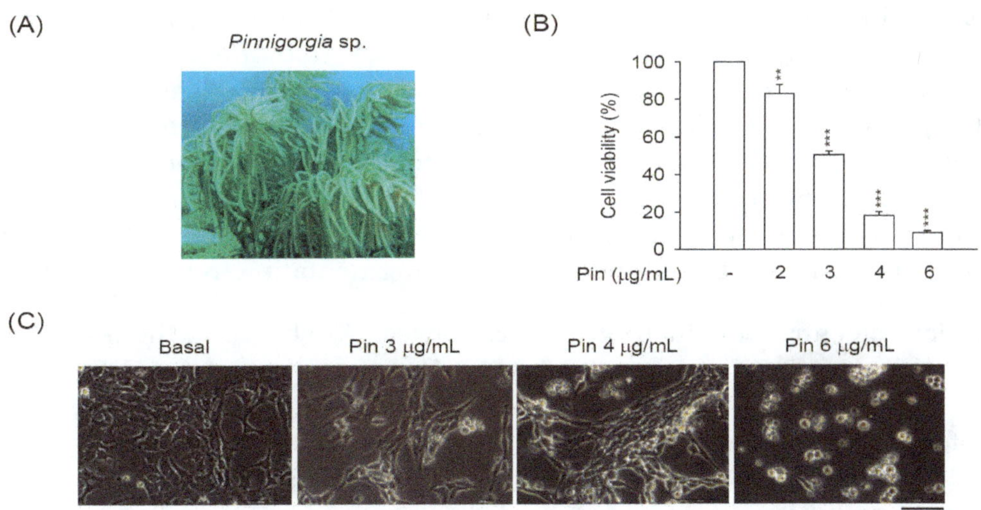

Figure 1. *Cont.*

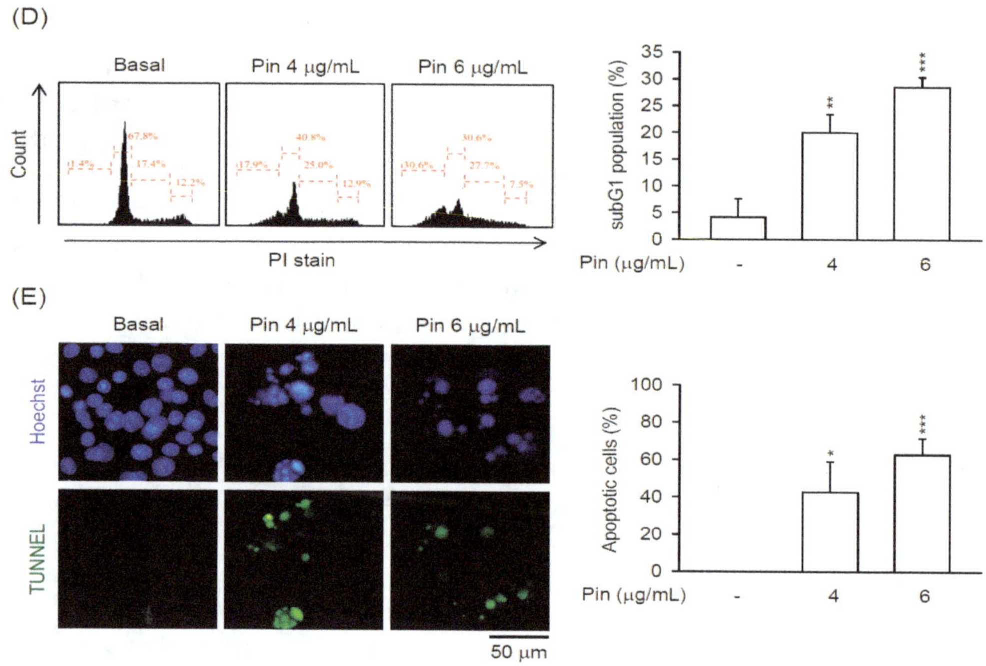

Figure 1. Pin elicits apoptosis in hepatic stellate cells (HSCs). HSC-T6 cells were treated with Pin (0–6 μg/mL) for 24 h. (**A**) Gorgonian coral *Pinnigorgia* sp.; (**B**) Cytotoxicity assay was monitored spectrophotometrically at 450 nm; (**C**) Cell retraction, bubbling, and apoptotic bodies were observed using microscopy; (**D**) SubG1 population was examined by propidium iodide (PI) staining and flow cytometry; (**E**) The Pin-induced apoptosis of HSC-T6 cells was determined by terminal deoxynucleotidyl transferase dUTP nick end labeling (TUNEL) assay (green). Hoechst 33,342 (blue) was used to visualize the cell nucleus. All data are expressed as the mean ± S.E.M. ($n = 3$). * $p < 0.05$, ** $p < 0.01$, *** $p < 0.001$ compared with the basal.

2. Results

2.1. Pin Exhibits Caspase-3-Dependent Apoptosis in HSC-T6 Cells

Recently, the extract from a gorgonian coral *Pinnigorgia* sp. (Pin) was isolated and found to suppress the cell viability of rat HSC-T6 cells [11]. However, the pharmacological mechanism of Pin-induced suppression of HSC-T6 cell viability is still undiscovered. Here, we studied the detailed mechanism of Pin-inhibited viability in HSCs. Pin inhibited the cell viability of HSC-T6 cells in a concentration-dependent manner (2–6 μg/mL) (Figure 1B). To monitor the Pin-induced cell death in HSC-T6 cells, we observed the changes in cellular morphology. Pin (3–6 μg/mL) gradually led to the apoptotic changes of HSC-T6 cells, including cell shrinkage and the formation of membrane blebs, apoptotic body, and cell debris (Figure 1C). To further determine the apoptotic features, flow cytometry and terminal deoxynucleotidyl transferase (TdT) dUTP nick-end labeling (TUNEL) staining were assayed. Pin (4 and 6 μg/mL) apparently increased the subG1 population, which was as an indicator of apoptosis. Also, Pin (4 and 6 μg/mL) induced DNA fragmentation in HSC-T6 cells (Figure 1D,E).

Caspase-3 plays a central role in apoptotic responses. As shown in the results, the expression of cleaved caspase-3 was significantly increased in Pin (6 μg/mL)-treated HSC-T6 cells during 9–24 h (Figure 2A). Moreover, the Pin-inhibited cell viability in HSC-T6 cells was blocked by pre-treatment of the general caspase inhibitor, Z-VAD-FMK, or the specific caspase-3 inhibitor, Z-DEVD-FMK (Figure 2B), suggesting that Pin-induced apoptosis in HSC-T6 cells occurs through caspase-3-dependent pathway.

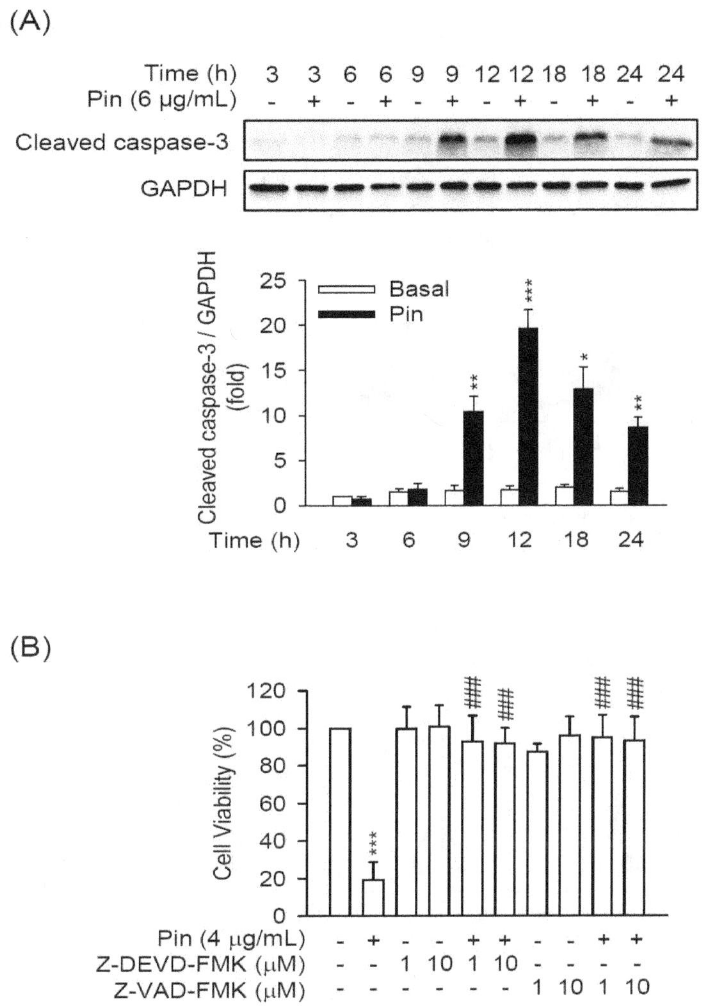

Figure 2. Pin-induced apoptosis is dependent on caspase-3 activation in HSCs. (**A**) HSC-T6 cells were treated with Pin (6 μg/mL) for 3–24 h. Cleaved caspase-3 and glyceraldehyde-3-phosphate dehydrogenase (GAPDH) were analyzed by immunoblot analysis using antibodies against cleaved caspase-3 or GAPDH. Quantitation of the cleaved caspase-3/GAPDH ratio is shown; (**B**) HSC-T6 cells were pretreated with Z-DEVD-FMK (caspase-3 inhibitor) or Z-VAD-FMK (general caspase inhibitor) for 1 h. Subsequently, HSC-T6 was incubated with Pin (4 μg/mL) for 24 h. The cytotoxicity assay was monitored spectrophotometrically at 450 nm. All data are expressed as the mean ± S.E.M. ($n = 3$). $^{*}p < 0.05$, $^{**}p < 0.01$, $^{***}p < 0.001$ compared with the basal; $^{\#\#\#}p < 0.001$ compared with the Pin alone.

2.2. Pin-Induced Apoptosis Is Dependent on Intracellular ROS Production in HSC-T6 Cells

Until now, GSH depletion-induced ROS accumulation is known to cause caspase-3-dependent apoptosis in HSCs [18,19]. To investigate whether Pin causes oxidative stress in HSCs, the intracellular ROS production was determined. Pin induced ROS production in HSC-T6 cells in a dose-dependent (3–6 μg/mL) manner (Figure 3A). Furthermore, the thiol-antioxidant, NAC, inhibited the Pin-induced ROS generation in HSC-T6 cells (Figure 3B). Importantly, both NAC and a permeable membrane derivative of GSH, glutathione monoethyl ester (GSH-MEE), apparently attenuated the Pin-induced caspase-3 activation, cell death, and DNA fragmentation in HSC-T6 cells (Figures 3C,D and S1), suggesting that the Pin-induced ROS production is a cause of cell death in HSC-T6 cells.

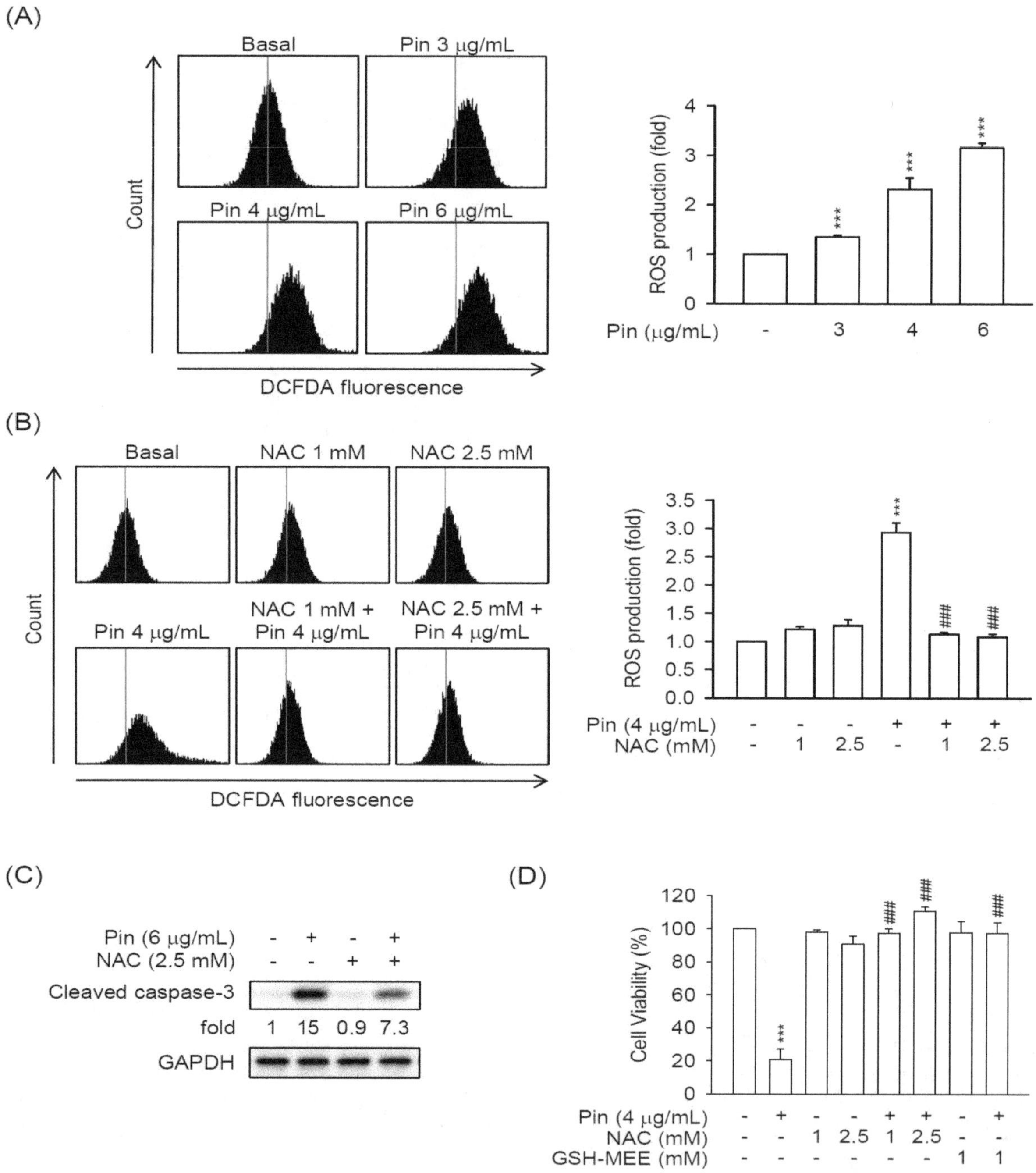

Figure 3. Pin-induced apoptosis relies on intracellular reactive oxygen species (ROS) production in HSCs. (**A**) HSC-T6 cells were treated with Pin (3–6 μg/mL) for 6 h. Intracellular ROS was determined by 2′,7′-dichlorofluorescein diacetate (DCFDA) assay using flow cytometry; (**B**) HSC-T6 cells were pretreated with *N*-acetylcysteine (NAC; 1 and 2.5 mM for 1 h) before the addition of Pin (4 μg/mL for 6 h). Intracellular ROS was determined by DCFDA assay using flow cytometry; (**C**) HSC-T6 cells were pretreated with NAC (2.5 mM) for 1 h and then exposed to Pin (6 μg/mL) for 12 h. Cleaved caspase-3 and GAPDH was analyzed by immunoblot analysis using antibodies against cleaved caspase-3 or GAPDH; (**D**) HSC-T6 cells were pretreated with NAC (1 and 2.5 mM) or glutathione reduced ethyl ester (GSH-MEE) (1 mM) for 1 h and then exposed to Pin (4 μg/mL) for 24 h. The cytotoxicity assay was monitored spectrophotometrically at 450 nm. All data are expressed as the mean ± S.E.M. ($n = 3$). *** $p < 0.001$ compared with the basal. ### $p < 0.001$ compared with the Pin alone.

2.3. Pin-Induced Cell Death of HSC-T6 Cells Is through ERK and JNK Pathway

The significance of MAPKs pathway in cell growth and apoptosis has been well established [24]. Therefore, we next examined whether MAPKs is involved in the Pin-induced apoptosis in HSC-T6 cells. Pin (6 μg/mL) significantly induced the phosphorylation of ERK and JNK but not p38 MAPK in HSC-T6 cells for 3–12 h (Figure S2A). In addition, Pin led to ERK and JNK activation in HSC-T6 cells in a dose-dependent manner. The pharmacological inhibitors of JNK (SP600125) and ERK (PD98059) completely blocked the Pin-repressed cell viability in HSC-T6 cells (Figure 4), suggesting the critical role of ERK and JNK activation in Pin-induced apoptosis in HSCs. In agreement with the inactivation of p38 MAPK in Pin-treated HSC-T6 cells, the inhibitors of p38 (SB202190 and 203580) failed to restrict the Pin-induced cell death (Figure S2B).

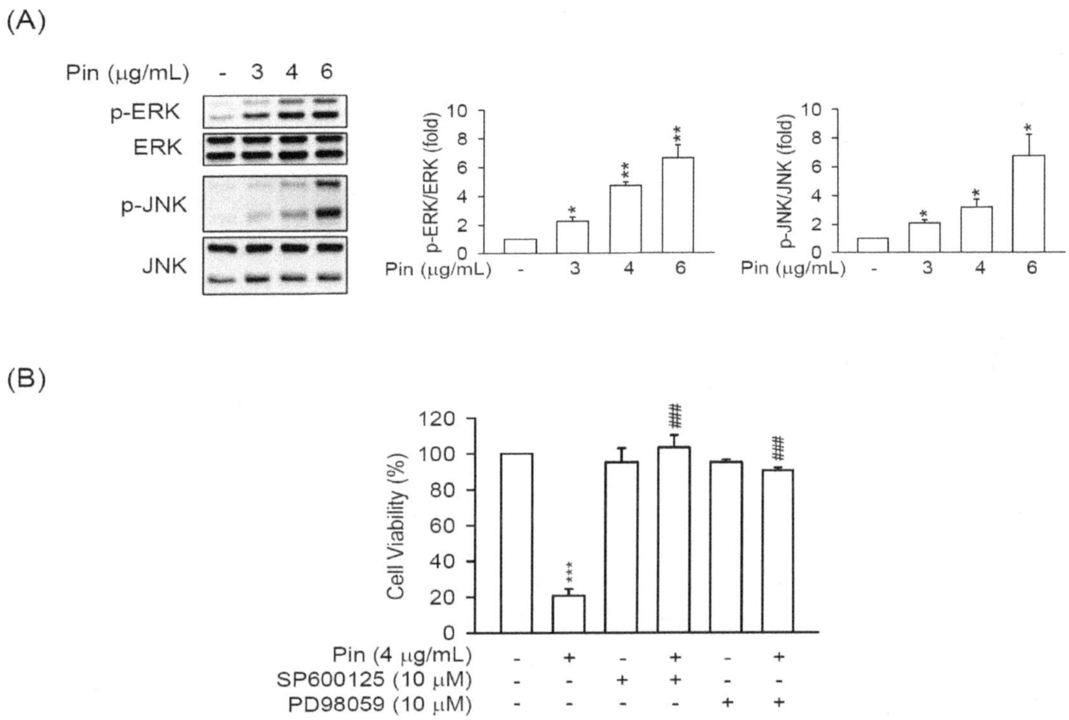

Figure 4. Pin-induced apoptosis is mediated through JNK and ERK pathway in HSCs. (**A**) HSC-T6 cells were treated with Pin (3–6 μg/mL) for 6 h. Phosphorylation of ERK and JNK were analyzed by immunoblot analysis using antibodies against p-JNK or p-ERK. Quantitation of the p-JNK/JNK and p-ERK/ERK ratio was shown; (**B**) HSC-T6 cells were pretreated with SP600125 (JNK inhibitor; 10 μM) or PD98059 (ERK inhibitor; 10 μM) for 1 h and then exposure to Pin (4 μg/mL) for 24 h. Cytotoxicity assay was monitored spectrophotometrically at 450 nm. All data are expressed as the mean ± S.E.M. ($n = 3$). * $p < 0.05$, ** $p < 0.01$, *** $p < 0.001$ compared with the basal. ### $p < 0.001$ compared with the Pin alone.

2.4. Pin-Activated ERK and JNK Pathway Act as Downstream Signals of ROS Production in HSC-T6 Cells

It has been documented that ERK may be an upstream regulator of ROS-induced apoptosis [25], however, different studies have reported conflicting findings [26]. To clarify the relationship between ROS and ERK/JNK in Pin-treated HSC-T6 cells, the HSC-T6 cells were pre-treated with inhibitors of ERK/JNK or thiol-antioxidant to examine it. As shown in the results, NAC evidently restrained the Pin-induced ERK and JNK activation in HSC-T6 cells (Figure 5A). In contrast, the inhibitors of JNK (SP600125) and ERK (PD98059) failed to alter Pin-induced ROS production in HSC-T6 cells (Figure 5B). Taken together, we propose that Pin stimulates the ROS production and subsequently activates ERK/JNK signaling leading to caspase-3-dependent cell death in HSC-T6 cells.

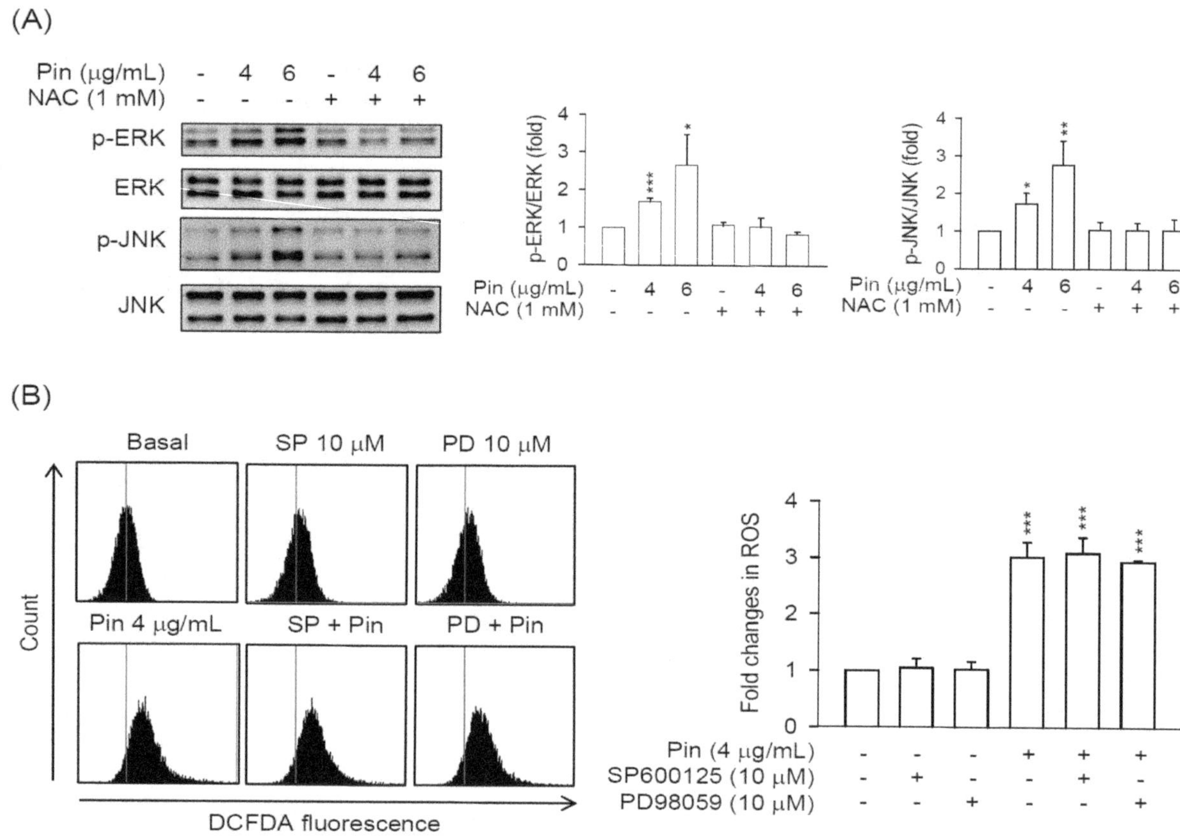

Figure 5. Pin-activated ERK and JNK signaling is triggered by ROS production in HSCs. (**A**) HSC-T6 cells were pretreated with or without NAC (1 mM) for 1 h and then exposed to Pin (4 or 6 μg/mL) for 6 h. Phosphorylation of ERK and JNK were analyzed by immunoblot analysis using antibodies against p-JNK or p-ERK. Quantitation of the p-JNK/JNK and p-ERK/ERK ratio was shown; (**B**) HSC-T6 cells were pretreated with SP600125 (JNK inhibitor; 10 μM) or PD98059 (ERK inhibitor; 10 μM) for 1 h and then exposed to Pin (4 μg/mL) for 6 h. Intracellular ROS was determined by DCFDA assay using flow cytometry. All data are expressed as the mean ± S.E.M. ($n = 3$). * $p < 0.05$, ** $p < 0.01$, *** $p < 0.001$ compared with the basal.

2.5. Pinnigorgiol a Serves as a Bioactive Component of Pin to Trigger the ROS-Dependent Apoptosis in HSC-T6 Cells

Three novel 9,11-secosterols, pinnigorgiol A–C, were isolated from Pin to test the viability of HSC-T6 cells. Among them, pinnigorgiol A and B displayed inhibitory effect on the cell viability with an IC_{50} value of 5.77 ± 0.27 and 7.89 ± 0.52 μM, respectively, but pinnigorgiol C had no effect on cell viability [16]. Pinnigorgiol A (Figure 6A) exhibited the maximum inhibitory effect on the cell viability of HSC-T6 cells; however, the pharmacological mechanism is still unknown. As shown in Figure 6B, pinnigorgiol A (1–10 μM) inhibited the cell viability of HSC-T6 cells in a dose-dependent manner. Pinnigorgiol B (3–10 μM) also dose-dependently repressed the cell viability of HSC-T6 cells (Figure S3); however, the inhibitory effect was weaker than pinnigorgiol A. Further, pinnigorgiol A induced ROS production and DNA fragmentation in HSC-T6 cells. Furthermore, the pinnigorgiol A-induced apoptotic effect and cell death were significantly attenuated by the thio-antioxidant NAC in HSC-T6 cells (Figure 6C–E), suggesting that the cytotoxic effect of Pin and pinnigorgiol A is comparable in HSCs. In summary, we propose that pinnigorgiol A may be a representative bioactive component of Pin that elicits apoptosis in HSCs through ROS-ERK/JNK-caspase-3 signal pathway and may offer a possible medical application in liver pathogenesis.

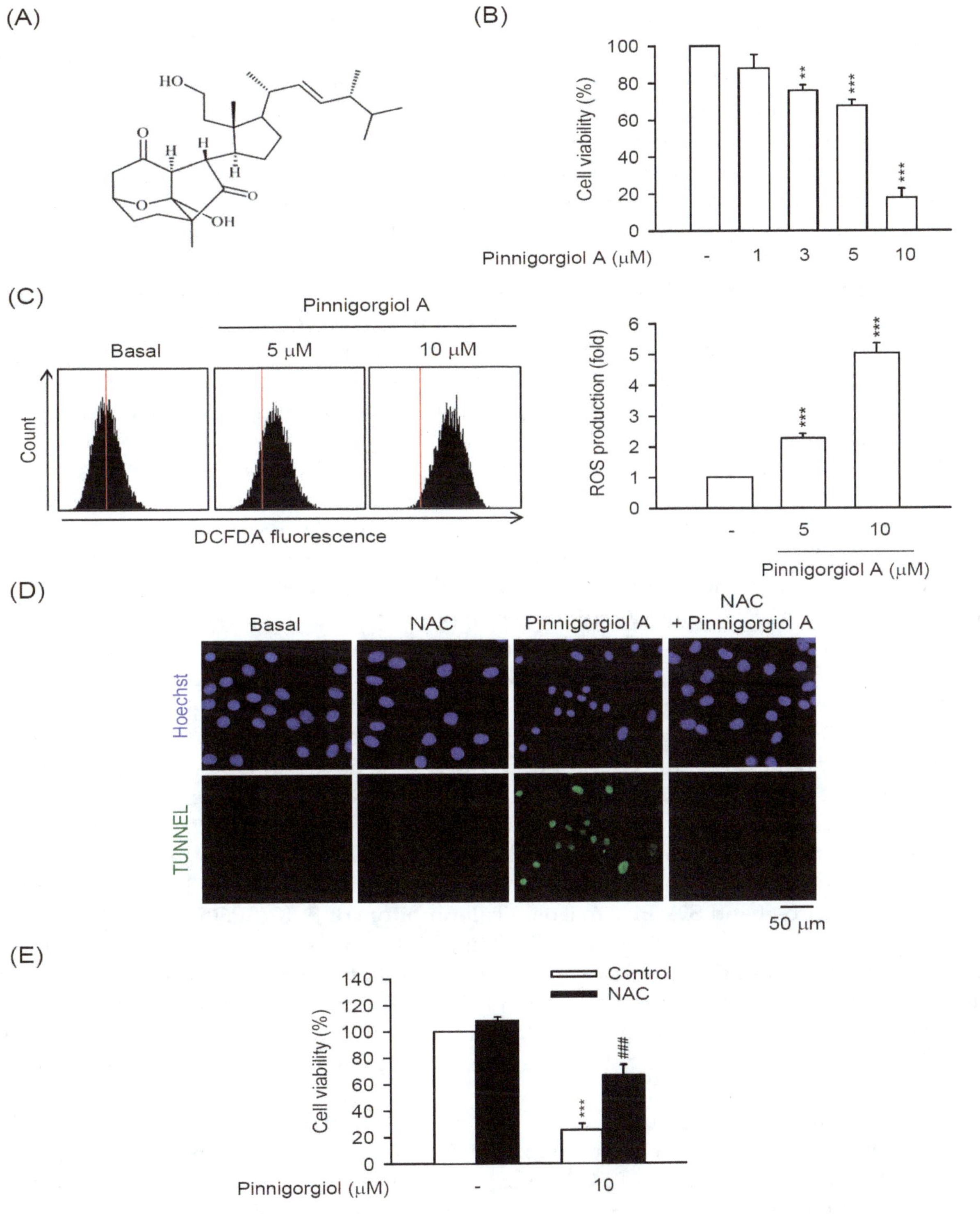

Figure 6. Pinnigorgiol A exhibits ROS-dependent apoptosis in HSCs. (**A**) Chemical structure of pinnigorgiol A; (**B**) HSC-T6 cells were treated with pinnigorgiol A (1–10 μM) for 24 h. Cytotoxicity assay was monitored spectrophotometrically at 450 nm; (**C**) HSC-T6 cells were treated with pinnigorgiol A (5 or 10 μM) for 6 h. Intracellular ROS was determined by DCFDA assay and flow cytometry; (**D**) HSC-T6 cells were treated with pinnigorgiol A (10 μM) for 12 h. Apoptotic effect of pinnigorgiol A was determined by TUNEL assay (green). Hoechst 33,342 (blue) was used to visualize the cell nucleus; (**E**) HSC-T6 cells were pretreated with NAC (2.5 mM) for 1 h and then incubated with pinnigorgiol A (10 μM) for 24 h. Cytotoxicity assay was monitored spectrophotometrically at 450 nm. All data are expressed as the mean ± S.E.M. (n = 3). ** $p < 0.01$; *** $p < 0.001$ compared with the basal. ### $p < 0.001$ compared with the pinnigorgiol A alone.

3. Discussion

The activation of HSCs is one of the major contributors to hepatic fibrosis. Emerging evidences show that promoting cell death of HSCs is a potential strategy in the remission of liver fibrosis [4,5,27,28]. In the present study, our data revealed that Pin significantly induced cell apoptosis in HSCs in a concentration-dependent way. Pin significantly exhibited an inhibitory effect on the cell viability in HSC-T6 cells with apparent apoptotic changes, including cell shrinkage, chromatin condensation, and membrane blebs and apoptotic bodies formation (Figure 1). Moreover, it has been proven that DNA fragmentation usually accompanies increased sub-G1 population and activated caspase-3 in apoptotic cells [29–31]. We also found that Pin increased the sub-G1 population, DNA fragmentation, and caspase-3 activation in HSC-T6 cells (Figures 1 and 2A), suggesting that the Pin-repressed HSCs viability is dependent on caspase-3-mediated apoptosis. In agreement with this proposal, the apoptotic effects of Pin were completely reversed by Z-DEVD-FMK, a specific caspase-3 inhibitor (Figure 3B). Activation of caspase-3 has a pivotal role in the apoptotic responses. Thus, Pin stimulated the apoptotic process in HSCs through caspase-3-dependent pathway. These findings suggest a possibility of Pin to restrict HSCs activation during liver pathogenesis.

Oxidative stress can induce the execution of the apoptotic pathway and excessive ROS production will lead to aggravation of apoptosis [32–34]. So far, ROS generation has been documented to cause apoptosis in HSCs [18,20,35]. In support of this theory, intracellular ROS was increased by treatment of Pin in HSC-T6 cells that was significantly reversed by a thiol-based antioxidant, NAC (Figure 3). In addition, GSH is another intracellular antioxidant that regulates the cell viability in HSCs and GSH displays an inhibitory effect against ROS-induced apoptotic cell death [17,18]. In addition, NAC and cell-permeable GSH (GSH-MEE) significantly blocked the Pin-inhibited cell viability in HSC-T6 cells, suggesting that the Pin-induced apoptosis is based on ROS production in HSCs.

MAPKs (ERK, JNK, and p38 MAPK) are important mediators of signal transduction under oxidative stress in HSCs to control cell growth, differentiation, survival, and apoptosis [18,36–38]. In our previous study, the apoptotic effect of oridonin-induced ROS in HSC-T6 cells was not affected by specific inhibitors of p38 MAPK, JNK, and ERK, respectively [20]. However, Huang and colleagues found that the oridonin-induced apoptosis and ROS production in HepG2 cells occurred through MAPK signaling pathways [37]. Thus, the role of MAPKs in the oxidative stress-elicited HSCs apoptosis is still uncertain. As the results showed, Pin induced the phosphorylation of ERK and JNK but not p38 MAPK in HSCs (Figures 4 and S2). Pharmacological inhibitors of JNK (SP600125) and ERK (PD98059) rescued the Pin-induced cell apoptosis in HSCs, suggesting that the apoptotic effects of Pin in HSC were mediated by ERK and JNK. It has been documented that blocking the p38 MAPK by a specific inhibitor, SB203580, increased the proliferation in HSCs [39], whereas activation of p38 induced HSC apoptosis [10,40]. This may explain the selective inhibition of Pin on the activation of ERK and JNK but not p38 MAPK in HSCs, which may also serve as a means to explore the relationship between MAPKs and apoptosis in HSCs.

Three pure compounds, pinnigorgiol A-C, were isolated from Pin to decrease the viability of HSC-T6 cells at 10 μM. Among them, pinnigorgiol A displayed the maximum inhibitory effect on the cell viability with an IC_{50} value of 5.77 ± 0.27 μM [16]. In the present study, we unraveled that pinnigorgiol A-induced apoptosis of HSCs was also mediated by increasing ROS production (Figure 6), suggesting that pinnigorgiol A may be the representative bioactive compound of Pin leading to cell death in HSCs. To date, marine bioactive compounds have been characterized and have therapeutic potential to treat human disorders; however, the studies investigating their role in treating liver diseases are still limited [10]. Therefore, pinnigorgiol A may provide a therapeutic opportunity to retrain HSCs activation in liver fibrosis. Activation of HSCs is mediated by various mechanisms and some of them exhibit the therapeutic specificity for restricting HSC activation but not affecting hepatocytes [2]. In this study, the proof of whether Pin or pinnigorgiol A leads to apoptosis in hepatocytes is not carried out yet. The possible liver injuries by Pin or pinnigorgiol A still should be carefully dissected in the future.

In summary, our findings reveal an important example of how a novel coral extract from *Pinnigorgia* sp. (Pin) leads to a caspase-3-dependent apoptosis in HSCs via inducing ROS-mediated ERK/JNK signaling. Pinnigorgiol A may be a bioactive compound of Pin that possibly attenuates HSCs activation in liver fibrosis.

4. Materials and Methods

4.1. Reagents

Glutathione monoethyl ester (GSH-MEE) was purchased from Calbiochem (La Jolla, CA, USA). Z-DEVD-FMK and Z-VAD-FMK were obtained from BioVision (Mountain, PA, USA). The cell proliferation reagent WST-1 and RNase A were obtained from Roche Applied Sciences (Mannheim, Germany). Antibodies against cleaved caspase-3, phospho-ERK1/2, ERK1/2, phospho-JNK, and JNK were purchased from Cell Signaling (Beverly, MA, USA). Antibodies against phospho-p38 and p38 MAPK were obtained from Santa Cruz Biotechnology (Santa Cruz, CA, USA). The other chemicals were purchased from Sigma (St. Louis, MO, USA). The extraction and isolation of crude extract from *Pinnigorgia* sp. (Pin) and pinnigorgiol A were carried out as described previously [11,16]. The ^{1}H and ^{13}C NMR spectrum of pinnigorgiol A–C have been identified previously [16]. When Pin and pinnigorgiol A were dissolved in dimethyl sulfoxide (DMSO) (Sigma-Aldrich), the final concentration of DMSO in the cell experiments was 0.1% and did not affect the parameters measured.

4.2. Cell Culture

HSC-T6, a rat HSC cell line, was kindly provided by Professor Scott L. Friedman (Mount Sinai School of Medicine, NY, USA). HSC-T6 cells were cultured at 37 °C in Dulbecco's minimum essential medium (DMEM; Gibco, Grand Island, NY, USA) supplemented with 10% fetal bovine serum (FBS) and antibiotics (100 U/mL penicillin, 100 μg/mL streptomycin, and 2.5 μg/mL amphotericin B) in a humidified atmosphere with 5% CO_2.

4.3. Cell Viability Assay

Cell viability was measured using WST-1 assay. HSC-T6 cells were cultured in DMEM containing 0.5% FBS for 24 h. After incubation, cells were incubated with indicated concentrations of Pin or pinnigorgiol A for 24 h. Subsequently, the WST-1 reagent was added and incubated at 37 °C for 2 h. The absorbance was measured spectrophotometrically at 450 nm (Thermo Labsystems, Waltham, MA, USA).

4.4. Analysis of SubG1 Population

HSC-T6 cells were treated with Pin for 24 h and then the cells were harvested and fixed in 70% ethanol for 1 h. After that, the cells were washed with PBS twice and incubated in propidium iodide staining buffer (50 μg/mL propidium iodide, 0.1 mg/mL DNase-free RNase A, and 0.5% Triton X-100) for 30 min at 37 °C. The subG1 population was determined by measuring DNA content using flow cytometry.

4.5. Measurement of Intracellular ROS Generation

The intracellular ROS levels were examined using 2′,7′-dichlorofluorescein diacetate (DCF-DA; Sigma) reagent and analyzed by flow cytometry (BD Biosciences, San Jose, CA, USA).

4.6. Western Blotting

Cell lysates were suspended in lysis buffer (50 mM HEPES, 100 mM NaCl, 1 mM EDTA, 2 mM Na_3VO_4, 5% 2-mercaptoethanol, and 1% Triton-X-100), and then centrifuged at 14,000× *g* for 20 min at 4 °C. Proteins were separated by sodium dodecyl sulfate-polyacrylamide gel electrophoresis (SDS-PAGE) and electrophoresed onto a nitrocellulose membrane. Indicated primary antibodies and horseradish peroxidase-conjugated secondary antibodies were used to determine the protein levels using an enhanced chemiluminescence system. Signals were detected and quantified using a densitometer (UVP, Upland, CA, USA).

4.7. TUNEL Assay

The DNA fragmentation in apoptosis was detected using terminal deoxyribonucleotidyl transferase-mediated dUTP-digoxigenin nick end labeling (TUNEL) apoptosis detection kit (Roche, Mannheim, Germany). The nuclei were counterstained with DAPI. Visual images were analyzed using an OLYMPUS IX 81 microscope (Olympus, Tokyo, Japan).

4.8. Statistical Analysis

Data were expressed as the mean ± standard error of mean (SEM). Statistical comparisons were made between two groups using Student's *t*-test. A value of $p < 0.05$ was considered statistically significant.

5. Conclusions

Clearance of activated HSCs is a potential strategy to treat liver fibrosis by pharmacologically prompting apoptosis. In the present study, we found that the extract from a gorgonian coral *Pinnigorgia* sp. (Pin) led to caspase-3-dependent apoptosis in HSCs that is modulated via ROS production and subsequent ERK/JNK activation. Moreover, the Pin-derived pure compound, pinnigorgiol A, was identified as a bioactive component which elicited apoptosis and ROS production in HSCs. Altogether, we uncovered the molecular mechanisms of the marine natural products, Pin and pinnigorgiol A, and predicted their therapeutic potential eliminating HSCs in liver diseases.

Acknowledgments: This research was financial supported by the grants from the Ministry of Science Technology (MOST 106-2320-B-255-003-MY3 and MOST 104-2320-B-255-004-MY3), Ministry of Education (EMRPD1G0231), and Chang Gung Memorial Hospital (CMRPG660201, CMRPG670421, CMRPG6D0081~3, CMRPF1F0011~3, CMRPF1F0061~3, and BMRP450), Taiwan. The funders had no role in study design, data collection and analysis, decision to publish, or preparation of the manuscript.

Author Contributions: L.-M.K., P.-J.C., C.-T.H. and Y.-H.W. designed, performed and analyzed experiments. P.-J.S. and Y.-C.C. provided Pin and pinnigorgiol A. P.-J.C. and T.-L.H. wrote and completed the manuscript. T.-L.H. supervised the entire study.

References

1. Yin, C.; Evason, K.J.; Asahina, K.; Stainier, D.Y. Hepatic stellate cells in liver development, regeneration, and cancer. *J. Clin. Investig.* **2013**, *123*, 1902–1910. [CrossRef] [PubMed]
2. Tsuchida, T.; Friedman, S.L. Mechanisms of hepatic stellate cell activation. *Nat. Rev. Gastroenterol. Hepatol.* **2017**, *14*, 397–411. [CrossRef] [PubMed]
3. Tacke, F.; Trautwein, C. Mechanisms of liver fibrosis resolution. *J. Hepatol.* **2015**, *63*, 1038–1039. [CrossRef] [PubMed]
4. Friedman, S.L. Evolving challenges in hepatic fibrosis. *Nat. Rev. Gastroenterol. Hepatol.* **2010**, *7*, 425–436. [CrossRef] [PubMed]
5. Huang, Y.; Deng, X.; Liang, J. Modulation of hepatic stellate cells and reversibility of hepatic fibrosis. *Exp. Cell Res.* **2017**, *352*, 420–426. [CrossRef] [PubMed]
6. Zhang, C.Y.; Yuan, W.G.; He, P.; Lei, J.H.; Wang, C.X. Liver fibrosis and hepatic stellate cells: Etiology, pathological hallmarks and therapeutic targets. *World J. Gastroenterol.* **2016**, *22*, 10512–10522. [CrossRef] [PubMed]
7. Fallowfield, J.A. Therapeutic targets in liver fibrosis. *Am. J. Physiol. Gastrointest. Liver Physiol.* **2011**, *300*, G709–G715. [CrossRef] [PubMed]
8. Molinski, T.F.; Dalisay, D.S.; Lievens, S.L.; Saludes, J.P. Drug development from marine natural products. *Nat. Rev. Drug Discov.* **2009**, *8*, 69–85. [CrossRef] [PubMed]

9. Fitton, J.H. Therapies from fucoidan; multifunctional marine polymers. *Mar. Drugs* **2011**, *9*, 1731–1760. [CrossRef] [PubMed]
10. Nair, D.G.; Weiskirchen, R.; Al-Musharafi, S.K. The use of marine-derived bioactive compounds as potential hepatoprotective agents. *Acta Pharmacol. Sin.* **2015**, *36*, 158–170. [CrossRef] [PubMed]
11. Chang, Y.C.; Kuo, L.M.; Hwang, T.L.; Yeh, J.; Wen, Z.H.; Fang, L.S.; Wu, Y.C.; Lin, C.S.; Sheu, J.H.; Sung, P.J. Pinnisterols A–C, New 9,11-Secosterols from a Gorgonian *Pinnigorgia* sp. *Mar. Drugs* **2016**, *14*, 12. [CrossRef] [PubMed]
12. Chang, H.H.; Chang, Y.C.; Chen, W.F.; Hwang, T.L.; Fang, L.S.; Wen, Z.H.; Chen, Y.H.; Wu, Y.C.; Sung, P.J. Pubinernoid A and Apo-9′-fucoxanthinone, Secondary Metabolites from a Gorgonian Coral *Pinnigorgia* sp. *Nat. Prod. Commun.* **2016**, *11*, 707–708. [PubMed]
13. Chang, Y.C.; Hwang, T.L.; Sheu, J.H.; Wu, Y.C.; Sung, P.J. New Anti-Inflammatory 9,11-Secosterols with a Rare Tricyclo [5,2,1,1] decane Ring from a Formosan Gorgonian *Pinnigorgia* sp. *Mar. Drugs* **2016**, *14*, 218. [CrossRef] [PubMed]
14. Chang, Y.C.; Hwang, T.L.; Chao, C.H.; Sung, P.J. New Marine Sterols from a Gorgonian *Pinnigorgia* sp. *Molecules* **2017**, *22*, 393. [CrossRef] [PubMed]
15. Chang, Y.C.; Hwang, T.L.; Kuo, L.M.; Sung, P.J. Pinnisterols D–J, New 11-Acetoxy-9,11-secosterols with a 1,4-Quinone Moiety from Formosan Gorgonian Coral *Pinnigorgia* sp. (Gorgoniidae). *Mar. Drugs* **2017**, *15*, 11. [CrossRef] [PubMed]
16. Chang, Y.; Kuo, L.; Su, J.; Hwang, T.; Kuo, Y.; Lin, C.; Wu, Y.; Sheu, J.; Sung, P. Pinnigorgiols A–C, 9,11-secosterols with a rare ring arrangement from a gorgonian coral *Pinnigorgia* sp. *Tetrahedron* **2016**, *72*, 999–1004. [CrossRef]
17. Brunati, A.M.; Pagano, M.A.; Bindoli, A.; Rigobello, M.P. Thiol redox systems and protein kinases in hepatic stellate cell regulatory processes. *Free Radic. Res.* **2010**, *44*, 363–378. [CrossRef] [PubMed]
18. Dunning, S.; Ur Rehman, A.; Tiebosch, M.H.; Hannivoort, R.A.; Haijer, F.W.; Woudenberg, J.; van den Heuvel, F.A.; Buist-Homan, M.; Faber, K.N.; Moshage, H. Glutathione and antioxidant enzymes serve complementary roles in protecting activated hepatic stellate cells against hydrogen peroxide-induced cell death. *Biochim. Biophys. Acta* **2013**, *1832*, 2027–2034. [CrossRef] [PubMed]
19. Circu, M.L.; Aw, T.Y. Glutathione and apoptosis. *Free Radic. Res.* **2008**, *42*, 689–706. [CrossRef] [PubMed]
20. Kuo, L.M.; Kuo, C.Y.; Lin, C.Y.; Hung, M.F.; Shen, J.J.; Hwang, T.L. Intracellular glutathione depletion by oridonin leads to apoptosis in hepatic stellate cells. *Molecules* **2014**, *19*, 3327–3344. [CrossRef] [PubMed]
21. Dong, H.; Guo, H.; Liang, Y.; Wang, X.; Niu, Y. Astragaloside IV synergizes with ferulic acid to suppress hepatic stellate cells activation in vitro. *Free Radic. Res.* **2017**, *51*, 167–178. [CrossRef] [PubMed]
22. Huang, Y.; Li, X.; Wang, Y.; Wang, H.; Huang, C.; Li, J. Endoplasmic reticulum stress-induced hepatic stellate cell apoptosis through calcium-mediated JNK/P38 MAPK and Calpain/Caspase-12 pathways. *Mol. Cell. Biochem.* **2014**, *394*, 1–12. [CrossRef] [PubMed]
23. Brenner, C.; Galluzzi, L.; Kepp, O.; Kroemer, G. Decoding cell death signals in liver inflammation. *J. Hepatol.* **2013**, *59*, 583–594. [CrossRef] [PubMed]
24. Takeda, K.; Naguro, I.; Nishitoh, H.; Matsuzawa, A.; Ichijo, H. Apoptosis signaling kinases: From stress response to health outcomes. *Antioxid. Redox Signal.* **2011**, *15*, 719–761. [CrossRef] [PubMed]
25. Sun, X.; Zhang, X.; Hu, H.; Lu, Y.; Chen, J.; Yasuda, K.; Wang, H. Berberine inhibits hepatic stellate cell proliferation and prevents experimental liver fibrosis. *Biol. Pharm. Bull.* **2009**, *32*, 1533–1537. [CrossRef] [PubMed]
26. Wasmuth, H.E.; Tacke, F.; Trautwein, C. Chemokines in liver inflammation and fibrosis. *Semin. Liver Dis.* **2010**, *30*, 215–225. [CrossRef] [PubMed]
27. Puche, J.E.; Saiman, Y.; Friedman, S.L. Hepatic stellate cells and liver fibrosis. *Compr. Physiol.* **2013**, *3*, 1473–1492. [PubMed]
28. Ray, K. Liver: Hepatic stellate cells hold the key to liver fibrosis. *Nat. Rev. Gastroenterol. Hepatol.* **2014**, *11*, 74. [CrossRef] [PubMed]
29. Kim, S.Y.; Kang, K.L.; Lee, J.C.; Heo, J.S. Nicotinic acetylcholine receptor alpha7 and beta4 subunits contribute nicotine-induced apoptosis in periodontal ligament stem cells. *Mol. Cells* **2012**, *33*, 343–350. [CrossRef] [PubMed]

30. Pamenter, M.E.; Perkins, G.A.; Gu, X.Q.; Ellisman, M.H.; Haddad, G.G. DIDS (4,4-diisothiocyanatostilbene disulphonic acid) induces apoptotic cell death in a hippocampal neuronal cell line and is not neuroprotective against ischemic stress. *PLoS ONE* **2013**, *8*, e60804. [CrossRef] [PubMed]
31. Posadas, I.; Santos, P.; Cena, V. Acetaminophen induces human neuroblastoma cell death through NFKB activation. *PLoS ONE* **2012**, *7*, e50160. [CrossRef] [PubMed]
32. Ricci, C.; Pastukh, V.; Leonard, J.; Turrens, J.; Wilson, G.; Schaffer, D.; Schaffer, S.W. Mitochondrial DNA damage triggers mitochondrial-superoxide generation and apoptosis. *Am. J. Physiol. Cell Physiol.* **2008**, *294*, C413–C422. [CrossRef] [PubMed]
33. Crosas-Molist, E.; Fabregat, I. Role of NADPH oxidases in the redox biology of liver fibrosis. *Redox Biol.* **2015**, *6*, 106–111. [CrossRef] [PubMed]
34. Wang, K. Autophagy and apoptosis in liver injury. *Cell Cycle* **2015**, *14*, 1631–1642. [CrossRef] [PubMed]
35. Siegmund, S.V.; Qian, T.; de Minicis, S.; Harvey-White, J.; Kunos, G.; Vinod, K.Y.; Hungund, B.; Schwabe, R.F. The endocannabinoid 2-arachidonoyl glycerol induces death of hepatic stellate cells via mitochondrial reactive oxygen species. *FASEB J.* **2007**, *21*, 2798–2806. [CrossRef] [PubMed]
36. Chowdhury, A.A.; Chaudhuri, J.; Biswas, N.; Manna, A.; Chatterjee, S.; Mahato, S.K.; Chaudhuri, U.; Jaisankar, P.; Bandyopadhyay, S. Synergistic apoptosis of CML cells by buthionine sulfoximine and hydroxychavicol correlates with activation of AIF and GSH-ROS-JNK-ERK-iNOS pathway. *PLoS ONE* **2013**, *8*, e73672. [CrossRef] [PubMed]
37. Huang, J.; Wu, L.; Tashiro, S.; Onodera, S.; Ikejima, T. Reactive oxygen species mediate oridonin-induced HepG2 apoptosis through p53, MAPK, and mitochondrial signaling pathways. *J. Pharmacol. Sci.* **2008**, *107*, 370–379. [CrossRef] [PubMed]
38. Szuster-Ciesielska, A.; Mizerska-Dudka, M.; Daniluk, J.; Kandefer-Szerszen, M. Butein inhibits ethanol-induced activation of liver stellate cells through TGF-beta, NFkappaB, p38, and JNK signaling pathways and inhibition of oxidative stress. *J. Gastroenterol.* **2013**, *48*, 222–237. [CrossRef] [PubMed]
39. Schnabl, B.; Bradham, C.A.; Bennett, B.L.; Manning, A.M.; Stefanovic, B.; Brenner, D.A. TAK1/JNK and p38 have opposite effects on rat hepatic stellate cells. *Hepatology* **2001**, *34*, 953–963. [CrossRef] [PubMed]
40. Jameel, N.M.; Thirunavukkarasu, C.; Wu, T.; Watkins, S.C.; Friedman, S.L.; Gandhi, C.R. p38-MAPK- and caspase-3-mediated superoxide-induced apoptosis of rat hepatic stellate cells: Reversal by retinoic acid. *J. Cell. Physiol.* **2009**, *218*, 157–166. [CrossRef] [PubMed]

14

Cytotoxic and Antimicrobial Constituents from the Essential Oil of *Lippia alba* (Verbenaceae)

Nara O. dos Santos [1], Renata C. Pascon [1], Marcelo A. Vallim [1], Carlos R. Figueiredo [2], Marisi G. Soares [3], João Henrique G. Lago [1,4,*] and Patricia Sartorelli [1,*]

1. Instituto de Ciências Ambientais, Químicas e Farmacêuticas, Universidade Federal de São Paulo, Diadema 09972-270, SP, Brazil; nara.oshiro@gmail.com (N.O.d.S.); renata.pascon@gmail.com (R.C.P.); marcelo.vallim@gmail.com (M.A.V.)
2. Disciplina de Biologia Celular, Departamento de Micro, Imuno e Parasitologia, Universidade Federal de São Paulo, Sao Paulo 04021-001, SP, Brazil; rogernty@hotmail.com
3. Instituto de Química, Universidade Federal de Alfenas, Alfenas 37130-000, MG, Brazil; marisigs@gmail.com
4. Centro de Ciências Naturais e Humanas, Universidade Federal do ABC, Santo Andre 09210-180, SP, Brazil

* Correspondence: joao.lago@unifesp.br (J.H.G.L.); psartorelli@unifesp.br (P.S.)

Academic Editor: James D. Adams

Abstract: Backgroud: *Lippia alba* (Verbenaceae) is a plant widely used in folk medicine to treat various diseases. The present work deals with the chemical composition of the crude essential oil extracted from leaves of *L. alba* and evaluation of its antimicrobial and cytotoxic activities. **Methods:** Leaves of *L. alba* were extracted by hydrodistillation and analyzed by gas chromatography/mass spectrometry (GC/MS) as well as by nuclear magnetic resonance (NMR) spectroscopy. Cytotoxic and antimicrobial activities of crude essential oil were evaluated in vitro using MTT and broth microdilution assays, respectively. **Results:** Chemical analysis afforded the identification of 39 substances corresponding to 99.45% of the total oil composition. Concerning the main compounds, monoterpenes nerol/geraniol and citral correspond to approximately 50% of crude oil. The cytotoxic activity of obtained essential oil against several tumor cell lines showed IC_{50} values ranging from 45 to 64 μg/mL for B16F10Nex2 (murine melanoma) and A549 (human lung adenocarcinoma). In the antimicrobial assay, was observed that all tested yeast strains, except *C. albicans*, were sensitive to crude essential oil. MIC values were two to four-folds lower than those determined to bacterial strains. **Conclusion:** Analysis of chemical composition of essential oils from leaves of *L. alba* suggested a new chemotype nerol/geraniol and citral. Based in biological evidences, a possible application for studied oil as an antifungal in medicine, as well as in agriculture, is described.

Keywords: *Lippia alba*; essential oil; cytotoxic activity; antimicrobial activity

---

1. Introduction

The Verbenaceae family, with tropical and subtropical distribution, is composed of approximately 90 genera, including *Lippia* [1], with more than 200 species of herbaceous plants, small shrubs, and trees [2,3]. Most of these species have traditionally been used in the treatment of gastrointestinal and respiratory diseases [4]. Several pharmacological aspects have been ascribed to the genus *Lippia*, including antimicrobial, antifungal, antimalarial, larvicidal, antispasmodic, analgesic, anti-inflammatory, and antipyretic activities. *Lippia alba* (Mill.) N.E. Brown is native to the Americas widely distributed across the Southern United States and Northern Argentina [5]. In Brazil, this plant is popularly known as lemon balm [6,7] and have been used in folk medicine for the treatment of various diseases, such as gastric diseases, diarrhea, fever, asthma, cough, and soothing, antispasmodic, and emenagoga [2,8–13]. As other species from the same genus, phytochemicals from *L. alba* exhibited antibacterial, antifungal, antiviral, antiprotozoal, analgesic, anti-inflammatory, cytotoxic, antioxidant, and acaricidal activities [5]. Essential oils obtained from the leaves of *L. alba* were previously studied and three different chemotypes were reported: myrcene/citral, limonene/citral and limonene/carvone [14]. Zoghbi et al. [15] classified three other chemotypes: eucalyptol/limonene, limonene/carvone, and citral/germacrene-D. In addition to these volatile compounds, other monoterpenes and phenylpropanoids have been described as main metabolites in the essential oils from *L. alba*: linalool, β-caryophyllene, tagetone, myrcene, γ-terpinene, camphor, estragole, eucalyptol, camphor, limonene, and piperitone [12–18]. This variability has been explained due to factors such as seasons, flowering time, plant age, amount of precipitation, geographic and climatic factors [8,12,19], as well as the part of the studied plant, extraction method, soil characteristics, and the genetic variability of these plants [12,20–23]. These differences may lead to a different oil composition and, therefore, to different pharmacological effects [9,12]. As part of our continuous study with volatile oils from Brazilian species [24–26], the present work deals with the chemical composition of the essential oil from leaves of the Brazilian species of *L. alba*, as well as the cytotoxic and antimicrobial evaluation of crude essential oil.

2. Materials and Methods

2.1. General Experimental Procedures

^1H and ^{13}C NMR spectra of crude oil were registered, respectively, at 300 and 75 MHz into a Ultrashield 300 Advance III spectrometer (Bruker, Fremont, CA, USA) using $CDCl_3$ (Aldrich, St. Louis, MO, USA) as solvent and tetramethylsilane (TMS) as internal standard. Gas chromatograms were obtained on a GC-2010 gas chromatograph (Shimadzu, Kyoto, Japan) equipped with an FID-detector and AOC-20i automatic injector (Shimadzu, Kyoto, Japan) using a RtX-5 (5% phenyl, 95% polydimethylsiloxane-30 m × 0.32 mm × 0.25 μm film thickness, Restek (Bellefonte, PA, USA)) capillary column. These analyses were performed by injecting 1.0 μL of a 1.0 mg/mL solution of volatile oil in CH_2Cl_2 in a split mode (1:10) employing helium as the carrier gas (1 mL/min) under the following conditions: injector and detector temperatures of 220 °C and 250 °C, respectively; oven programmed temperature from 40 to 240 °C at 3 °C/min, holding 5 min at 240 °C. The percentage compositions of the oil samples were computed by internal normalization from the flame ionization detector gas chromatography (GC-FID) peak areas without using correction for response factors. Gas chromatography coupled to low resolution electronic impact mass spectrometry (GC-LREIMS) analysis was conducted in a GC-17A chromatograph interfaced with a MS-QP-5050A mass spectrometer (Shimadzu, Kyoto, Japan). The LREIMS operating conditions were an ionization voltage of 70 eV and an ion source temperature of 230 °C with the same conditions described above. The identification of the individual compounds was performed by comparison of retention indexes (determined relatively to the retention times of a series of *n*-alkanes) and comparison of recorded mass spectra with those available in the system [27].

2.2. Plant Material

Leaves of *L. alba* were collected at Instituto Plantarum de Estudos da Flora in Nova Odessa city (coordinates 22°46′46″ S e 47°18′49″ O), São Paulo State, Brazil in 2014. Botanical identification was performed by Dr. Harri Lorenzi. The voucher of the studied species has been deposited in the Herbarium Plantarum (HPL) at number Lorenzi 1.713.

2.3. Essential Oil Extraction and Analysis

Fresh leaves (150 g) of *L. alba* were submitted to a steam distillation in a Clevenger-type apparatus over 5 h to afford 931 mg of the crude essential oil. The obtained oil was immediately analyzed by GC-FID and GC-LREIMS.

2.4. Cell Lines

The murine melanoma cell line B16F10 was originally obtained from the Ludwig Institute for Cancer Research (São Paulo, Brazil). The melanotic B16F10Nex2 subline, characterized at the Experimental Oncology Unit (UNIFESP-Federal University of São Paulo), is characterized by low immunogenicity and moderate virulence. Human breast cancer cell line (MCF-7), human lung adenocarcinoma (A549), and human umbilical vein endothelial (HUVEC) were obtained from the Ludwig Institute for Cancer Research.

2.5. In Vitro Cytotoxic Activity

The essential oil extracted from leaves of *L. alba* was dissolved in dimethyl sulfoxide (DMSO) to the final concentration of 10 mg/mL, diluted in RPMI medium containing 10% fetal calf serum ranging from 100 to 0 µg/mL and incubated with 1×10^4 cells in a 96-well plate. After 18 h of incubation, cell viability was measured using the Cell Proliferation Kit I (MTT) (Sigma, St. Louis, MI, USA), an MTT-based colorimetric assay [27,28]. Readings were made with a plate reader at 570 nm. All experiments were performed in triplicate.

2.6. Media, Antibiotics, and Growth Conditions

Yeast were cultivated on agar plates containing YPD (1% yeast extract, 2% peptone, 2% dextrose, and 2% agar) or RPMI1640 (Sigma). Gram-negative bacteria were grown in LB (0.5% yeast extract, 1% tryptone, 1% NaCl, and 2% agar) and Gram-positive bacteria were tested in BHI (Himedia, Mumbai, India). Fluconazole (Sigma) was used as the positive control for yeast and chloramphenicol (Sigma) was the positive control for bacteria. Crude essential oil from *L. alba* was diluted in DMSO or saline (0.9%) plus Tween 80 (0.5%) and spotted on 5 mm sterile filter paper [25].

2.7. Microorganisms Strains

The bacteria and yeast species used in this work are described in the Table 1.

Table 1. Target strains used for antimicrobial activity assays.

Species	Designation
Yeast	
Candida dubliniensis	ATCC 7978
Candida tropicalis	ATCC 13803
Candida glabrata	ATCC 90030
Candida parapsilosis	Clinical isolate 68
Candida krusei	Clinical isolate 9602
Candida albicans	CBMAI * 560
Cryptococcus grubii (A)	ATCC 208821
Cryptococcus gattii (B)	ATCC MYA-4563
Cryptococcus gattii (C)	ATCC MYA-4560
Cryptococcus neoformans (D)	ATCC MYA-4567
Saccharomyces cerevisiae	ATCC 201389
Bacteria	
Escherichia coli	-
Serratia marcescens	CBMAI * 469
Pseudomonas aeruginosa	CBMAI * 602
Staphylococcus epidermidis	CBMAI * 604
Enterococcus faecalis	-

* CBMAI: Coleção Brasileira de Microrganismos do Ambiente e Indústria.

2.8. Disk Diffusion Assay

Antimicrobial activity of essential oil from leaves of *L. alba* was evaluated using the disk diffusion method according to the Clinical and Laboratory Standards Institute (CLSI, OPAS M2-A8) with modifications. Thin agar plates were prepared with 10 mL of YPD (yeast), LB (Gram-negative) and BHI (Gram-positive) media. Three milliliters of liquid cultures were grown at 30 °C with aeration

(150 rpm) overnight on YPD (yeast), LB (Gram-negative), or BHI (Gram-positive). A top agar was prepared by mixing 100 μL of each culture with 10 mL of soft agar medium for confluent plates (YPD, LB or BHI plus 1% agar) and poured on top of the thin agar (2% agar medium). Sterilized 5 mm filter paper disks were then impregnated with 20 μL of crude essential oil diluted in DMSO. The disks were placed on top of agar plates and incubated at 30 °C for 24 or 48 h depending on the microorganism. Fluconazole (1 mg) and chloramphenicol (200 μg) were used as positive controls for yeast and bacteria, respectively. Negative control was prepared by impregnating the paper disks with the same amount of DMSO used to dilute the essential oil. All tests were performed in triplicate. Tested strains were selected since they represent clinical important microbes and were previously tested in other studies conducted by our research group [25].

2.9. Minimum Inhibitory Concentration

Microdilution tests were conducted according to the Clinical and Laboratory Standards Institute (CLSI), OPAS1 M27-A2 for yeasts and OPAS M7-A6 for bacteria according to literature [25] with slight modifications. Briefly, minimum inhibitory concentration (MIC) values were determined using microtiter plates (96 wells) with a total volume of 100 μL. Microorganisms were cultured in test tubes filled with 3 mL medium RPMI 1640 (Sigma, St. Louis, MI, USA) for yeast and BHI (Sigma, St. Louis, MI, USA) for bacteria, overnight at 30 °C in a rotary shaker (150 rpm). The cultures were diluted and adjusted to 1–2 × 10^2 CFU/mL, which was confirmed by viability counts on YPD and BHI plates (100 μL of diluted cells). Crude essential oil and reference standards were serial diluted (two-fold) and added to each well. A sterilization control containing medium only and growth control containing cell, DMSO (10 μL), or saline (10 μL), and Tween 80 were included as negative and positive controls, respectively. Depending on the microorganism the microtiter plates were then incubated at 30 °C for 24 or 48 h. Microorganism growth was determined by reading the absorbance at 530 nm in a plate reader Logen MT-960 (Tecan, Männedorf, Switzerland) and the minimum inhibitory concentration was considered the lowest concentration at which at least 80% of growth was inhibited. All tests were performed in triplicate.

3. Results and Discussion

3.1. Chemical Composition of Essential Oil from *L. alba*

The yield of the essential oil extracted from *L. alba* was 0.21% based on the weight of the fresh leaves used in the distillation procedure. Analysis of the crude oil by gas chromatography with flame ionization detector (GC-FID) and by gas chromatography coupled to low resolution electronic impact mass spectrometry (GC-LREIMS), followed by calculation of Kovats indices, and comparison with the literature data [27] allowed the identification of 39 compounds corresponding to 99.45% (Table 2) of the crude essential oil.

Among the identified compounds, approximately 67% corresponds to monoterpenes and 19% to sesquiterpenes. The main characterized components were the isomeric monoterpenes nerol/geraniol (27.09%) and citral (21.87%), as well as 6-methyl-5-heptene-2-one (11.98%) and *E*-caryophyllene (9.25%), as showed in Figure 1. These compounds were previously found as minor metabolites in the essential oil from leaves of *L. alba* [29], suggesting the new chemotype nerol/geraniol and citral to the studied oil.

To confirm the identification of these main monoterpenes, the ^{13}C NMR spectrum of crude oil was recorded and exhibited peaks assigned to carbonyl groups of aldehydes (C-1) at δ 191.5 and 190.9 of geranial and neral, respectively. The peaks at δ 127.4/128.6 and δ 122.5/122.2 were assigned to double bonds (C-2 and C-6), whereas those at δ 164.2/164.2 and δ 132.9/133.7 were attributed to C-3 and C-7 of geranial and neral, respectively. The secondary carbons C-4 and C-5 were represented by signals δ 40.6/25.7 and 32.6/27.0. The signals of carbons C-8 (δ 17.7) and C-9 (δ 25.6) displayed the same chemical shift for neral and geranial, but the peaks observed to C-10 were observed at δ 25.1 to neral and δ 17.6 to geranial, according to literature data [30,31]. Finally, analysis of ^{1}H NMR spectrum indicated a ratio of 5:3 of geranial:neral based in the integration of the doublets at δ 9.99 (J = 9.0 Hz) and 9.89 (J = 9.0 Hz), assigned to aldehyde hydrogens (H-1).

Table 2. Chemical composition of the essential oil obtained from leaves of *L. alba*.

Compound	IK	Relative Amount
α-pinene	939	0.15
Sabinene	976	0.41
6-methy-5-hepten-2-one	985	11.98
α-phelandrene	1005	3.25
α-terpinene	1018	0.23
β-phelandrene	1031	1.67
Z-β-ocimene	1040	0.18
E-β-ocimene	1050	2.70
γ-terpinene	1062	0.03
cis-sabinene hydrate	1068	0.04
Terpinolene	1088	0.02
Linalol	1098	2.14
cis-oxide rose	1111	0.80
Dihydrolinalol	1134	0.14
Citronelal	1153	0.45
Borneol	1165	0.33
α-terpineol	1189	1.15
Citronelol	1228	4.43
nerol/geraniol	1252	27.09
citral (neral/geranial)	1267	21.87
geranyl formate	1300	1.48
Longicyclene	1373	0.11
Longifolene	1402	1.65
α-cedrene	1409	0.62
E-caryophyllene	1418	9.25
cis-thujopsene	1429	0.12
α-humulene	1454	0.82
allo-aromadendrene	1461	0.25
α-acoradiene	1463	0.04
Chamigrene	1475	0.04
germacrene-D	1480	1.67
Ar-curcumene	1483	0.38
α-zingiberene	1495	0.97
germacrene-A	1503	0.98
β-bisabolene	1509	0.20
Z-γ-bisabolene	1515	0.18
epi-longipinanol	1561	0.03
Longipinanol	1566	1.53
(6*R*,7*R*)-bisabolone	1737	0.07
Monoterpenes		67.08
Sesquiterpenes		18.91
Other compounds		13.46
Total		99.45

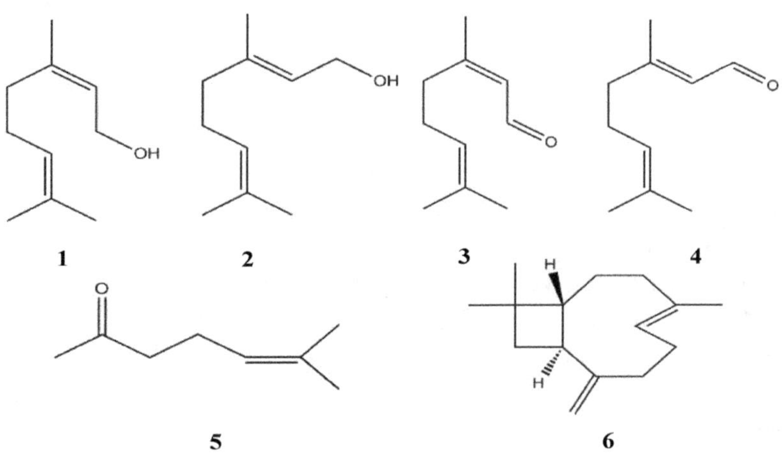

Figure 1. Structures of main compounds identified in essential oil from *L. alba*: nerol (**1**), geraniol (**2**), neral (**3**), geranial (**4**), 6-methy-5-hepten-2-one, (**5**) and *E*-caryophyllene (**6**).

3.2. Cytotoxic Activity

The essential oil from leaves of *L. alba* was evaluated for its cytotoxic activity in vitro against the lines B16F10Nex2 and A549 with IC_{50} of 45.8 μg/mL and 63.9 μg/mL, respectively, and IC_{50} higher than 100 μg/mL to the MCF-7 cell line. Comparatively, positive control cisplatin displayed IC_{50} of 52.8 μg/mL (B16F10Nex2), whereas paclitaxel showed IC_{50} of 84.3 μg/mL (A549) and 171.5 μg/mL (MCF), as showed in Table 3. Based in the obtained results, the essential oil from *L. alba* could be considered as a source of antitumor compounds, since it showed lower IC_{50} values in comparison to standard drugs in the tested cells. Additionally, the essential oil from *L. alba* was non-toxic to non-tumorigenic in HUVEC, in opposition to the cisplatin positive control, which displayed an IC_{50} value of 42.6 μg/mL.

Table 3. IC_{50} (μg/mL) values to the essential oil from leaves of *L. alba* and to positive control (cisplatin and paclitaxel) against cell lines.

Cell Line	IC_{50} (μg/mL)		
	Essential Oil	**Cisplatin**	**Paclitaxel**
B16F10Nex2	45.82 ± 4.16	52.8 ± 4.50	-
A549	63.98 ± 6.76	-	84.3 ± 6.83
MCF-7	>100	-	171.5 ± 16.39
HUVEC	>100	42.6 ± 2.25	-

In a previous study concerning the cytotoxic activity of essential oils from *L. alba* against cell lines CT26WT (murine colon carcinoma), A549 (human lung adenocarcinoma), MDA-MB-231 (human breast adenocarcinoma), CACO 2 (human colon carcinoma), and CHO (normal hamster ovary cells) no activity was observed to chemotype geraniol, whereas chemotype carvone inhibited A549 cells with IC_{50} of 47.80 μg/mL [32,33]. Otherwise, citral and carvone chemotypes of *L. alba* displayed dose-dependent cytotoxicity effect against HeLa (human cervical carcinoma) cells [34]. Regarding the major component citral, this compound exhibited antitumor activity. The effect of citral combined with retinoic acid showed inhibition of proliferation of A549 (lung carcinoma epithelial) in a dose dependent manner [35]. Additionally, antitumor properties was detected to micelle formulation of citral [36], whereas cytotoxicity against colon adenocarcinoma (HCT) and lung adenocarcinoma was described for citral, administrated as a mixture of monoterpenes neral + geranial and in a combination with lysine [37]. Geraniol, another main compound found in the studied essential oil from *L. alba*, was described as an inhibitor of prostate cancer growth by targeting cell cycle and apoptosis pathways [38].

3.3. Antimicrobial Activity

Initially, disk diffusion assays were conducted with the yeasts and bacterial strains listed in Table 1 in order to screen for antimicrobial activity. Four bacterial strains (two Gram-negative and two Gram-positive) were sensitive to the essential oil from *L. alba*. In sequence, the species listed in Table 4 were tested to determine the MICs. The results showed that yeasts are considerably more sensitive to essential oil from *L. alba* than bacterial strains. At 4 mg/mL only *E. coli* showed a growth inhibition over 80%; all other strains showed an MIC of 4.0 mg/mL with growth inhibitions below 70%. Conversely, all yeast strains tested were sensitive to the essential oil from *L. alba* and the MICs calculated for them was two- to four-fold lower than those found for bacterial strains. *C. dubliniensis* was the microbial strain most sensitive to essential oil from *L. alba* (0.5 mg/mL). All yeast strains tested showed, at least, 90% of growth inhibition.

Table 4. Minimum inhibitory concentrations (MIC) for essential oil from *L. alba*. Concentrations are given in mg/mL. Numbers in parentheses denote the percentage of growth inhibition and its standard deviation.

Species	Essential Oil	Positive Control
E. coli	4.0 (98% ± 1%)	0.01 [a]
S. marcescens	4.0 (42% ± 3%)	0.01 [a]
E. faecalis	4.0 (64% ± 2%)	0.02 [a]
S. epidermidis	4.0 (56% ± 2%)	0.04 [a]
C. albicans	2.0 (99% ± 2%)	0.025 [b]
C. dubliniensis	0.5 (93% ± 2%)	0.006 [b]
C. tropicalis	2.0 (99% ± 1%)	0.05 [b]
C. glabrata	2.0 (99% ± 1%)	0.05 [b]
C. parapsilosis	2.0 (99% ± 1%)	0.006 [b]
C. krusei	2.0 (99% ± 1%)	0.05 [b]
C. grubii (A)	1.0 (99% ± 2%)	0.013 [b]
C. gattii (B)	2.0 (97% ± 2%)	0.025 [b]
C. gattii (C)	2.0 (98% ± 1%)	0.006 [b]
C. neoformans (D)	1.0 (98% ± 2%)	0.006 [b]
S. cerevisiae	2.0 (99% ± 1%)	0.013 [b]

[a] chloramphenicol; [b] fluconazole.

There are many reports in the literature about the antimicrobial effects of essential oils from *L. alba*. In our investigation the activity of this oil on bacterial growth was modest, suggesting that the tested crude oil does not play an important role as an antibacterial. However, future studies with purified fractions from this oil could uncover more significant biological activities against bacteria, as shown before by Klein et al. [39]. Essential oils from *L. alba* have been extensively reported as antifungal, especially against phyto [40–43] and human pathogens [43]. In summary, these results hold a promise of possible applications for *L. alba* essential oil as an antifungal in medicine, as well as in agriculture.

Acknowledgments: The authors wish to thank MSc. Harri Lorenzi for the collection of *Lippia alba*. Also the authors would like to thank Fundação de Amparo a Pesquisa do Estado de São Paulo-FAPESP (Project 2015/11936-2) and Conselho Nacional de Desenvolvimento Científico e Tecnológico-CNPq for providing financial support to this study. Nara O. dos Santos obtained a fellowship from Coordenação de Aperfeiçoamento de Pessoal de Nível Superior-CAPES. Patricia Sartorelli and João Henrique G. Lago received a scientific research award from CNPq.

Author Contributions: N.O.d.S., R.C.P., M.A.V., C.R.F., M.G.S. performed the experiments, contributed reagents/materials/analysis tools and wrote the manuscript. J.H.G.L. and P.S. conceived, designed the project, analyze the results and wrote the paper.

References

1. Trease, G.E.; Evans, W.C. *Pharmacognosy*, 12th ed.; Bailliere & Tindall: London, UK, 1983.
2. Pascual, M.E.; Slowing, K.; Carretero, E.; Mata, D.S.; Villar, A. *Lippia*: Traditional uses, chemistry and pharmacology: A review. *J. Ethnopharmacol.* **2001**, *76*, 201–214. [CrossRef]
3. Terblanché, F.C.; Kornelius, G. Essential oil constituents of the genus *Lippia* (Verbenaceae)—A literature review. *J. Essent. Oil Res.* **1996**, *8*, 471–485. [CrossRef]
4. Morton, J.F. *Atlas of medicinal plants of middle America: Bahamas to Yucatan*; Charles, C., Ed.; Thomas: Springfield, IL, USA, 1981.
5. Hennebelle, T.; Sahpaz, S.; Joseph, H.; Bailleul, F. Ethnopharmacology of *Lippia alba*. *J. Ethnopharmacol.* **2008**, *116*, 211–222. [CrossRef] [PubMed]
6. Jannuzzi, H.; Mattos, J.K.A.; Silva, D.B.; Gracindo, L.A.M.; Vieira, R.F. Avaliação agronômica e química de dezessete acessos de erva-cidreira (*Lippia alba* (Mill.) N.E. Brown)—Quimiotipo citral, cultivados no Distrito Federal. *Rev. Bras. Plantas Med.* **2011**, *13*, 258–264. (In Portuguese)
7. Matos, F.J.A. *Plantas Medicinais: Guia de seleção e emprego de plantas usadas em fitoterapia no Nordeste do Brasil*, 2nd ed.; UFC: Fortaleza, Brazil, 2000. (In Portuguese)

8. Corrêa, C.B.V. Contribuição ao estudo de *Lippia alba* (Mill.) N.E. Br. ex Britt & Wilson—Erva-cidreira. *Rev. Bras. Farmacogn.* **1992**, *73*, 57–64. (In Portuguese)
9. Matos, F.J.A. As ervas cidreiras do Nordeste do Brasil—Estudo de três quimiotipos de *Lippia alba* (Mill.) N.E. Brown (Verbenaceae). Parte II—Farmacoquímica. *Rev. Bras. Farm.* **1996**, *77*, 137–141. (In Portuguese)
10. Gupta, M. *270 Plantas Medicinales Iberoamericanas*, 1st ed.; Convenio Andrés Bello: Santafé de Bogotá, Colombia, 1995.
11. Morais, S.M.; Dantas, J.D.P.; Silva, A.R.A.; Magalhães, E.F. Plantas medicinais usadas pelos índios Tapebas do Ceará. *Rev. Bras. Farmacogn.* **2005**, *15*, 169–177. (In Portuguese) [CrossRef]
12. Tavares, E.S.; Julião, L.S.; Lopes, D.; Bizzo, H.R.; Lage, C.L.S.; Leitão, S.G. Análise do óleo essencial de folhas de três quimiotipos de *Lippia alba* (Mill.) N.E. Br. (Verbenaceae) cultivados em condições semelhantes. *Rev. Bras. Farmacogn.* **2005**, *15*, 1–5. (In Portuguese) [CrossRef]
13. Pinto, E.P.P.; Amorozo, M.C.M.; Furlan, A. Conhecimento popular sobre plantas medicinais em comunidades rurais de mata atlântica-Itacaré, BA, Brasil. *Acta Bot. Bras.* **2006**, *20*, 751–762. (In Portuguese) [CrossRef]
14. Matos, F.J.A.; Machado, M.I.L.; Craveiro, A.A.; Alencar, J.W. Essential oil composition of two chemotypes of *Lippia alba* grown in Northeast Brazil. *J. Essent. Oil Res.* **1996**, *8*, 695–698. [CrossRef]
15. Zoghbi, M.G.B.; Andrade, E.H.A.; Santos, A.S.; Silva, M.H.L.; Maia, J.G. Essential oils of *Lippia alba* (Mill.) N.E. Br. growing wild in the Brazilian Amazon. *Flavour Fragr. J.* **1998**, *13*, 47–48. [CrossRef]
16. Hennebelle, T.; Sahpaz, S.; Joseph, H.; Bailleul, F. Phenolics and iridoids of *Lippia alba*. *Nat. Prod. Commun.* **2006**, *1*, 727–730.
17. Dellacassa, E.; Soler, E.; Menéndez, P.; Moyna, P. Essential oils from *Lippia alba* (Mill.) N.E. Brown and *Aloysia chamaedrifolia* Cham. (Verbenaceae) from Uruguay. *Flavour Fragr. J.* **1990**, *5*, 107–108. [CrossRef]
18. Senatore, F.; Rigano, D. Essential oil of two *Lippia* spp. (Verbenaceae) growing wild in Guatemala. *Flavour Fragr. J.* **2001**, *16*, 169–171. [CrossRef]
19. Machado, T.F.; Pereira, R.C.A.; Batista, V.C.V. Seasonal variability of the antimicrobial activity of the essential oil of *Lippia alba*. *Rev. Ciênc. Agron.* **2014**, *45*, 515–519. [CrossRef]
20. Alea, J.A.P.; Luis, A.G.O.; Pérez, A.R.; Jorge, M.R.; Baluja, R. Composición y propriedades antibacterianas del aceite esencial de *Lippia alba* (Mill.) N.E. Brown. *Rev. Cuba. Farm.* **1996**, *30*, 1–8. (In Spanish)
21. Stashenko, E.E.; Jaramillo, B.E.; Martínez, J.R. Comparison of different extraction methods for the analysis of volatile secondary metabolites of *Lippia alba* (Mill.) N.E. Brown, grown in Colombia, and evaluation of its in vitro antioxidant activity. *J. Chromatogr. A* **2004**, *1025*, 93–103. [CrossRef] [PubMed]
22. Castro, D.M.; Ming, L.C.; Marques, M.O.M. Composição fitoquímica dos óleos essenciais de folhas da *Lippia alba* (Mill). N.E. Br. em diferentes épocas de colheita e partes do ramo. *Rev. Bras. Plantas Med.* **2002**, *4*, 75–79. (In Portuguese)
23. Viccini, L.F.; Silveira, R.S.; Vale, A.A.; Campos, J.M.S.; Reis, A.C.; Santos, M.O.; Campos, V.R.; Carpanez, A.G.; Grazul, R.M. Citral and linalool content has been correlated to DNA content in *Lippia alba* (Mill.) N.E. Brown (Verbenaceae). *Ind. Crop. Prod.* **2014**, *59*, 14–19.
24. Bou, D.D.; Lago, J.H.G.; Figueiredo, C.R.; Matsuo, A.L.; Guadagnin, R.C.; Soares, M.G.; Sartorelli, P. Cytotoxicity evaluation of essential oil, zingiberene and derivatives from leaves of *Casearia sylvestris* (Salicaceae). *Molecules* **2013**, *18*, 9477–9487. [CrossRef] [PubMed]
25. Santos, N.O.; Mariane, B.; Lago, J.H.G.; Sartorelli, P.; Rosa, W.; Soares, M.G.; da Silva, A.M.; Lorenzi, H.; Vallim, M.A.; Pascon, R.C. Assessing the chemical composition and antimicrobial activity of essential oils from Brazilian plants—*Eremanthus erythropappus* (Asteraceae), *Plectrantuns barbatus*, and *P. amboinicus* (Lamiaceae). *Molecules* **2015**, *20*, 8440–8452. [CrossRef] [PubMed]
26. Grecco, S.S.; Martins, E.G.; Girola, N.; de Figueiredo, C.R.; Matsuo, A.L.; Soares, M.G.; Bertoldo, B.C.; Sartorelli, P.; Lago, J.H.G. Chemical composition and in vitro cytotoxic effects of the essential oil from *Nectandra leucantha* leaves. *Pharm. Biol.* **2015**, *53*, 133–137. [CrossRef] [PubMed]
27. Adams, R.P. *Identification of Essential Oil Components by Gas Chromatography/Mass Spectrometry*, 4th ed.; Allured Publishing: Carol Stream, IL, USA, 2007.
28. Mosmann, T. Rapid colorimetric assay for cellular growth and survival: Application to proliferation and cytotoxicity assays. *J. Immunol. Meth.* **1983**, *65*, 55–63. [CrossRef]
29. Soares, L. Estudo tecnológico, fitoquímico e biológico de *Lippia alba* (Miller) N.E. Brown Ex Britt. & Wils. (falsa-melissa) Verbenaceae. Master's Thesis, Federal University of Santa Catarina, Florianópolis, Brazil, 2001. (In Portuguese)

30. Glamoclija, J.; Sokovic, M.; Tesevic, V.; Linde, G.A.; Colauto, N.B. Chemical characterization of *Lippia alba* essential oil: An alternative to control green molds. *Braz. J. Microbiol.* **2011**, *42*, 1537–1546. [PubMed]
31. Ragasa, C.Y.; Ha, H.K.; Hasika, M.; Maridable, J.B.; Gaspillo, P.D.; Rideout, J.A. Antimicrobial and Cytotoxic Terpenoids from *Cymbopogon citratus* Stapf. *Philipp. Scient. J.* **2008**, *45*, 111–122. [CrossRef]
32. Jeon, J.H.; Lee, C.H.; Lee, H.S. Food protective effect of geraniol and its congeners against stored food mites. *J. Food Prot.* **2009**, *72*, 1468–1471. [PubMed]
33. Gomide, M.S.; Lemos, F.O.; Lopes, M.T.P.; Alves, T.M.A.; Viccini, L.F.; Coelho, C.M. The effect of the essential oils from five different *Lippia* species on the viability of tumor cell lines. *Rev. Bras. Farmacogn.* **2013**, *23*, 895–902. [CrossRef]
34. Mesa-Arango, A.C.; Montiel-Ramos, J.; Zapata, B.; Durán, C.; Betancur-Galvis, L.; Stashenko, E. Citral and carvone chemotypes from the essential oils of Colombian *Lippia alba* (Mill.) N.E. Brown: Composition, cytotoxicity and antifungal activity. *Mem. Inst. Oswaldo Cruz* **2009**, *104*, 878–884. [CrossRef] [PubMed]
35. Farah, I.O.; Trimble, Q.; Ndebele, K.; Mawson, A. Retinoids and citral modulated cell viability, metabolic stability, cell cycle progression and distribution in the A549 lung carcinoma cell line. *Biomed. Sci. Instrum.* **2010**, *46*, 410–421. [PubMed]
36. Zeng, S.; Kapur, A.; Patankar, M.S.; Xiong, M.P. Formulation, Characterization, and Antitumor Properties of Trans- and Cis-Citral in the 4T 1 Breast Cancer Xenograft Mouse Model. *Pharm. Res.* **2015**, *32*, 2548–2558. [PubMed]
37. Shi, C.; Zhao, X.; Liu, Z.; Meng, R.; Chen, X.; Guo, N. Antimicrobial, antioxidant, and antitumor activity of epsilon-poly-L-lysine and citral, alone or in combination. *Food Nutr. Res.* **2016**, *60*, 31891–31898. [CrossRef] [PubMed]
38. Kim, S.H.; Bae, H.C.; Park, E.J.; Lee, C.R.; Kim, B.J.; Lee, S.; Park, H.H.; Kim, S.J.; So, I.; Kim, T.W.; et al. Geraniol inhibits prostate cancer growth by targeting cell cycle and apoptosis pathways. *Biochem. Biophys. Res. Commun.* **2011**, *407*, 129–134. [CrossRef] [PubMed]
39. Klein, G.; Rüben, C.; Upmann, M. Antimicrobial activity of essential oil components against potential food spoilage microorganisms. *Curr. Microbiol.* **2013**, *67*, 200–208. [CrossRef] [PubMed]
40. Tomazoni, E.Z.; Pansera, M.R.; Pauletti, G.F.; Moura, S.; Ribeiro, R.T.; Schwambach, J. In vitro antifungal activity of four chemotypes of *Lippia alba* (Verbenaceae) essential oils against *Alternaria solani* (Pleosporeaceae) isolates. *An. Acad. Bras. Cienc.* **2016**, *31*, 999–1010. [CrossRef] [PubMed]
41. Anaruma, N.D.; Schmidt, F.L.; Duarte, M.C.; Figueira, G.M.; Delarmelina, C.; Benato, L.A.; Sartoratto, A. Control of *Colletotrichum gloeosporioides* (Penz.) Sacc. in yellow passion fruit using *Cymbopogon citratus* essential oil. *Braz. J. Microbiol.* **2010**, *41*, 66–73. [CrossRef] [PubMed]
42. Shukla, R.; Kumar, A.; Singh, P.; Dubey, N.K. Efficacy of *Lippia alba* (Mill.) N.E. Brown essential oil and its monoterpene aldehyde constituents against fungi isolated from some edible legume seeds and aflatoxin B1 production. *Int. J. Food Microbiol.* **2009**, *135*, 165–170. [CrossRef] [PubMed]
43. Singh, R.K. Fungitoxicity of some higher plants and synergistic activity of their essential oils against *Sclerotium rolfsii* Sacc. causing foot-rot disease of barley. *Hind. Antibiot. Bull.* **2005**, *47*, 45–51.

15

Successful Pregnancy after Treatment with Chinese Herbal Medicine in a 43-Year-Old Woman with Diminished Ovarian Reserve and Multiple Uterus Fibrosis

Benqi Teng [1,2], Jie Peng [1,3], Madeleine Ong [1] and Xianqin Qu [1,*]

1. School of Life Sciences, University of Technology Sydney, NSW 2007, Australia; tengbq@mail.sysu.edu.cn (B.T.); PengJie528@outlook.com (J.P.); Madeleine.L.Ong@student.uts.edu.au (M.O.)
2. Department of Obstetrics, The Third Affiliated Hospital of Sun Yat-sen University, 600 Tianhe Road, Guangzhou 510630, China
3. Department of Gynaecology and Obstetrics, Suzhou Wuzhong People's Hospital, Suzhou 215128, China

* Correspondence: Xianqin.Qu@uts.edu.au

Academic Editor: James D. Adams

Abstract: Objective: To highlight a natural approach to coexisting oligomenorrhea, subfertility, luteal phase insufficiency and multiple fibroids cohesively when in vitro fertilisation (IVF) has failed. **Case Presentation:** A 43-year-old woman with diminished ovarian reserve and multiple uterine fibroids had previously been advised to discontinue IVF treatment. According to Chinese Medicine diagnosis, herbal formulae were prescribed for improving age-related ovarian insufficiency as well as to control the growth of fibroids. After 4 months of treatment, the patient's menstrual cycle became regular and plasma progesterone one week after ovulation increased from 10.9 nmol/L to 44.9 nmol/L. After 6 months, she achieved a natural conception, resulting in a live birth of a healthy infant at an estimated gestational age of 40 weeks. **Conclusions:** The successful treatment with Chinese Herbal Medicine for this case highlights a natural therapy to manage infertility due to ovarian insufficiency and multiple fibroids after unsuccessful IVF outcome.

Keywords: Chinese herbal medicine; diminished ovarian reserve; infertility; in vitro fertilization; uterus fibrosis

1. Introduction

Advanced maternal age contributes to subfertility due to diminished ovarian reserve (DOR) and decreased oocyte quality [1]. Reduced fertility potential may also be attributable to uterine fibroids which are more prevalent in women aged over 30 [2] depending on their size and location, which can affect embryo implantation [3]. Indeed, women with DOR and fibroids have a significantly low fertility rate despite advanced in vitro fertilization (IVF) techniques [4]. Given the limited treatment options after failure in IVF with DOR, these women often seek alternative therapy, such as Traditional Chinese medicine (TCM) to reserve adoption or using donor's egg as the last option.

Chinese medicinal herbs have been used for more than two thousand years to treat gynaecological disorders including infertility. In the last decades, experimental and clinical studies have shown that these herbal ingredients can regulate gonadotropin-releasing hormone and ovarian sex hormone levels to induce ovulation and promote blood flow to the ovaries to improve ovarian reserve [5]. TCM is unique as it applies a formula with multiple natural ingredients that are capable of counteracting complex endocrine and reproductive disorders. Here, we present a successful live birth with Chinese herbal medicine (CHM) treatment to a 43-year-old nulliparous woman with DOR and uterus fibroids after failed conception from IVF.

2. Case Presentation

A 43-year-old woman visited our clinic for CHM treatment of infertility. She reached menarche at 13 years of age and at this time her menstrual cycle was regular with a normal menstrual flow. Oral contraceptive pills were taken from age 21–23 and she had no previous pregnancies prior to our treatment. She started trying to conceive at age 40 and her husband, aged 41, had no remarkable health problems and normal semen analysis as defined by the World Health Organization 2010 criteria [6]. After two years of trying to achieve natural conception, she was referred to a fertility specialist for IVF treatment. Prior to the initiation of treatment, a pelvic ultrasound showed that the right ovary was not visible and the left ovary measured 2.7 mL with only 3 antral follicles and both fallopian tubes were clearly patent. The uterus was bulky measuring at 103 × 125 × 68 mm with multiple fibroids including two larger subserosal fibroids. Serum anti-mullerian hormone (AMH) level of <3 pmol/L was within the <25% percentile for correlated age. Hormone testing on day 5 of her menstrual cycle identified follicle stimulating hormone (FSH) levels of 1.9 IU/L (normal range 1.5–10), luteinising hormone (LH) levels of 2.8 IU/L (normal range 2.0–12), Oestradiol (E2) levels of 913 pmol/L (normal range <320) and Progesterone (P) levels of <0.5 nmol/L (normal range 0.3–4.0). According to the ESHRE criteria this patient had suspected poor ovarian response [7]. Therefore, controlled ovarian hyperstimulation (COH) with daily FSH injections from day 3 of her cycle was applied for oocyte retrieval, however, only one mature oocyte was collected, and she failed to conceive after fertilized embryo transferring. The fertility specialist therefore advised her to seek egg donation or cease IVF. The patient consequently sought out treatment at our Chinese Medicine clinic in hope of achieving fertility.

At the time the patient visited the clinic her menstrual cycles ranged between 24 and 42 days. According to the diagnosis, basic formula containing 10 herbs was prescribed (Table 1), aiming to (1) improve diminished ovarian function and regulate the menstrual cycle and (2) restrain the growth of uterus fibroids which corresponds to tonifying vital essence and regulating and nourishing blood in TCM.

Table 1. Description of Chinese Herbal Formula and Possible Pharmacological Effects [8,9].

Herb Name	TCM Action	Possible Pharmacological Effects
Shu Di Huang (Radix *Rehmannia glutinosa*)	Tonifies Qi and Blood.	Improves blood supply to reproductive tissue.
Dang Gui (Radix *Angelicae sinensis*)	Tonifies and moves blood.	Improves blood supply to reproductive tissue and organs. Improves ovarian function.
Tu Si Zi (Semen *Cuscutae chinensis*)	Consolidates vital essence.	Promotes fertility by improving the quality of oocyte.
Sang Shen Zi (*Fructus mori*)	Strengthens vital essence.	Anti-oxidant and improves the quality of the oocyte. Anti-ageing properties.
Gou Qi Zi (*Fructus lycii*)	Nourishes blood.	Scavenges free radicals, increases DNA synthesis in reproductive tissue.
Ba Ji Tian (Radix *Morindae officinalis*)	Supports the vital essence.	Stimulates pituitary gland to improve ovulation.
Dan Shen (Radix *Salvia miltiorrhizae*)	Dissolves blood stasis.	Anti-inflammatory, promotes microcirculation to reproductive organs.
Bai Shao (Radix *Paeoniae lactiflorae*)	Nourish blood, regulate qi.	Anti-inflammatory.
Xia Ku Cao (Spica *Prunellae vulgaris*)	Dissolves mass formation.	Anti-fibrotic.
E Zhu (Rhizoma *Curcuma phaeocaulis*)	Dissolves blood stasis.	Anti-fibrotic.

Abbreviations: TCM: Traditional Chinese Medicine. Possible pharmacological effects were derived from.

The herbal mixture was decocted into 500 mL and divided into two drinks daily. Ovulation was monitored by basal body temperature (BBT) and ovulation prediction kit. Plasma progesterone was measured one week of ovulation revealed by BBT chart and LH surge. Following initial consult and first month treatment with CHM, the patient underwent hormone testing one week after ovulation: P was 10.9 nmol/L, LH was 0.8 IU/L (normal range 2.0–12), FSH was 2.0 IU/L (normal range 1.5–10), E2 was 184 pmol/L (normal range 125–1300). After 12 weeks of treatment, the patient's menstrual cycle became regular with cycle lengthen between 30 and 35 days. Pelvic ultrasound on day 9 of cycle indicated ovaries of both sides were normal in size and uterine size was reduced with measuring 84 × 62 × 56 mm as well as decreased sizes of intramural and subserosal fibroids. A blood test was also performed at day 23 of her menstrual cycle (about one week after ovulation) and revealed improvement of progesterone levels from 10.9 up to 28.1 nmol/L.

From week 13, the formula was slightly modified according to the follicular phase by adding Radix *Polygoni multiflori* (*He Shou Wu*) 10 g to nourish blood, and in the luteal phase by adding Radix Dipsaci (*Xu Duan*) 12 g and Cortex *Eucommiae ulmoidis* (*Du Zhong*) 9 g to assist in embryo implantation. Anti-fibrosis herb, *Prunellae vulgaris* and Rhizoma *Curcuma phaeocaulis* had been ceased after 4 months of treatment. After 5 months of taking CHM, although AMH was at 1.3 pmol/L, plasma progesterone levels after one week of ovulation went from 10.9 nmol/L to 44.9 nmol/L, suggesting that the quality of oocyte and function of corpus luteum had been improved. After 6 months of treatment with CHM, she achieved natural conception, resulting in a live birth of a healthy female infant weighing 3350 g at an estimated gestational age of 40 weeks through caesarean section. No modifications to the lifestyle of the patient were made during this period.

3. Discussion

The conventional approaches to sterility include ovulation induction, intrauterine insemination and IVF. In this case, woman with advanced maternal age, IVF may be the most successful technique to achieve conception. However, because of the DOR, this patient presented a very poor response to COH, resulting in unsuccessful IVF. Consequently, the patient turned to CHM. Our treatment achieved pregnancy and a healthy live birth with Chinese herbal formulae containing herbs supporting the folliculogenesis cycle, invigorating blood, improving microcirculation, and resolving masses to benefit both ovary and uterus.

Chinese herbal medicines have long been used for the treatment of infertility. Numerous studies demonstrated that CHM could regulate the gonadotropin-releasing hormone (GnRH) to induce ovulation and improve the uterus blood flow and menstrual changes of endometrium [10,11]. An advantage of CHM treatment is that it utilizes individualized formulas tailored to a patient's condition. In this case, non-invasive treatment with CHM targeted two major causes underlying her infertility simultaneously, including poor quality of oocyte due to diminished ovarian reserve and uterine fibroids. The successful pregnancy eventually achieved through improvement of uterus environment and enhanced ovarian function.

It is generally accepted that submucousal fibroids but not subserosal fibroids have a negative impact on fertility by the virtue of their involvement in the endometrial cavity. This patient had multiple large subserosal and intramural fibroids of equal proportions. It has also been confirmed that myomas have higher levels of aromatase converting estrogens to estradiol, resulting in an imbalance of estradiol and progesterone, which is detrimental to embryo implantation and contributes to miscarriage [3]. In this infertility case, uterine fibroids have been considered as a treatment target because the estradiol levels of 913 pmol/L (normal range <320) was significantly high at follicular phase and there was also evidence of a bulky uterus caused by multiple fibroids. The large subserosal and intramural fibroids affect the endometrium homogeneous and may have negative impact on the embryo implantation on her natural conception and during IVF procedure. It is also a concern that these fibroids may aggressively grow during the pregnancy because of the ovarian hormone surge, subsequently affecting foetus development.

The herbal formula used in this case is able to balance *yin* and *yang*, nourish blood and invigorate blood circulation from a TCM perspective. In medical science, the CHM formula may restore ovarian function through improving blood flow to reproductive organs, regulating hormone secretions, lowering systemic inflammation as well as having anti-tumour properties. Among of them, Radix *Salvia miltiorrhizae*, Radix *Paeoniae lactiflorae*, Spica *Prunellae vulgaris* and Rhizoma *Curcuma phaeocaulis* have strong effects on blood stasis which is involved in mass (fibroids) formation in the reproductive system. Pharmacological studies have shown that these herbs reduce inflammation and inhibit neoplasia [12,13]. Meanwhile, the combination of Radix *Rehmannia glutinosa*, Semen *Cuscutae chinensis*, *Fructus mori*, *Fructus lycii*, Radix *Morindae officinalis* are commonly used in infertility due to ovarian factors, such as PCOS and primary ovarian insufficiency [13–16]. However, the precise mechanisms of Chinese herbs remain unclear with further research warranted.

After one month of treatment, day 6 oestradiol levels of 930 pmol/L reduced to 387 pmol/L. At the month five of the treatment, plasma progesterone from 10.9 nmol/L raised to 44.9 nmol/L, indicating improved ovarian function. Meanwhile, the size of the fibroids had shrunk with an overall reduced size of the uterus. These results indicate that CHM treatment inhibited fibroid growth and improved ovarian function, and may suggest enhanced quality of oocyte, evidenced by regularity of menstrual cycle, mid-cycle ovulation and elevated progesterone levels at luteal phase. Evidence suggests that oocyte quality profoundly affects fertilisation and embryo development [17]. The treatment achieved this woman's natural pregnancy, suggesting the improvement of oocyte quality. The limitation in this case observation is that other assessments for oocyte quality such as morphological character of oocyte and corpus luteum and other biomarkers, such as mitochondrial status and glucose-6-phosphate dehydrogenase 1 activity and apoptosis of follicular cells, were not measured.

Infertility is a life-altering burden and the disorder affects a couple's emotional health and wellness. Given the limited treatment options after failure in IVF, women with DOR who intend to get pregnant have to rely on assisted reproductive technology using donor eggs. The procedure is costly and only has a live birth rate of ~30% [4] and contributes to psychological distress. The results of this case demonstrate that CHM is capable of targeting multiple reproductive abnormalities involved in infertility. More specifically, herbal medicine can improve ovarian function and prevent inevitable miscarriage related to luteal phase defect and multiple fibroids. The successful treatment with CHM for this case highlights the potential of a natural approach to coexisting oligomenorrhea, subfertility, luteal phase insufficiency and multiple fibroids cohesively. CHM therapy offers a hope for aged women who have failed IVF cycles and decide to pursue parenthood with their own oocytes. The repeatability of CHM on infertility should be warranted through rigorously designed clinical trials.

Acknowledgments: We are thankful to our patient for her willingness to use her anonymized data for this publication.

References

1. Gurtcheff, S.E.; Klein, N.A. Diminished ovarian reserve and infertility. *Clin. Obstet. Gynecol.* **2011**, *54*, 666–674. [CrossRef] [PubMed]
2. Purohit, P.; Vigneswaran, K. Fibroids and Infertility. *Curr. Obstet. Gynecol. Rep.* **2016**, *5*, 81–88. [CrossRef] [PubMed]
3. Vitale, S.G.; Padula, F.; Gulino, F.A. Management of uterine fibroids in pregnancy: Recent trends. *Curr. Opin. Obstet. Gynecol.* **2015**, *27*, 432–437. [CrossRef] [PubMed]
4. Nelson, L.M. Clinical practice. Primary ovarian insufficiency. *N. Engl. J. Med.* **2009**, *360*, 606–614. [CrossRef] [PubMed]
5. Zhang, C.; Xu, X. Advancement in the treatment of diminished ovarian reserve by traditional Chinese and Western medicine. *Exp. Ther. Med.* **2016**, *11*, 1173–1176. [CrossRef] [PubMed]

6. Coope, T.G.; Noonan, E.; von Eckardstein, S.; Auger, J.; Baker, G.; Behre, H.M.; Haugen, T.B.; Kruger, T.; Wang, C.; Mbizvo, M.T.; et al. World Health Organization Reference Values for Human Semen Characteristics. *Hum. Reprod. Update* **2010**, *16*, 231–245. [CrossRef] [PubMed]
7. Ferraretti, A.P.; La Marca, A.; Fauser, B.C.; Tarlatzis, B.; Nargund, G.; Gianaroli, L.; ESHRE Working Group on Poor Ovarian Response Definition. ESHRE consensus on the definition of 'poor response' to ovarian stimulation for in vitro fertilization: The Bologna criteria. *Hum. Reprod.* **2011**, *26*, 1616–1624. [CrossRef] [PubMed]
8. Chen, J.K.; Chen, T.T. *Chinese Medical Herbology and Pharmacology*, 1st ed.; Art of Medicine Press Inc.: City of Industry, CA, USA, 2001.
9. Shen, Y.J. *Pharmacology of Chinese Herbal Medicine*, 1st ed.; People's Medical Publishing House: Beijing, China, 2000.
10. Huang, S.T.; Chen, A.P. Traditional Chinese medicine and infertility. *Curr. Opin. Obstet. Gynecol.* **2008**, *20*, 211–215. [CrossRef] [PubMed]
11. Lee, S.H.; Kwak, S.C.; Kim, D.K.; Park, S.W.; Kim, H.S.; Kim, Y.S.; Kim, Y.; Lee, D.; Lee, J.W.; Lee, C.G.; et al. Effects of Huang Bai (*Phellodendri Cortex*) and Three Other Herbs on GnRH and GH Levels in GT1–7 and GH3 Cells. *Evid. Based Complement. Alternat. Med.* **2016**, *2016*, 9389028. [CrossRef] [PubMed]
12. Chen, X.X.; Lin, W.L.; Yeung, W.F.; Song, T.H.; Lao, L.X.; Zhang, Y.B.; Meng, W. Quality and safety control of Tumor-Shrinking Decoction (TSD), a Chinese herbal preparation for the treatment of uterine fibroids. *Biotechnol. Appl. Biochem.* **2015**. [CrossRef] [PubMed]
13. Hu, Q.; Noor, M.; Wong, Y.F.; Hylands, P.J.; Simmonds, M.S.; Xu, Q.; Jiang, D.; Hendry, B.M.; Xu, Q. In vitro anti-fibrotic activities of herbal compounds and herbs. *Nephrol. Dial. Transplant.* **2009**, *24*, 3033–3041. [CrossRef] [PubMed]
14. Hung, Y.C.; Kao, C.W.; Lin, C.C.; Liao, Y.N.; Wu, B.Y.; Hung, I.L.; Hu, W.L. Chinese Herbal Products for Female Infertility in Taiwan: A Population-Based Cohort Study. *Medicine (Baltimore)* **2016**, *95*, e3075. [CrossRef] [PubMed]
15. Ong, M.; Peng, J.; Jin, X.L.; Qu, X. Chinese Herbal Medicine for the Optimal Management of Polycystic Ovary Syndrome. *Am. J. Chin.* **2017**, in press.
16. Chao, S.L.; Huang, L.W.; Yen, H.R. Pregnancy in premature ovarian failure after therapy using Chinese herbal medicine. *Chang. Gung Med. J.* **2003**, *26*, 449–452. [PubMed]
17. Wang, Q.; Sun, Q.Y. Evaluation of oocyte quality: Morphological, cellular and molecular predictors. *Reprod. Fertil. Dev.* **2007**, *19*, 1–12. [CrossRef] [PubMed]

16

Pharmacokinetics of Jaspine B and Enhancement of Intestinal Absorption of Jaspine B in the Presence of Bile Acid in Rats

Min-Koo Choi [1], Jihoon Lee [2], So Jeong Nam [2], Yun Ju Kang [2], Youjin Han [2], Kwangik Choi [2], Young A. Choi [1], Mihwa Kwon [2], Dongjoo Lee [3] and Im-Sook Song [2,*]

[1] College of Pharmacy, Dankook University, Cheon-an 31116, Korea; minkoochoi@dankook.ac.kr (M.-K.C.); ayha06@gmail.com (Y.A.C.)
[2] College of Pharmacy and Research Institute of Pharmaceutical Sciences, Kyungpook National University, Daegu 41566, Korea; legadema0905@naver.com (J.L.); goddns159@nate.com (S.J.N.); yun-ju6895@nate.com (Y.J.K.); gksdbwls2@nate.com (Y.H.); reggirchoi@naver.com (K.C.); mihwa_k@naver.com (M.K.)
[3] College of Pharmacy, Ajou University, Suwon 16499, Korea; dongjoo@ajou.ac.kr
* Correspondence: issong@knu.ac.kr

Abstract: We aimed to investigate the pharmacokinetics and the underlying mechanisms of the intestinal absorption, distribution, metabolism, and excretion of Jaspine B in rats. The oral bioavailability of Jaspine B was 6.2%, but it decreased to 1.6% in bile-depleted rats and increased to 41.2% (normal) and 23.5% (bile-depleted) with taurocholate supplementation (60 mg/kg). Consistent with the increased absorption in the presence of bile salts, rat intestinal permeability of Jaspine B also increased in the presence of 10 mM taurocholate or 20% bile. Further studies demonstrated that the enhanced intestinal permeability with bile salts was due to increased lipophilicity and decreased membrane integrity. Jaspine B was designated as a highly tissue-distributed compound, because it showed large tissue to plasma ratios in the brain, kidney, heart, and spleen. Moreover, the recovery of Jaspine B from the feces and urine after an intravenous administration was about 6.3%, suggesting a substantial metabolism of Jaspine B. Consistent with this observation, 80% of the administered Jaspine B was degraded after 1 h incubation with rat liver microsomes. In conclusion, the facilitated intestinal permeability in the presence of bile salts could significantly increase the bioavailability of Jaspine B and could lead to the development of oral formulations of Jaspine B with bile salts. Moreover, the highly distributed features of Jaspine B in the brain, kidney, heart, and spleen should be carefully considered in the therapeutic effect and toxicity of this compound.

Keywords: Jaspine B; bile salts; intestinal permeability; bioavailability; metabolic instability

1. Introduction

The development of anticancer drugs with effective therapeutic mechanisms is most interesting [1]. In that sense, various herbal and marine compounds have emerged as potential alternative medicines because of their structural diversity and safety, which was demonstrated by their long history of dietary use [2,3]. Marine natural products have been isolated since 1950s and marine sponges are one of the richest sources of bioactive compounds, showing the anti-proliferative effect through the inhibition of microtubule formation, the promotion of cell growth arrest, and stimulation of the cells death program [1]. Of these, the discovery of the sponge-derived nucleoside such as spongothymidine and spongouridine was made and three marine-based, anti-cancer drugs are currently being marketed [4]. Cytarabine was the first marine-derived anticancer drug approved in 1998 for the treatment of acute myelogenous leukemia. It was isolated from the marine sponge, Cryptotethya crypta, and induced apoptotic signals by inhibiting the NF-κB/Rel nuclear factor and binding to Bcl-2, and resulting in growth arrest at the G1/S phase [5]. Trabectedin, isolated from Ecteinascidia turbinata, was an approved anti-cancer drug against metastatic soft tissue carcinoma and ovarian cancer in 2009 in Europe [1]. Another approved marine drug is eribulin, an analog of halichondrin B, extracted from the marine sponge, Halichondria okadai [6], in 2010 from the FDA for the treatment of metastatic breast cancer. It also showed Bcl-2 inactivation and inhibition of microtubule polymerization [1,6].

Metabolites of sphingolipids such as ceramide, sphingosine, and sphingosine-1-phosphate (S1P), have been emerged as modulators for cancer progression [7]. Several studies addressing the effectiveness of sphingosine kinase SphK1 inhibition for cancer therapy have been reported [8–11]. The mRNA levels of SphK1 were significantly increased in breast, colon, lung, ovary, uterus, and kidney cancer patients, as well as in acute leukemia patients [12–14], and the downregulation of SphK1 decreased the epidermal growth factor and reduced prolactin- and E2-induced migration in metastatic breast cancer [7].

Jaspine B (pachastrissamine) (Figure 1) is an anhydrophytosphingosine, which is extracted from the marine sponge, *Pachastrissa* spp. [15]. It showed effective anti-cancer activity against several human carcinomas. Owing to its structural similarity with sphingosine, Jaspine B inactivated SphK1 and induced apoptotic signals [16]. In addition, Jaspine B inhibited melanoma cell growth by inhibiting the phosphorylation of Forkhead box O3 (FOXO3) [17] and by inducing apoptosis [18].

Previously, we had reported the anti-tumor activity of Jaspine B against various tumor cells that overexpressed sphingosine kinase. The results showed that Jaspine B was the most effective against breast cancer cells (MCF-7, IC_{50} = 2.31 μM) and showed differential cytotoxicity towards human breast adenocarcinoma (MDA-MB-231, IC_{50} > 100 μM), renal carcinoma (786-O, IC_{50} = 29.4 μM), melanoma (MDA-MB-435, IC_{50} = 2.60 μM), ovarian (SK-OV3, IC_{50} = 4.78 μM), and hepatoma (HepG2, IC_{50} = 5.69 μM) cells. The steady-state cellular concentration of Jaspine B was associated with the cytotoxic effect [19].

However, there have been few studies determining the absorption, disposition, and pharmacokinetic properties of Jaspine B, despite the importance of understanding these properties of the active, natural components. Therefore, in this study, we aimed to evaluate the pharmacokinetics, absorption, disposition, and excretion profile of Jaspine B and to investigate the underlying mechanisms related to its pharmacokinetic properties.

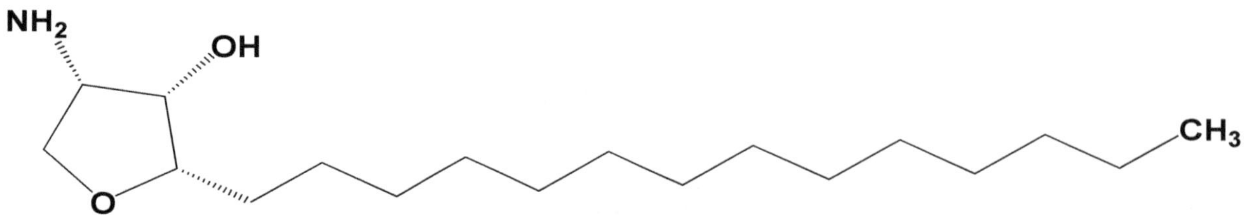

Figure 1. Structure of Jaspine B.

2. Results

2.1. LC/MS-MS Analysis of Jaspine B in the Biological Samples

We developed an analytical method of Jaspine B in the rat plasma, urine, bile, and various tissue homogenates using a liquid chromatography tandem-mass spectrometry (LC-MS/MS) system. Figure 2A showed the representative multiple reaction monitoring (MRM) chromatograms obtained from the analysis of blank rat plasma and rat plasma samples at 1 h after the oral dose of 30 mg/kg Jaspine B. In addition, representative MRM chromatograms obtained from other resources such as urine, bile, and tissue homogenates of brain, kidney, liver, heart, and spleen were also shown in Figure 2B–H. Although the concentration range of Jaspine B varied depending on the biological samples used, the analyses of Jaspine B in other resources such as urine, bile, and tissue homogenates of brain, kidney, liver, heart, and spleen did not show any interference at the retention times of Jaspine B (Figure 2).

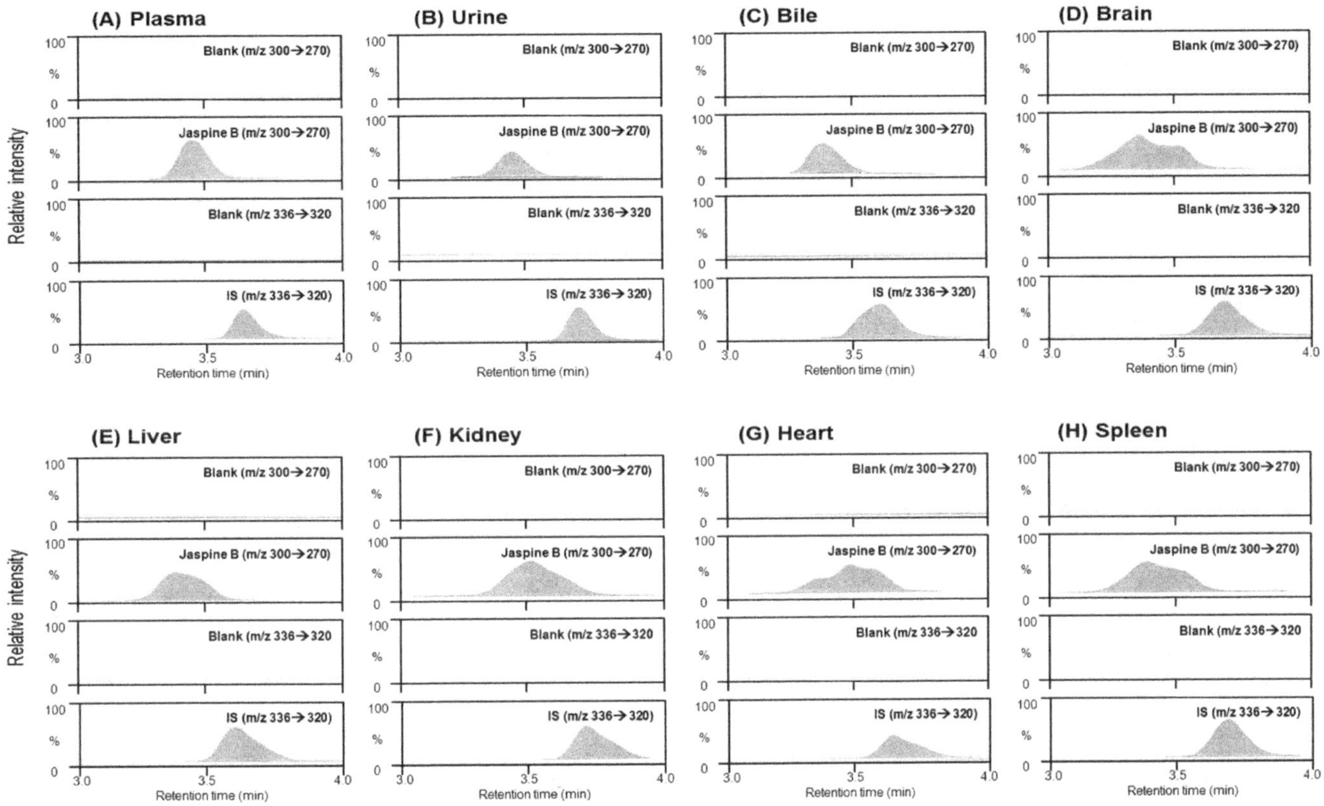

Figure 2. Representative multiple reaction monitoring (MRM) chromatograms of rat (**A**) plasma, (**B**) urine, (**C**) bile, and tissue homogenates of (**D**) brain, (**E**) liver, (**F**) kidney, (**G**) heart, and (**H**) spleen samples. In each panel from A to H, the chromatograms represent the MRM of Jaspine B (m/z 300→270) and internal standard (IS) (berberine, m/z 336→320) from blank and biological samples, respectively.

2.2. Pharmacokinetics of Jaspine B Following Intravenous Injection of 10 mg/kg Jaspine B

The mean plasma concentration–time profiles of Jaspine B after IV administration at a dose of 10 mg/kg in rats are shown in Figure 3A and the relevant pharmacokinetic parameters are listed in Table 1. The plasma concentration of Jaspine B after a IV administration declined, with a bi-exponential elimination process, and the terminal half-life was calculated as 6.7 h. The distribution half-life, which was calculated from the distribution phase in Figure 3A, was 1.4 h, and the volume of distribution at steady-state was calculated as 21.2 L/kg, suggesting a fast distribution of this compound into the second compartment.

The excreted amounts of Jaspine B via the urinary and biliary routes are shown in Figure 3B. After 10 mg/kg of Jaspine B was administered, 0.4 ± 0.2% and 2.4 ± 0.8% of the IV dose were recovered in the urine and bile, respectively (Table 1), suggesting that there was substantial metabolism of Jaspine B during its disposition. This was also supported by the large systemic clearance (CL_{total}) of Jaspine B, 98.3 mL/min/kg and low CL_{bile} and CL_{urine} of Jaspine B compared with CL_{total}. The contribution of CL_{bile} and CL_{urine} was about 4% of CL_{total} (Table 1).

Table 1. Pharmacokinetic parameters of Jaspine B after intravenous injection of Jaspine B at a dose of 10 mg/kg in rats.

	Parameters	IV (10 mg/kg)
Plasma	$T_{1/2}$ (h)	6.7 ± 1.6
	MRT (h)	3.6 ± 0.5
	AUC_{12h} (ng·h/mL)	1286.9 ± 165.6
	AUC_{∞} (ng·h/mL)	1701.9 ± 137.1
	Vss (L/kg)	21.2 ± 2.6
	CL_{total} (mL/min/kg)	98.3 ± 7.7
Bile	X_{bile} (% of dose)	2.4 ± 0.8
	CL_{bile} (mL/min/kg)	3.1 ± 0.6
Urine	X_{urine} (% of dose)	0.4 ± 0.2
	CL_{urine} (mL/min/kg)	0.5 ± 0.3

Data are expressed as the means ± S.D. from four different rats.

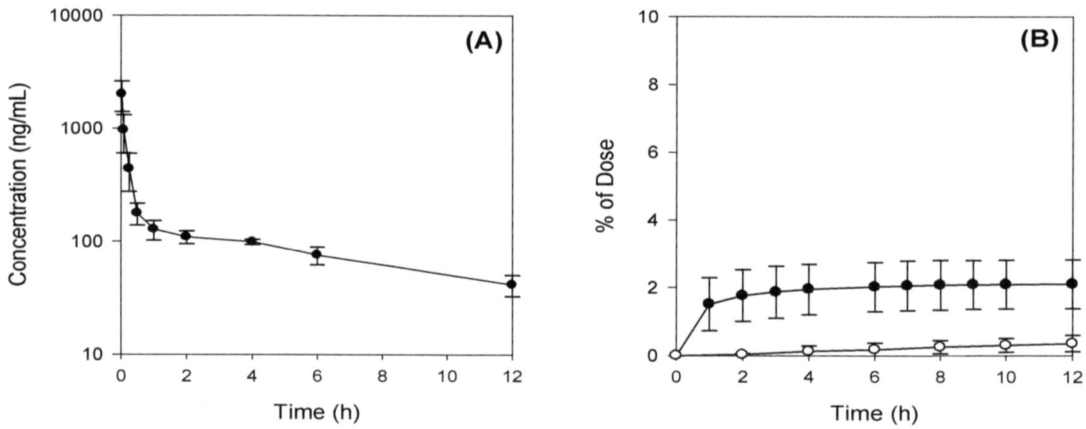

Figure 3. (**A**) Plasma concentration-time profile and (**B**) biliary (●) and urinary (○) excretion of Jaspine B after intravenous injection of Jaspine B (10 mg/kg) in rats. The means ± S.D. from four different rats.

The cumulative excreted amounts of Jaspine B were measured for 72 h using a metabolic cage. After 10 mg/kg of Jaspine B was intravenously administered, 1.6 ± 0.7% and 4.7 ± 0.8% of the dose were recovered after 72 h from the urine and feces, respectively. Therefore, over the 72 h period, the recovery of unaltered Jaspine B was estimated to be 6.3% of the single IV dose from the combined feces and urine samples, suggesting that a large amount of Jaspine B was metabolized in vivo.

2.3. Metabolic Instability of Jaspine B

Given the evidence of the substantial metabolism of Jaspine B, its microsomal stability was measured using rat liver microsomes. The percentage remaining after incubating for 30 min and 60 min was 59.8% and 20.4%, respectively, and the degradation half-life was calculated as 24 min (Figure 4). These results suggest the metabolic instability of Jaspine B in the liver, which is consistent with the previous results of the low contribution of biliary and urinary excretion of Jaspine B to the large clearance of this compound.

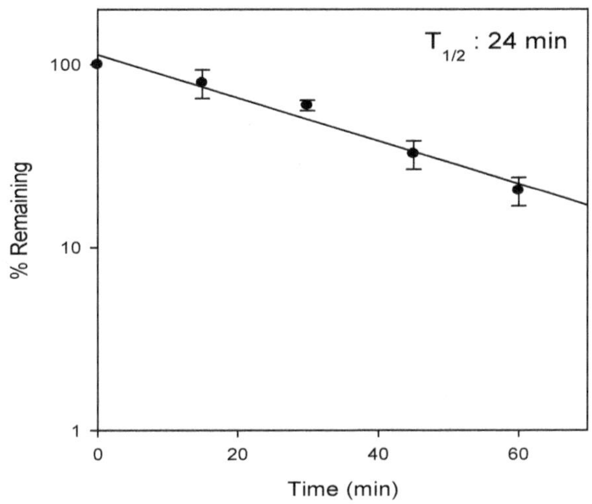

Figure 4. Metabolic instability of Jaspine B with rat liver microsomes. Jaspine B (1 μM) was incubated with 0.25 mg rat liver microsomes in the presence of a β-nicotinamide adenine dinucleotide 2′-phosphate reduced (NADPH)-generating system (1.3 mM β-NADP, 3.3 mM glucose-6-phosphate, 3.3 mM $MgCl_2$, and 1.0 unit/mL glucose-6-phosphate dehydrogenase) for 60 min at 37 °C in a shaking water bath. The half-life ($T_{1/2}$) was calculated from the first-order degradation rate constant.

2.4. Bile Acid Facilitates the Intestinal Absorption of Jaspine B

The mean plasma concentration–time profiles of Jaspine B after oral administration at a dose of 30 mg/kg in rats are shown in Figure 5A, and the relevant pharmacokinetic parameters are listed in control group (Table 2). Absolute bioavailability (BA), calculated by dividing the oral AUC by the intravenous AUC, was calculated as 6.2%.

Interestingly, the plasma concentration of Jaspine B decreased in the rats with bile depletion (Figure 5B) compared with that of the control group (Figure 5A). In our study, bile depletion was accomplished with 4 h drainage of bile through the bile cannula, which was cannulated to the bile duct using PE-10 tubing. After this bile drainage, the concentration of total bile salts in the bile sample decreased from 50.1 $\pm$ 6.5 mM to 15.3 $\pm$ 5.7 mM (i.e., 70% decrease), which was measured using an enzymatic-fluorometric assay with the slight modifications reported by Choi et al. [20].

However, the co-administration of taurocholate (TC, 60 mg/kg) with Jaspine B in bile-depleted rats prevented the decrease in plasma Jaspine B and elevated the levels above those of controls (Figure 5C). This was also observed when TC was administered to the control rats; in this situation, the plasma concentration of Jaspine B was higher than that of the control group (Figure 5D vs. Figure 5A). The addition of TC increased the C_{max} and AUC of orally administered Jaspine B without changing the terminal half-life ($T_{1/2}$) (Table 2). These results suggest that the increase in C_{max} and AUC by the addition of TC was attributed to the absorption phase rather than the disposition phase, and consequently, the addition of TC increased the oral bioavailability of this compound from 6.2% to 41.2% (Table 2). In case of bile-depleted rats, AUC_∞ and $T_{1/2}$ were not calculated because the elimination rate constant could not be obtained. Therefore, the oral bioavailability of Jaspine B was calculated as $AUC_{12h,PO}/AUC_{12h,IV}$.

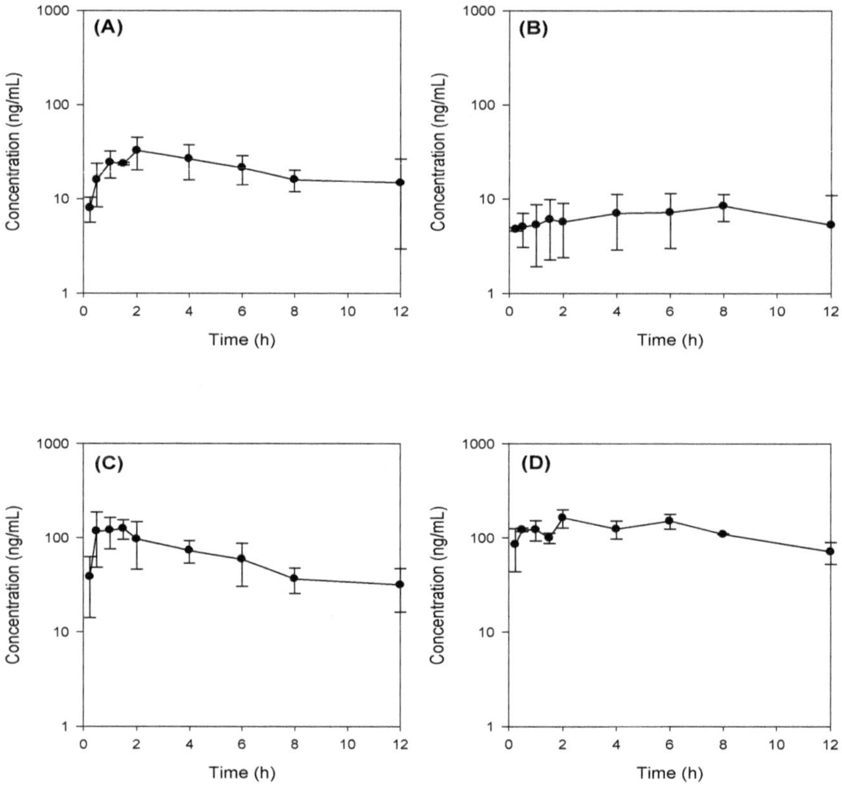

Figure 5. Plasma concentration-time profile of Jaspine B in rats after oral administration of Jaspine B (30 mg/kg) with or without taurocholate (TC; 60 mg/kg) in control and bile-depleted rats. (**A**) Control group; (**B**) bile-depleted group; (**C**) bile-depletion + TC; (**D**) Control + TC group. Data are expressed as the means ± S.D. from three to five different rats.

Table 2. Pharmacokinetic parameters of Jaspine B after oral administration of Jaspine B at a dose of 30 mg/kg in rats.

Parameters	Control (n = 3)	Bile Depletion (n = 3)	Bile Depletion + TC (n = 5)	Control + TC (n = 3)
C_{max} (ng/mL)	36.3 ± 11.3	8.5 ± 2.8 *	163.4 ± 28.4 *	174.1 ± 13.0 *
T_{max} (h)	2.5 ± 1.3	9.3 ± 2.3 *	1.0 ± 0.5	3.3 ± 2.3
$T_{1/2}$ (h)	5.5 ± 1.1	–	7.2 ± 1.5	6.4 ± 2.8
MRT (h)	4.9 ± 0.4	6.1 ± 0.3 *	4.9 ± 0.5	5.5 ± 0.03
AUC_{12h} (ng·h/mL)	240.6 ± 57.8	80.3 ± 42.7 *	828.3 ± 180 *	1406.3 ± 4.3 *,#
AUC_{∞} (ng·h/mL)	314.4 ± 76.1	–	1201.7 ± 254 *	2100.9 ± 419 *,#
BA (%)	6.2	1.6	23.5	41.2

Each value represents the mean ± S.D. * $p < 0.05$, significant versus control group; # $p < 0.05$, significant versus Bile depletion + TC group.

To confirm the role of bile salts in intestinal absorption, we measured intestinal permeability in rat intestinal segments using an Ussing chamber system. At first, to determine the optimized bile salt concentration, we monitored the permeability of Lucifer yellow, a marker compound for paracellular permeation and cell integrity [21,22], with various concentrations of TC (0.1–100 mM). The permeability of Lucifer yellow increased gradually until 10 mM TC and then showed a sharp increase at 100 mM TC (Figure 6A), suggesting that the cell integrity was disrupted between 10 and 100 mM TC.

To determine whether the intestinal absorption was increased by the addition of 10 mM TC, we measured the absorptive (A to B direction) and secretory (B to A direction) permeability of Jaspine B with 10 mM TC. The addition of 10 mM TC increased both absorptive and secretory permeability approximately 5-fold. The increased Jaspine B permeability (~5-fold) was greater than the increased Lucifer yellow permeability caused by tight junction opening (~2.8-fold), which was 56% of the increased Jaspine B permeability (Figure 6B). Therefore, the facilitated intestinal permeability in the presence of TC was caused partly by tight junction opening and partly by another unidentified mechanism. Since the absorptive and secretory permeabilities were almost identical, the intestinal transport mechanism such as efflux pump or uptake transport process may not contribute to the intestinal absorption of this compound [23]. The addition of 20% bile also increased the permeability of Jaspine B (Figure 6B) where the concentration of total bile salts in 20% bile was 10.1 $\pm$ 2.3 mM, which is similar to the concentration of bile salts in the intestinal lumen [24] as well as equilvalent to 10 mM TC. Thus the increased Jaspine B permeability in the presence of 10 mM TC and 20% bile was not statistically different.

Next, to unveil other mechanisms of increased Jaspine B permeability, we investigated whether the lipophilicity of Jaspine B increased in the presence of TC, since tertiary amines and quaternary ammonium can interact with endogenous bile to form lipophilic ion-pair complexes of Jaspine B and TC [25–27]. The partition coefficient of Jaspine B increased 10-fold in the presence of 10 mM TC compared with that in the absence of TC (Figure 6C).

Collectively, these results show that the enhancement of Jaspine B absorption in the presence of 20% bile and 10 mM TC could be attributed to the increased passive diffusion by the formation of lipophilic ion-pair complexes of Jaspine B-bile salts, as well as increased paracellular permeation through the tight junction opening by bile or bile salts [22,25]. As consequence, the increased absorption of Jaspine B in the presence of bile salts would lead to the increased BA of Jaspine B.

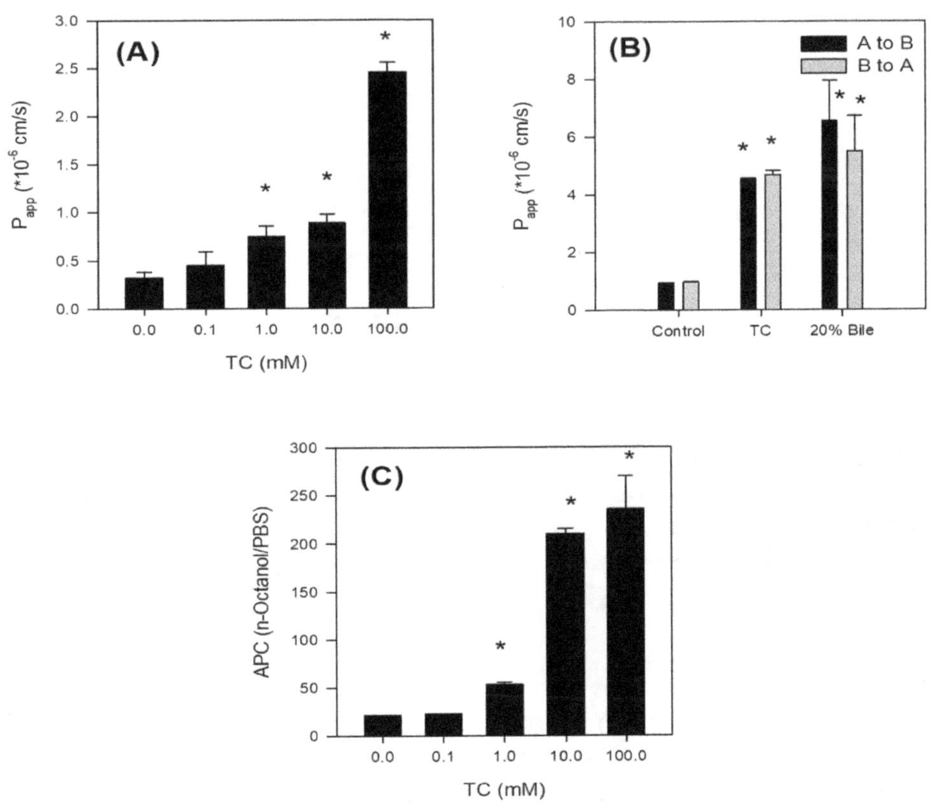

Figure 6. (**A**) Effect of taurocholate (TC) on the permeability of Lucifer yellow in the rat ileum. Permeability (P_{app}) of Lucifer yellow (10 μM) in the presence of TC (0, 0.1, 1, 10, and 100 mM) was measured in the rat ileum using the Ussing chamber system. (**B**) Effect of TC and bile on the permeability of Jaspine B in the rat ileum. Permeability (P_{app}) of Jaspine B (10 μM) in the presence of TC (10 mM) and bile (20%) was measured in the rat ileum using the Ussing chamber system. (**C**) Effect of TC on the lipophilicity of Jaspine B. Apparent partition coefficient (APC) of Jaspine B between *n*-octanol and PBS phases was measured in the presence of TC (0, 0.1, 1, 10, or 100 mM).Each data point represents the mean $\pm$ S.D. of three independent experiments. * $p < 0.05$, statistically significant versus the corresponding control group.

2.5. Tissue Distribution of Jaspine B

To investigate the tissue distribution of Jaspine B, its concentrations in the brain, liver, kidney, heart, spleen, and plasma were measured at 0.5 h and 12 h after IV administration of 10 mg/kg. The liver, kidney, heart, and spleen were selected as major organs that show high distribution, and the brain was selected as an organ that shows limited distribution. To calculate the drug concentration ratios of tissue to plasma (T/P ratio) of Jaspine B, 0.5 h and 12 h were selected to represent the distribution and elimination phases, respectively. As shown in Figure 7, the T/P ratios of Jaspine B in the brain, kidney, heart, and spleen were significantly higher than that in the plasma at 0.5 h (i.e., 6.2-, 11.1-, 14.4-, and 18.5-fold greater in the brain, kidney, heart, and spleen, respectively, than in the plasma). The significantly higher concentrations of Jaspine B in the brain, kidney, heart, and spleen were maintained 12 h after administration (i.e., 1.8-, 4.7-, 3.2-, and 3.9-fold greater in the brain, kidney, heart, and spleen, respectively, than in the plasma). These results were consistent with the large volume of distribution of Jaspine B, 21.2 L/kg. Interestingly, the concentration of Jaspine B in the liver was lower than in the other tissues (i.e., 2.3- and 1.2-fold higher than plasma levels at 0.5 and 12 h, respectively), which may be attributed to the substantial metabolism of this compound in the liver.

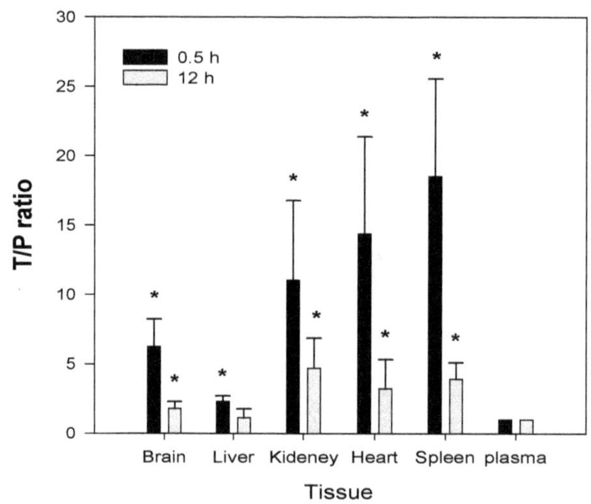

Figure 7. Tissue to plasma (T/P) ratios of Jaspine B recovered from tissues at 0.5 h and 12 h after intravenous (10 mg/kg) administration of Jaspine B to rats. At 0.5 h and 12 h after dosing, plasma, liver, kidney, heart, spleen, and brain samples were collected and the concentrations of Jaspine B in the samples were measured. The bars represent the means ± S.D. of the results from four rats. * $p < 0.05$, significant versus plasma ratio.

3. Discussion

Jaspine B is an anhydrophytosphingosine, extracted from the marine sponge, *Pachastrissa* spp. It shows meaningful inhibitory activity against sphingosine kinases (SphK1 and SphK2), which is an important mechanism of action for its anti-proliferative effect [28]. Jaspine B shows differential efficacy against a variety of tumor types of different tissue origins, and the cellular accumulation of Jaspine B at steady-state is a crucial determining factor of efficacy [19]. Moreover, the intravenous injection of Jaspine B (200 mg/mouse, equivalent to 6.7 mg/kg) on 4th, 8th, and 12th day dramatically decreased metastatic melanoma cell growth in the lungs of Jaspine B-injected mice on day 14 [18]. Although this in vivo and in vitro anti-proliferative effects of Jaspine B, the pharmacokinetics features of this compound was not investigated.

Therefore, the next step in understanding the anti-tumor activity of Jaspine B was to investigate its pharmacokinetic characteristics and the underlying mechanisms controlling the absorption, distribution, metabolism, and elimination of this compound.

The absorption of Jaspine B itself was limited, however, and the presence of bile salts increased the intestinal permeability of this compound over 5-fold by increasing partitioning of Jaspine B to lipophilic phase and tight junction opening (Figure 6). However, since the TC infusion to the rat liver did not significantly alter the metabolic activity of sulfobromophthalein [29], it is unlikely to conclude that concomitant administration of Jaspine B with TC inhibited metabolism of Jaspine B, and consequently increased BA of Jaspine B. To the contrary, the co-existence of Jaspine B with TC increased intestinal permeability and thereby increased the intestinal absorption and BA of Jaspine B. The results were consistent with a low oral BA of Jaspine B (6.2%) that decreased to 1.6% in bile-depleted rats, and after the co-addition of TC, oral BA increased to 23.5% in bile-depleted rats and 41.2% in control rats. Since the increased permeability of Jaspine B was the modulating factor that increased the low oral BA of Jaspine B and the permeability of Jaspine B in the rat intestine was very limited (0.11×10^{-6} cm/s), the important factors for the low BA of Jaspine B can be elucidated as low intestinal permeability. In addition, the low oral BA was known to be attributed to the limited permeability, the chemical and enzymatic degradation of a drug in the gut lumen, and the intestinal or hepatic first-pass effect [30]. The instability of Jaspine B in the gut lumen and the hepatic or intestinal first-pass effect also need to be investigated to elucidate the underlying mechanisms for the low BA of Jaspine B.

In our study, bile depletion was accomplished with 4 h drainage of bile through the bile cannula, which was evidenced by the 70% reduction of total bile salts concentration (from 50.1 ± 6.5 mM in control rats to 15.3 ± 5.7 mM) in bile drainage rats, which we named as bile-depleted rats. Since over 90% of bile salts were recirculated gut-liver-bile cycle [31], a 70% decrease of bile salts concentration in the bile implicated the significant decrease of bile salts in the gut as well, which resulted in the decreased absorption of Jaspine B in bile-depleted rats (Figure 5B). As a result of TC supplementation (60 mg/kg) with Jaspine B, which was suspended in 3 mL of DMSO: PEG400: saline solution, the TC concentration would be approximately 10 mM in the gut and could enhance the absorption of Jaspine B in rats from bile depletion + TC group and control + TC group (Figure 5C,D).

These results could be applied to the development of oral Jaspine B formulations consisting of bile salts and lipophilic phospholipids, i.e., mixed micelle formulations [32], to increase the permeability and lipophilicity of this compound. However, for the clinical and pharmaceutical application, the use of pharmaceutical excipients that enhance the transport without affecting tight junctions of intestine rather than high concentrations of TC would be the best approach. For example, SP1049C (Supratek Pharma Inc., Montreal, PQ, Canada), a doxorubicin-containing mixed-micelle formulation with Pluronic L61 and F127, showed increased cellular concentration of the doxorubicin in tumor cells and has reached clinical phase 3 study because of its superior antitumor activity compared with that of doxorubicin standard formulation [33]. A phospholipid-Tween 80 mixed micelle formulation of paclitaxel showed higher anti-tumor activity and reduced systemic toxicity than Taxol formulation did [34].

The second feature of Jaspine B is that it is highly distributed to tissues such as brain, kidney, heart, and spleen. The T/P ratios in these organs were 6.2, 11.1, 14.4, and 18.5, respectively, and remained elevated 2–4-fold 12 h after a single IV administration of Jaspine B (Figure 7). Since we previously reported that the steady-state drug concentration was important for the anti-cancer efficacy of this compound [19,35,36], the tissue distribution of Jaspine B is very important to predict the therapeutic efficacy of this compound. Moreover, this compound showed differential cytotoxicity depending on the cancer cell type, thus the highly tissue distributed features of this compound should be carefully considered in terms of drug response and toxicity. However, we should note that the use of PEG400 as a vehicle in the tissue distribution study (Figure 7) might change the tissue distribution profile of Jaspine B because PEG400 has an ability to entrap of this compound in the spleen's reticuloendothelial systems and thereby increase the in vivo metabolic stability compared with in vitro metabolic stability results (Figure 4).

In addition, the low the recovery from feces and urine (about 6.3% after IV administration) was consistent with the observed microsomal instability in the rat liver microsomes (Figure 4), although the involvement CYP enzymes as well as the proposed metabolite structures were not investigated in this study. Therefore, identification of metabolites and the elucidation of the metabolic enzyme(s) involved will be necessary for future investigation. Moreover, since the metabolites of Jaspine B may have pharmacological activities on the inhibition of SphK1 and the inhibition of FOXO3 phosphorylaiton, the evaluation of the pharmacological activity or toxicity of the proposed metabolite would be of importance.

4. Materials and Methods

4.1. Reagents

Jaspine B was synthesized by Dr. D. Lee (Ajou University, Suwon, Korea) with a purity of over 99% and was confirmed by nuclear magnetic resonance (NMR) and mass spectroscopy results [37]. Its structure is shown in Figure 1.

Hank's balanced salt solution (HBSS), taurocholate (TC), Lucifer yellow, dimethyl sulfoxide (DMSO), polyethylene glycol (PEG) 400, β-nicotinamide adenine dinucleotide (β-NAD), 3α-hydroxysteroid dehyrogenase (3α-HSD), EDTA, and Tris base were purchased from Sigma-Aldrich (St. Louis, MO, USA). Fetal bovine serum, Dulbecco's Modified Eagle's medium (DMEM), and penicillin-streptomycin were purchased from Hyclone Laboratories (Logan, UT, USA). All other reagents were reagent grade.

Rat liver microsomes (RLMs) from Sprague Dawley (SD) rats and the reaction solutions, including the NADH-generating system were purchased from BD-Corning (Corning, NY, USA).

A NaviCyte Ussing chamber system was obtained from Harvard Apparatus Co. (Holliston, MA, USA). Round metabolic cages for rats were purchased from Jungdo B&P Inc. (Seoul, Korea).

4.2. LC-MS/MS Analysis of Jaspine B

The concentrations of Jaspine B in the biological samples were analyzed using an Agilent 6430 Triple Quad LC/MS-MS system (Agilent, Wilmington, DE, USA) coupled with an Agilent Infinity 1290 series high performance liquid chromatography (HPLC) system. The separation was performed on a Synergi Polar RP column (2.0 mm i.d. $\times$ 150 mm, 4 µm, Phenomenex) using a mobile phase that consisted of acetonitrile and DDW (85:15, v/v) with 0.1% formic acid at a flow rate of 0.2 mL/min. Mass spectra were recorded by electrospray ionization in the positive mode. Quantification was performed using multiple reaction monitoring (MRM) at m/z 300.3$\rightarrow$270.2 for Jaspine B and m/z 336.1$\rightarrow$320.0 for berberine.

For the analytical validation of Jaspine B in plasma samples, the standard curve range was 25–5000 ng/mL and the concentrations of quality control (QC) samples were 75, 500, and 3000 ng/mL. The recovery of these spiked QC sample were in the range of 88.2–98.1%. Intra- and inter-day precision and accuracy had coefficients of variance of less than 10%. The stability of Jaspine B QC samples after 3 freeze thaw cycles were 83.9–94.4% and the short-term stability of these samples after standing for 6 h at room temperature was 94.3–100.1%.

The respective standard curve range and sample preparation methods in various biological samples from various experiments were described in detail in each experimental section.

4.3. Pharmacokinetics of Jaspine B

Male SD rats (aged 8–9 weeks, weighing 250–300 g) were obtained from Samtako Bio Korea, Inc. (Osan, Korea). The rats were acclimatized for 1 week in a temperature-controlled room (23 $\pm$ 2 °C) with a 12-h illumination cycle. Food and water were given *ad libitum*. All animal procedures were approved by the Animal Care and Use Committee of the Kyungpook National University (No. 2015-0064). The rats were fasted for at least 12 h before the oral administration of drugs.

The femoral artery, femoral vein, and bile duct were cannulated with polyethylene tubes (PE-50 and PE-10; Jungdo, Seoul, Korea) under light anesthesia with isoflurane.

For intravenous (IV) dosing, Jaspine B was dissolved in a vehicle containing DMSO: PEG400: saline (2:4:4, *v*/*v*/*v*) and was IV-injected via the femoral vein at 10 mg/kg (vehicle volume, 1 mL/kg). Blood samples were collected from the femoral artery at 0, 0.083, 0.167, 0.25, 0.5, 1, 2, 4, 6, 8, and 12 h following the IV administration of Jaspine B. Bile and urine samples were collected every 2 h for a total of 12 h. After centrifugation of blood samples at 13,200 rpm for 10 min, aliquots of 50 μL of plasma, bile, and urine were stored at −80 °C until the analysis of Jaspine B.

In the experiment using metabolic cages, feces were collected at 12, 24, 48, and 72 h following the IV administration of Jaspine B (10 mg/kg). Aliquots of 50 μL of urine and 10% feces homogenates were stored at −80 °C until the analysis.

Aliquots (50 μL) of plasma, bile, feces homogenates, and urine samples were added to 250 μL of acetonitrile containing 0.5 ng/mL of berberine (an internal standard). After vortexing for 10 min and centrifugation at 13,200 rpm for 5 min, an aliquot (2 μL) of the supernatant was injected directly into the LC-MS/MS system. For the analysis of plasma concentration, the standard curve range was 25–5000 ng/mL and the concentrations of quality control (QC) samples were 75, 500, and 3000 ng/mL, as described previously. Concentrations of Jaspine B in urine, bile, and feces homogenates were 5–300 ng/mL, 20–5000 ng/mL, and 20–5000 ng/mL, respectively. The concentrations of QC samples were 15, 100, and 300 ng/mL for urine samples and 75, 500, and 3000 ng/mL for bile and feces homogenates.

For oral dosing, Jaspine B was dissolved in a vehicle containing DMSO: PEG400: saline (2:4:4, *v*/*v*/*v*) and was administered by oral gavages at a single dose of 30 mg/kg of Jaspine B concomitantly with or without 60 mg/kg TC (vehicle volume, 3 mL/kg) to the control and bile-depleted rats. Bile depletion was accomplished with 4 h drainage of bile through the bile cannula, which was cannulated to the bile duct using PE-10 tubing.

Blood samples (approximately 250 μL each) were collected from the femoral artery at 0, 0.25, 0.5, 1, 1.5, 2, 4, 8, and 12 h following the oral administration of Jaspine B. After centrifugation of blood samples at 13,200 rpm for 10 min, plasma samples (50 μL) were collected and stored at −80 °C until the analysis by liquid chromatography tandem-mass spectrometry (LC-MS/MS). Aliquots (50 μL) of plasma samples were added to 250 μL of acetonitrile containing 0.5 ng/mL of berberine (an internal standard). After vortexing for 10 min and centrifugation at 13,200 rpm for 5 min, an aliquot (10 μL) of the supernatant was injected directly into the LC-MS/MS system. The standard curve range was 5–2000 ng/mL and the concentrations of quality control (QC) samples were 60, 300, and 2000 ng/mL. Standard curves showed good linearity ($R^2 > 0.999$) and the interday accuracy and precision was 99.0–105.1% and 0.3–6.9%, respectively.

4.4. Tissue Distribution of Jaspine B

Jaspine B was dissolved in a vehicle containing DMSO: PEG400: saline (2:4:4, *v*/*v*/*v*) and IV-injected via the femoral vein at a dose of 10 mg/kg (vehicle volume, 1 mL/kg). Blood samples were collected from the abdominal artery and animals were euthanized at 0.5 h and 12 h after IV dosing. The blood, brain, liver, kidney, heart, and spleen were immediately excised, gently washed with ice-cold saline, and weighed. The tissue samples were homogenized with 9 volumes of saline. Aliquots of 50 μL of tissue homogenates and plasma were stored at −80 °C until the analysis.

Aliquots (50 μL) of plasma and tissue homogenates were added to 250 μL of acetonitrile containing 0.5 ng/mL of berberine. After vortexing for 10 min and centrifugation at 13,200 rpm for 5 min, an aliquot (2 μL) of the supernatant was injected directly into the LC-MS/MS system. For the analysis of plasma and tissue concentration, the standard curves with a range of 5–1000 ng/mL in the blank plasma and 10% bank tissue homogenates from brain, liver, kidney, heart, and spleen were prepared, and the concentrations of quality control (QC) samples of respective plasma and tissue homogenates were 25 and 750 ng/mL. The recovery of these spiked QC samples were in the range of 73.6–112.2% in all tissue homogenates. Intra- and inter-day precision and accuracy had coefficients of variance of less than 15%.

4.5. Metabolic Stability of Jaspine B in Rat Liver Microsomes (RLMs)

Jaspine B (1 μM) was reconstituted in 100 mM potassium phosphate buffer (pH 7.4) containing 0.25 mg of RLMs and was pre-incubated for 5 min at 37 °C. The reaction was initiated by adding an NADPH-generating system (1.3 mM β-NADP, 3.3 mM glucose-6-phosphate, 3.3 mM $MgCl_2$, and 1.0 unit/mL glucose-6-phosphate dehydrogenase) and then incubated (final volume 100 μL) for 0, 15, 30, and 60 min at 37 °C in a shaking water bath. The reaction was stopped by placing the incubation tubes on ice and adding 200 μL of ice-cold acetonitrile containing 0.5 ng/mL of berberine. After vortexing for 10 min and centrifugation at 13,200 rpm for 5 min, 2 μL of the supernatant was injected directly into the LC-MS/MS system. We also determined the metabolic stability of 1 μM propranolol and 1 μM metformin as a positive and negative control, respectively, using the same procedure [38]. The remaining % of propranolol and metformin after 60 min incubation was 12.2% and 63.4% of initial concentration, indicating the feasibility of this system.

4.6. Determination of Bile Salts Concentration in Bile

Total bile salt concentrations in bile samples were determined by means of an enzymatic-fluorometric assay with the slight modification of Choi at al. [20]. Briefly, bile samples were collected. Fifty μL aliquots of standard TC solutions (5, 10, 25, 50, 100, 200 μM), bile samples were added to 950 μL of reaction buffer containing 1mM β-nicotinamide adenine dinucleotide (β-NAD), 50 μU 3α-hydroxysteroid dehyrogenase (3α-HSD), 0.385 mM EDTA and 760 mM Tris (pH 9.5), followed by incubation at 37 °C for 30 min. The reaction was quenched by the addition of 3 mL of ice cold water and the fluorescence was measured at an excitation wavelength of 340 nm and an emission wavelength of 465 nm.

4.7. Determination of the Intestinal Permeability of Jaspine B

For the measurement of the effect of TC on the tight junction of biological membranes, the permeability of 50 μM Lucifer yellow, a marker of paracellular permeation [21], was measured in the presence of TC (0, 0.1, 1, 10, 100 mM). Prior to the experiment, ileal segments from SD rats (about 20 cm) were placed in the chambers and were submerged in fresh, prewarmed (37 °C) HBSS for 15 min for acclimatization. The chambers were continuously bubbled with carbogen gas (5% CO_2/ 95% O_2) during the experiment. The experiments began by replacing the HBSS with HBSS containing 50 μM Lucifer yellow and various concentrations of TC on the apical side (A) and adding fresh HBSS to the basal side (B). Aliquots (400 μL) of media were withdrawn from the receiver compartment (B) after 0, 20, 40, 60, and 80 min, and the volume of liquid in the receiver compartment was replenished with fresh, prewarmed HBSS after each sampling. Aliquots (200 μL) of all samples were used for the determination of Lucifer yellow concentration. The fluorescence of Lucifer yellow in the samples was measured using a fluorescence spectrophotometer (Infinite 200 PRO, Tecan, Switzerland) with excitation at 425 nm and emission at 535 nm.

A to B and B to A permeability of Jaspine B was measured in the presence of TC and rat bile. One mL of HBSS containing 50 μM Jaspine B and 10 mM TC or 20% bile was added to the donor side and 1 mL of preheated fresh HBSS was added to the receiver side. Aliquots (400 μL) of media were withdrawn at 0, 20, 40, 60, and 80 min from the receiver compartment as described above. Aliquots (50 μL) of all samples were stored at −80 °C until analysis.

Aliquots (50 μL) of all samples were added to 250 μL of acetonitrile containing 0.5 ng/mL of berberine. After vortexing for 10 min and centrifugation at 13,200 rpm for 5 min, 2 μL of the supernatant was injected directly into the LC-MS/MS system.

4.8. Effect of TC on the Lipophilicity of Jaspine B

The effect of TC on the apparent partition coefficients (APC) of Jaspine B between aqueous and organic phases was investigated [26]. *n*-Octanol and phosphate-buffered saline (PBS, pH 7.4) were used as the organic and aqueous phases, respectively, in the partition study. *n*-Octanol and PBS were saturated with respect to one another prior to use. An equal volume of *n*-octanol was added to PBS (5 mL each) containing Jaspine B (10 mM) and TC (0, 0.1, 1, 10, or 100 mM) in a screw-capped test tube, and the mixture was vortexed vigorously for 5 min followed by shaking for 2 h at 25 °C in a temperature-controlled water bath. After standing for 1 h at 25 °C in the water bath, the mixture was separated into two phases by centrifugation at 3000 rpm for 10 min. The concentration of Jaspine B in a 50-μL aliquot of aqueous and organic phase was measured. Briefly, 50 μL of sample was added to 250 μL of acetonitrile containing 0.5 ng/mL of berberine. After vortexing for 10 min and centrifugation at 13,200 rpm for 5 min, an aliquot (2 μL) of the supernatant was injected directly into the LC-MS/MS system. The APC was calculated from the concentration ratio of each compound between the octanol and PBS phases.

4.9. Data Analysis

Pharmacokinetic parameters were determined using a non-compartmental analysis (WinNonlin® 2.0; Pharsight, Mountain View, CA, USA). Maximum plasma concentration (C_{max}) and time to reach C_{max} (T_{max}) values were obtained from plasma concentration-time curves. The area under the plasma concentration–time curve from zero to infinity (AUC) was calculated using the trapezoidal-extrapolation method. For extrapolation, the area from the last data point to infinity was estimated by dividing the terminal-phase rate constant by plasma concentration at the last time point. Oral bioavailability was calculated by dividing AUC_{PO}, which was normalized by Jaspine B dose (30 mg/kg) by AUC_{IV}, which was also normalized by IV dose of Jaspine B (10 mg/kg):

$$BA(\%) = \frac{\frac{AUC_{\infty,PO}}{Dose(30mg/kg)}}{\frac{AUC_{\infty,IV}}{Dose(10mg/kg)}} \times 100 \quad (1)$$

However, in the case of bile-depleted rats, AUC_∞ and $T_{1/2}$ were not calculated because the elimination rate constant could not be obtained. Therefore, the oral bioavailability of Jaspine B was calculated as follows:

$$BA(\%) = \frac{\frac{AUC_{12h,PO}}{Dose(30mg/kg)}}{\frac{AUC_{12h,IV}}{Dose(10mg/kg)}} \times 100 \quad (2)$$

Total systemic clearance (CL_{total}) was calculated by dividing IV dose by plasma AUC and the apparent volume of distribution at steady-state (Vss) was calculated by multiplying mean residence time (MRT) by CL_{total}. Urinary and biliary clearances of Jaspine B (CL_{urine} and CL_{bile}) were estimated by dividing the total amount of Jaspine B excreted into urine and bile, respectively, for the 0–12 h period by plasma AUC.

The apparent permeability (P_{app}) of the drug was calculated by dividing the initial drug transport rate (dQ/dt, pmol/min) by the initial drug concentration in the donor compartment of the insert (C_o) multiplied by the surface area of the insert (A, cm^2) [22]:

$$P_{app} = \frac{dQ}{dt} \times \frac{1}{AC_o} \quad (3)$$

Data are expressed as the means ± standard deviations (S.D.), and statistical significance was determined by *t*-test using SPSS software version 16.1.

Acknowledgments: This work was supported by a grant from the Korea Institute of Planning and Evaluation for Technology in Food, Agriculture, Forestry, and Fisheries (IPET) through Export Promotion Technology Development Program, funded by the Ministry of Agriculture, Food and Rural Affairs (MAFRA) (No 316017-3), Republic of Korea.

Author Contributions: Im-Sook Song and Min-Koo Choi designed the study, performed the experiments, analyzed the data, and wrote the manuscript. Jihoon Lee, So Jeong Nam, Yun Ju Kang, Youjin Han, Kwangik Choi, Young A. Choi, and Mihwa Kwon performed the pharmacokinetics and tissue distribution study and also performed intestinal permeability experiments and analyzed the Jaspine B concentrations from the various samples. Dongjoo Lee synthesized, purified, and confirmed the Jaspine B. All authors reviewed the manuscript.

References

1. Indumathy, S.; Dass, C.R. Finding chemo: The search for marine-based pharmaceutical drugs active against cancer. *J. Pharm. Pharmacol.* **2013**, *65*, 1280–1301. [CrossRef] [PubMed]
2. Haefner, B. Drugs from the deep: Marine natural products as drug candidates. *Drug Discov. Today* **2003**, *8*, 536–544. [CrossRef]
3. Sima, P.; Vetvicka, V. Bioactive substances with anti-neoplastic efficacy from marine invertebrates: Porifera and coelenterata. *World J. Clin. Oncol.* **2011**, *2*, 355–361. [CrossRef] [PubMed]
4. Singh, R.; Sharma, M.; Joshi, P.; Rawat, D.S. Clinical status of anti-cancer agents derived from marine sources. *Anticancer Agents Med. Chem.* **2008**, *8*, 603–617. [CrossRef] [PubMed]
5. Russo, P.; Nastrucci, C.; Cesario, A. From the sea to anticancer therapy. *Curr. Med. Chem.* **2011**, *18*, 3551–3562. [CrossRef] [PubMed]
6. Kuznetsov, G.; Towle, M.J.; Cheng, H.; Kawamura, T.; TenDyke, K.; Liu, D.; Kishi, Y.; Yu, M.J.; Littlefield, B.A. Induction of morphological and biochemical apoptosis following prolonged mitotic blockage by halichondrin b macrocyclic ketone analog e7389. *Cancer Res.* **2004**, *64*, 5760–5766. [CrossRef] [PubMed]
7. Shida, D.; Takabe, K.; Kapitonov, D.; Milstien, S.; Spiegel, S. Targeting SphK1 as a new strategy against cancer. *Curr. Drug Targets* **2008**, *9*, 662–673. [CrossRef] [PubMed]
8. Kunkel, G.T.; Maceyka, M.; Milstien, S.; Spiegel, S. Targeting the sphingosine-1-phosphate axis in cancer, inflammation and beyond. *Nat. Rev. Drug Discov.* **2013**, *12*, 688–702. [CrossRef] [PubMed]
9. Lim, K.G.; Gray, A.I.; Pyne, S.; Pyne, N.J. Resveratrol dimers are novel sphingosine kinase 1 inhibitors and affect sphingosine kinase 1 expression and cancer cell growth and survival. *Br. J. Pharmacol.* **2012**, *166*, 1605–1616. [CrossRef] [PubMed]
10. Lim, K.G.; Tonelli, F.; Li, Z.; Lu, X.; Bittman, R.; Pyne, S.; Pyne, N.J. Fty720 analogues as sphingosine kinase 1 inhibitors: Enzyme inhibition kinetics, allosterism, proteasomal degradation, and actin rearrangement in mcf-7 breast cancer cells. *J. Biol. Chem.* **2011**, *286*, 18633–18640. [CrossRef] [PubMed]
11. Pyne, S.; Bittman, R.; Pyne, N.J. Sphingosine kinase inhibitors and cancer: Seeking the golden sword of hercules. *Cancer Res.* **2011**, *71*, 6576–6582. [CrossRef] [PubMed]
12. French, K.J.; Schrecengost, R.S.; Lee, B.D.; Zhuang, Y.; Smith, S.N.; Eberly, J.L.; Yun, J.K.; Smith, C.D. Discovery and evaluation of inhibitors of human sphingosine kinase. *Cancer Res.* **2003**, *63*, 5962–5969. [PubMed]
13. Johnson, K.R.; Johnson, K.Y.; Crellin, H.G.; Ogretmen, B.; Boylan, A.M.; Harley, R.A.; Obeid, L.M. Immunohistochemical distribution of sphingosine kinase 1 in normal and tumor lung tissue. *J. Histochem. Cytochem.* **2005**, *53*, 1159–1166. [CrossRef] [PubMed]
14. Sobue, S.; Iwasaki, T.; Sugisaki, C.; Nagata, K.; Kikuchi, R.; Murakami, M.; Takagi, A.; Kojima, T.; Banno, Y.; Akao, Y.; et al. Quantitative rt-pcr analysis of sphingolipid metabolic enzymes in acute leukemia and myelodysplastic syndromes. *Leukemia* **2006**, *20*, 2042–2046. [CrossRef] [PubMed]
15. Kuroda, I.; Musman, M.; Ohtani, I.I.; Ichiba, T.; Tanaka, J.; Gravalos, D.G.; Higa, T. Pachastrissamine, a cytotoxic anhydrophytosphingosine from a marine sponge, *Pachastrissa* sp. *J. Nat. Prod.* **2002**, *65*, 1505–1506. [CrossRef] [PubMed]
16. Salma, Y.; Lafont, E.; Therville, N.; Carpentier, S.; Bonnafe, M.J.; Levade, T.; Genisson, Y.; Andrieu-Abadie, N. The natural marine anhydrophytosphingosine, Jaspine B, induces apoptosis in melanoma cells by interfering with ceramide metabolism. *Biochem. Pharmacol.* **2009**, *78*, 477–485. [CrossRef] [PubMed]
17. Stoica, B.A.; Movsesyan, V.A.; Lea, P.M.; Faden, A.I. Ceramide-induced neuronal apoptosis is associated with dephosphorylation of AKT, BAD, FKHR, GSK-3beta, and induction of the mitochondrial-dependent intrinsic caspase pathway. *Mol. Cell. Neurosci.* **2003**, *22*, 365–382. [CrossRef]
18. Yoo, H.; Lee, Y.S.; Lee, S.; Kim, S.; Kim, T.Y. Pachastrissamine from pachastrissa sp. Inhibits melanoma cell growth by dual inhibition of CDK2 and ERK-mediated FOXO3 downregulation. *Phytother. Res.* **2012**, *26* 1927–1933. [CrossRef] [PubMed]

19. Lee, J.; Choi, K.; Kwon, M.; Lee, D.; Choi, M.K.; Song, I.S. Differential cytotoxic effects of Jaspine B in various cancer cells. *J. Life Sci.* **2016**, *26*, 101–109. [CrossRef]
20. Choi, M.K.; Song, I.S.; Park, S.R.; Hong, S.S.; Kim, D.D.; Chung, S.J.; Shim, C.K. Mechanism of the stationary canalicular excretion of tributylmethyl ammonium in rats with a ccl4-induced acute hepatic injury. *J. Pharm. Sci.* **2005**, *94*, 317–326. [CrossRef] [PubMed]
21. Zhang, W.; Parniak, M.A.; Sarafianos, S.G.; Empey, P.E.; Rohan, L.C. In vitro transport characteristics of efda, a novel nucleoside reverse transcriptase inhibitor using caco-2 and mdckii cell monolayers. *Eur. J. Pharmacol.* **2014**, *732*, 86–95. [CrossRef] [PubMed]
22. Choi, Y.A.; Yoon, Y.H.; Choi, K.; Kwon, M.; Goo, S.H.; Cha, J.S.; Choi, M.K.; Lee, H.S.; Song, I.S. Enhanced oral bioavailability of morin administered in mixed micelle formulation with pluronicf127 and tween80 in rats. *Biol. Pharm. Bull.* **2015**, *38*, 208–217. [CrossRef] [PubMed]
23. Oude Elferink, R.P.; Meijer, D.K.; Kuipers, F.; Jansen, P.L.; Groen, A.K.; Groothuis, G.M. Hepatobiliary secretion of organic compounds; molecular mechanisms of membrane transport. *Biochim. Biophys. Acta* **1995**, *1241*, 215–268. [CrossRef]
24. Martinez-Augustin, O.; Sanchez de Medina, F. Intestinal bile acid physiology and pathophysiology. *World J. Gastroenterol.* **2008**, *14*, 5630–5640. [CrossRef] [PubMed]
25. Song, I.S.; Choi, M.K.; Shim, W.S.; Shim, C.K. Transport of organic cationic drugs: Effect of ion-pair formation with bile salts on the biliary excretion and pharmacokinetics. *Pharmacol. Ther.* **2013**, *138*, 142–154. [CrossRef] [PubMed]
26. Song, I.S.; Chung, S.J.; Shim, C.K. Contribution of ion pair complexation with bile salts to biliary excretion of organic cations in rats. *Am. J. Physiol. Gastrointest. Liver Physiol.* **2001**, *281*, 515–525.
27. Song, I.S.; Han, Y.H.; Chung, S.J.; Shim, C.K. Contribution of ion-pair complexation with bile salts to the transport of organic cations across llc-pk1 cell monolayers. *Pharm. Res.* **2003**, *20*, 597–604. [CrossRef] [PubMed]
28. Yoshimitsu, Y.; Oishi, S.; Miyagaki, J.; Inuki, S.; Ohno, H.; Fujii, N. Pachastrissamine (Jaspine B) and its stereoisomers inhibit sphingosine kinases and atypical protein kinase c. *Bioorg. Med. Chem.* **2011**, *19*, 5402–5408. [CrossRef] [PubMed]
29. Boyer, J.L.; Scheig, R.L.; Klatskin, G. The effect of sodium taurocholate on the hepatic metabolism of sulfobromophthalein sodium (bsp). The role of bile flow. *J. Clin. Investig.* **1970**, *49*, 206–215. [CrossRef] [PubMed]
30. Yang, J.; Jamei, M.; Yeo, K.R.; Tucker, G.T.; Rostami-Hodjegan, A. Prediction of intestinal first-pass drug metabolism. *Curr. Drug Metab.* **2007**, *8*, 676–684. [CrossRef] [PubMed]
31. Dawson, P.A. Role of the intestinal bile acid transporters in bile acid and drug disposition. *Handb. Exp. Pharmacol.* **2011**, *201*, 169–203.
32. Prabagar, B.; Yoo, B.K.; Woo, J.S.; Kim, J.A.; Rhee, J.D.; Piao, M.G.; Choi, H.G.; Yong, C.S. Enhanced bioavailability of poorly water-soluble clotrimazole by inclusion with beta-cyclodextrin. *Arch. Pharm. Res.* **2007**, *30*, 249–254. [CrossRef] [PubMed]
33. Valle, J.W.; Armstrong, A.; Newman, C.; Alakhov, V.; Pietrzynski, G.; Brewer, J.; Campbell, S.; Corrie, P.; Rowinsky, E.K.; Ranson, M. A phase 2 study of sp1049c, doxorubicin in p-glycoprotein-targeting pluronics, in patients with advanced adenocarcinoma of the esophagus and gastroesophageal junction. *Investig. New Drugs* **2011**, *29*, 1029–1037. [CrossRef] [PubMed]
34. Liang, H.; Yang, Q.; Deng, L.; Lu, J.; Chen, J. Phospholipid-tween 80 mixed micelles as an intravenous delivery carrier for paclitaxel. *Drug Dev. Ind. Pharm.* **2011**, *37*, 597–605. [CrossRef] [PubMed]
35. Adedokun, O.J.; Sandborn, W.J.; Feagan, B.G.; Rutgeerts, P.; Xu, Z.; Marano, C.W.; Johanns, J.; Zhou, H.; Davis, H.M.; Cornillie, F.; et al. Association between serum concentration of infliximab and efficacy in adult patients with ulcerative colitis. *Gastroenterology* **2014**, *147*, 1296–1307. [CrossRef] [PubMed]
36. Kuo, M.T.; Chen, H.H.; Song, I.S.; Savaraj, N.; Ishikawa, T. The roles of copper transporters in cisplatin resistance. *Cancer Metastasis Rev.* **2007**, *26*, 71–83. [CrossRef] [PubMed]
37. Kwon, Y.; Song, J.; Bae, H.; Kim, W.J.; Lee, J.Y.; Han, G.H.; Lee, S.K.; Kim, S. Synthesis and biological evaluation of carbocyclic analogues of pachastrissamine. *Mar. Drugs* **2015**, *13*, 824–837. [CrossRef] [PubMed]
38. Choi, M.K.; Kwon, M.; Ahn, J.H.; Kim, N.J.; Bae, M.A.; Song, I.S. Transport characteristics and transporter-based drug-drug interactions of tm-25659, a novel taz modulator. *Biopharm. Drug Dispos.* **2014**, *35*, 183–194. [CrossRef] [PubMed]

17

Heteromeles Arbutifolia, a Traditional Treatment for Alzheimer's Disease, Phytochemistry and Safety

Xiaogang Wang [1], Raphael Dubois [2], Caitlyn Young [2], Eric J. Lien [2] and James D. Adams [2,*]

[1] Tongji School of Pharmacy, Huazhong University of Science and Technology, Wuhan 430030, Hubei, China; wxg0122@163.com

[2] Department of Pharmacology and Pharmaceutical Sciences, School of Pharmacy, University of Southern California, Los Angeles, CA 90899-9121, USA; rd_820@usc.edu (R.D.); caitlyny@usc.edu (C.Y.); elien@usc.edu (E.J.L.)

* Correspondence: jadams@usc.edu

Academic Editor: Gerhard Litscher

Abstract: Background: This study examined the chemistry and safety of *Heteromeles arbutifolia*, also called toyon or California holly, which is a traditional California Indian food and treatment for Alzheimer's disease. **Methods:** Plant extracts were examined by HPLC/MS, NMR and other techniques to identify compounds. Volunteers were recruited to examine the acute safety of the plant medicine using a standard short-term memory test. **Results:** The plant was found to contain icariside E4, dihydroxyoleanenoic acid, maslinic acid, betulin, trihydroxyoxo-seco-ursdienoic acid, catechin, vicenin-2, farrerol, kaempferide and tetrahydroxyoleanenoic acid. These compounds are anti-inflammatory agents that may protect the blood-brain barrier and prevent inflammatory cell infiltration into the brain. The dried berries were ingested by six volunteers to demonstrate the safety of the medicine. **Conclusion:** The plant medicine was found to contain several compounds that may be of interest in the treatment of Alzheimer's disease. The plant medicine was found to be safe.

Keywords: *Heteromeles arbutifolia*; toyon; California holly; Alzheimer's disease; phytochemistry; safety

1. Introduction

Senile dementia, now commonly called Alzheimer's disease or vascular dementia, was known among California Indians before Europeans came to California [1]. The condition was commonly treated with a native plant, *Heteromeles arbutifolia*, also called toyon or California holly. The medicine consists of about 5 g of the dried berries which are slowly chewed and swallowed by the patient. The medicine slows down the progression of the disease and helps patients continue to have productive lives. The phytochemistry of the plant has not been adequately addressed, except for two publications that found cyanide in the plant [2,3]. There are reports of cyanide poisoning in insects and goats foraging on the leaves of the plant [3,4]. This indicates that the leaves of the plant may be toxic to some animal species. Most fruits from plants in the Rosaceae family contain cyanide, including apples, apricots, peaches, cherries and plums. The berries of *H. arbutifolia* are eaten fresh and cooked as foods by California Indians and other people [1]. The current study examined the chemistry and safety of the plant medicine.

Several plant-derived compounds are known to be protective in models of Alzhiemer's disease, including flavonoids, resveratrol, green tea polyphenols, curcumin and ferulic acid [5–9]. Ferulic acid is an antioxidant derived from fruits, vegetables and grains. It prevents beta-amyloid fibril formation and is neuroprotective.

2. Experimental Section

Plant material: The leaves of *H. arbutifolia* were collected in May in a canyon near Pasadena, CA, USA, and were used for phytochemical analysis. The fruit of the plant were collected in October in the same location and were made into the plant medicine. The leaves were stored frozen. The fruit were dehydrated with a food dehydrator and stored frozen.

Preparation of solvent extraction and isolation: The frozen leaves (123 g) were thawed and added to 275 mL of ultrapure water, finely chopped with a blender and extracted with 500 mL of ultrapure acetonitrile to make a preparation for phytochemical analysis. Column chromatography was performed with Silicagel 60 columns (EMD, Darmstadt, Germany) that were developed with the following solvents: ethyl acetate (20%, 30%, then 100%) in hexane. Six fractions were collected and checked by analytical TLC using 20% ethyl acetate in hexane. The plates were sprayed with 10% sulfuric acid and heated to visualize spots. Column purified fractions were further purified by preparative TLC (250 μm thick plates, EMD, Darmstadt, Germany) in 20% or 30% ethyl acetate/hexane. Several bands were scraped from each preparative TLC plate. Some bands were further purified by preparative TLC.

NMR spectra (^{1}H and ^{13}C NMR) were recorded at room temperature with a Varian Mercury Plus instrument at 400 MHz. Chemical shifts (δ) are reported in ppm relative to TMS. HPLC/MS analysis involved a Thermo Finnigan LCQ DECA (Waltham, MA, USA) with a reverse phase column. The solvent system consisted of 10% MeOH in water that increased at 2% per min to 100% MeOH.

Volunteers were recruited from the community by word of mouth and posters. Each volunteer claimed to be of normal health and no history of dementia. All six volunteers were male and ranged from 21 to 60 years old. Each volunteer was administered the modified mini-mental state test [10], which is routinely used to assess Alzheimer's disease in patients. They then chewed and swallowed 5 g of the dried berries. After 30 min, they were again administered the mini-mental state test. Each volunteer served as their own control since they were examined before and after ingesting the medicine. There was no blinding of the subjects or investigators, since the purpose was to examine the safety of the medicine.

This work was performed in accordance with the Declaration of Helsinki. Each volunteer signed an informed consent document. All personal information on each volunteer was kept confidential.

3. Results

Several known compounds were identified in the plant extract by HPLC/MS, UV and NMR. Despite reports of cyanide in the leaves of the plant, no cyanogenic compounds were found. The identified compounds were all known compounds. Data for each compound matched published data: icariside E4 [11], 2A,3β-dihdroxyolean 13(18)-en-28-oic acid [12], maslinic acid [13–15], betulin [16,17], trihydroxy19-oxo-18,19-seco-urs-11,13(18)-dien-28-oic acid [12], catechin [18], vicenin-2 [18], farrerol [19,20], kaempferide [21], 2A,3α,19α,23-tetrahydroxyolean-12-en-28-oic acid [12], lupeol acetate [22]. The data found in this study are shown below.

3.1. Icariside E4

UV/Vis λmax (MeOH) nm (logε): 230, 280.

MS (CI, 70 eV): m/z (%) = 507 [M + H^+] (100).

2A,3β-Dihdroxyolean13(18)-en-28-oic acid.

UV/Vis λmax (MeOH) nm (logε): 235, 280.

MS (CI, 70 eV): m/z (%) = 495 [M + Na^+] (60), 391 (100), 383, 149.

3.2. Maslinic Acid

UV/Vis λmax (MeOH) nm (logε): 232, 275.

MS (EI, 70 eV): *m/z* (%) = 471 [M^+] (20), 419 (100).

3.3. Betulin

UV/Vis λmax (MeOH) nm (logε): 235, 265.

^{1}H NMR (400 MHz, CDCl3): 0.89, 1.66 (2H, m, CH2), 1.52, 1.57 (2H, m, CH2), 3.0 (1H, m, CH), 1.07 (1H, m, CH), 1.34, 1.47 (2H, m, CH2), 1.36, 1.42 (2H, m CH2), 1.11 (1H, m, CH), 1.21, 1.45 (2H, m, CH2), 1.48, 1.51 (2H, m, CH2), 1.67 (1H, s, CH), 1.07, 1.7 (2H, m, CH2), 1.23, 1.92 (2H, m, CH2), 1.32 (1H, m, CH), 2.2 (1H, m, CH), 1.4, 2.0 (2H, m, CH2), 1.06, 1.86 (2H, m, CH2), 0.96 (3H, s, Me), 0.75 (3H, s, Me), 0.81 (3H, s, Me), 0.91 (3H, s, Me), 0.96 (6H, s, 2Me), 3.2 (2H, m, CH2), 3.66 (3H, s, Me), 4.6, 4.75 (2H, d, CH2, J = 15 Hz).

^{13}C NMR (400 MHz, CDCl3): 12.3 (C23), 19.9 (C29), 20.3 (C26), 20.7 (C6), 20.9 (C11), 22.5 (C25), 23.3 (C24), 24.0 (C22), 26.5 (C2), 28.0 (C12), 28.7 (C15), 29.6 (C20), 30.2 (C16), 34.6 (C21), 34.9 (C7), 35.8 (C1), 38.1 (C4), 38.4 (C10), 39.0 (C13), 39.4 (C8), 41.4 (C14), 47.1 (C17), 47.8 (C18), 48.1 (C19), 48.8 (C9), 54.0 (C5), 68.3 (C27), 78.3 (C3), 110.4 (C30), 150.7 (C28).

MS (CI, 70 eV): *m/z* (%) = 443 [$M+H^+$] (50), 429 [$MH\text{-}CH_2{}^+$] (100).

Trihydroxy19-oxo-18,19-seco-urs-11,13(18)-dien-28oic acid.

UV/Vis λmax (MeOH) nm (logε): 240.

MS (CI, 70 eV): *m/z* (%) = 523 [$M+Na^+$], 501 [$M+H^+$], 439.

3.4. Catechin

UV/Vis λmax (MeOH) nm (logε): 240, 280.

MS (CI, 70 eV): *m/z* (%) = 291 [$M+H^+$], 161, 147, 139, 123.

3.5. Vicenin-2

UV/Vis λmax (MeOH) nm (logε): 230, 270, 340.

MS (EI, 70 eV): *m/z* (%) = 593 [M^+], 455, 358, 295

3.6. Farrerol

UV/Vis λmax (MeOH) nm (logε): 291, 337.

MS (CI, 70 eV): *m/z* (%) = 301 [$M+H^+$], 282, 152, 120.

3.7. Kaempferide

UV/Vis λmax (MeOH) nm (logε): 289, 337.

MS (EI, 70 eV): *m/z* (%) = 301 [$M+H^+$], 258, 210.

2A,3α,19α,23-Tetrahydroxyolean-12-en-28-oic acid.

UV/Vis λmax (MeOH) nm (logε): 233, 283.

MS (EI, 70 eV): *m/z* (%) = 503 [M^-], 451.

3.8. Lupeol Acetate

UV/Vis λmax (MeOH) nm (logε): 233, 399.

MS (EI, 70 eV): *m/z* (%) = 469 [$M+H^+$], 443, 425 [M-Ac], 409, 184.

The safety of the plant medicine was demonstrated in six volunteers. Each volunteer scored 100% on the modified mini-mental state test before and after ingesting 5 g of the berries. No volunteer complained of any adverse effects from eating the berries, which were reported to taste like sweet apples. There were no obvious signs of cyanide poisoning in any individual. The berries of the plant are a traditional food and medicine of California Indians [1].

4. Discussion

Several compounds that may be beneficial in the treatment of Alzheimer's disease were found. A recent paper suggests that Alzheimer's disease may be caused by damage to the blood-brain barrier which allows macrophages and other inflammatory cells to invade the brain and increase the formation of amyloid plaques and neurofibrillary tangles [23].

Icariside compounds, similar to icariside E4, were found in *H. arbutifolia* and are known to protect the blood-brain barrier, prevent the infiltration of inflammatory cells into the brain and prevent neuronal damage [19,24]. An unknown that is either maslinic acid [8–10] or pomolic acid [13,25] was found. Maslinic acid is well known to occur in plants in the Rosaceae family, whereas pomolic acid is not. This implies that the compound found in the current study is maslinic acid. Maslinic acid suppresses nuclear factor kappa B which decreases the secretion of tumor necrosis factor α by astrocytes [26]. This is an anti-inflammatory effect that protects the blood-brain barrier since tumor necrosis factor α is involved in stimulating the production of vascular endothelial adhesion factors that increase the adhesion and transmigration of inflammatory cells across the blood-brain barrier [27].

Flavonoids seem to be beneficial in the prevention of Alzheimer's disease [28]. Flavonoids such as catechin were found in the plant and stimulate the non-amyloidogenic cleavage of amyloid precursor protein. Vicenin-2 inhibits the glycation of proteins, an anti-inflammatory effect [29]. Farrerol protects the blood-brain barrier by inhibiting the destruction of endothelial cells through apoptosis [30]. Kaempferide is 4′-methylkaempferol. Kaempferol is neuroprotective in a model of Alzheimer's disease and reverses amyloid beta–induced neuronal impairment [31]. It remains to be shown if kampferide has similar actions.

Betulin was a major component in the plant and it prevents sterol regulatory element binding protein activation [32]. It improves insulin resistance and decreases fat build-up in atherosclerosis. By the inhibition of the sterol regulatory element binding protein, it inhibits genes involved in fat accumulation. This may prevent the accumulation of perivascular fat that secretes adipokines such as visfatin. Visfatin may be involved in damaging the blood-brain barrier in Alzheimer's disease [23].

Lupeol acetate was found in the plant and is a triterpene that has anti-inflammatory properties through the modulation of the brain opioid system and tumor necrosis factor α [33]. This is potentially useful in the treatment of Alzheimer's disease.

H. arbutifolia must not be confused with English holly, *Ilex aquifolium*. Although both plants have red berries and spiny leaves, *I. aquifolium* berries are poison, whereas *H. arbutifolia* berries are not.

5. Conclusions

The traditional medicine *H. arbutifolia* has a number of active compounds that are potentially beneficial in Alzheimer's disease. This plant medicine may provide new leads for drug therapy in the disease. The phytochemistry of the plant indicates that protection of the blood-brain barrier and prevention of inflammatory cell infiltration into the brain may be important targets in the treatment of Alzheimer's disease. It may be worthwhile to investigate the use of the plant medicine itself in Alzheimer's disease.

Acknowledgments: This work was supported by a Visiting Scholar Fellowship from the government of China awarded to Xiaogang Wang.

Author Contributions: All authors conceived and designed the experiments; Xiaogang Wang, Raphael Dubois, Caitlyn Young and James D. Adams performed the experiments; all authors analyzed the data; James D. Adams contributed reagents/materials/analysis tools; all authors contributed to writing the paper.

References

1. Garcia, C.; Adams, J. *Healing with Medicinal Plants of the West Cultural and Scientific Basis for Their Use*, 3rd ed.; Abedus Press: La Crescenta, CA, USA, 2012; pp. 123–125.
2. Dement, W.; Mooney, H. Seasonal variation in the production of tannins and cyanogenic glucosides in the chaparral shrub *Heteromeles arbutifolia*. *Oecologia* **1974**, *15*, 65–76. [CrossRef]
3. Dahlman, D.; Johnson, V. *Heteromeles arbutifolia* (Rosaceae: Pomoideae) found toxic to insects. *Entomol. News* **1980**, *91*, 141–142.
4. Teqzes, J.; Puschner, B.; Melton, L. Cyanide toxicosis in goats after ingestion of California Holly (*Heteromeles arbutifolia*). *J. Vet. Diagn. Investig.* **2003**, *15*, 478–480. [CrossRef]
5. Pocernich, C.; Lange, M.; Sultana, R.; Butterfield, D. Nutritional approaches to modulate oxidative stress in Alzheimer's disease. *Curr. Alzheimer Res.* **2011**, *8*, 452–469. [CrossRef] [PubMed]
6. Picone, P.; Bondi, M.; Montana, G.; Bruno, A.; Pitarresi, G.; Giammona, G.; di Carlo, M. Ferulic acid inhibits oxidative stress and cell death induced by Ab oligomers: Improved delivery by solid lipid nanoparticles. *Free. Radic. Res.* **2009**, *43*, 1133–1145. [CrossRef] [PubMed]
7. Ono, K.; Hirohata, M.; Yamada, M. Ferulic destabilizes preformed beta-amyloid fibrils in vitro. *Biochem. Biophys. Res. Commun.* **2005**, *336*, 444–449. [CrossRef] [PubMed]
8. Sgarbossa, A.; Giacomazza, D.; di Carlo, M. Ferulic acid: A hope for Alzheimer's disease therapy from plants. *Nutrients* **2015**, *7*, 5764–5782. [CrossRef] [PubMed]
9. Jung, J.; Yan, J.; Li, H.; Sultan, M.; Yu, J.; Lee, H.; Shin, K.; Song, D. Protective effects of a dimeric derivative of ferulic acid in animal models of Alzheimer's disease. *Eur. J. Pharmacol.* **2016**, *782*, 30–34. [CrossRef] [PubMed]
10. Teng, E.; Chui, H. The modified mini-mental state (3MS) examination. *J. Clin. Psychiatry* **1987**, *48*, 314–318. [PubMed]
11. Miyase, T. Ionone and lignan glycosides from *Epimedium diphyllum*. *Phytochemistry* **1989**, *28*, 3483–3485. [CrossRef]
12. Zeng, N.; Shen, Y.; Li, L.; Jiao, W.; Gao, P.; Song, S.; Chen, W.; Lin, H. Antiinflammatory triterpenes from the leaves of *Rosa laevigata*. *J. Nat. Prod.* **2011**, *74*, 732–738. [CrossRef] [PubMed]
13. Numata, A. Cytotoxic triterpenes from a Chinese medicine, Goreishii. *Chem. Pharm. Bull.* **1989**, *37*, 648–651. [CrossRef] [PubMed]
14. Hossain, M.; Ismail, Z. Isolation and characterization of triterpenes from the leaves of *Orthosiphon stamineus*. *Arab. J. Chem.* **2013**, *6*, 295–298. [CrossRef]
15. Chaudhuri, P.; Singh, D. A new triterpenoid from the rhizomes of *Nelumbo nucifera*. *Nat. Prod. Res.* **2013**, *27*, 532–536. [CrossRef] [PubMed]
16. Hayek, E.; Jordis, U.; Moche, W.; Sauter, F. A bicentennial of betulin. *Phytochemistry* **1989**, *28*, 2229–2242. [CrossRef]
17. Kim, D.; Chen, Z.; Nguyen, V.; Pezzuto, J.; Qiu, S.; Lu, Z. A concise semi-synthetic approach to betulinic acid from betulin. *Synth. Commun.* **1997**, *27*, 1607–1612. [CrossRef]
18. Grayer, R.; Kite, G.; Abou-Zaid, M.; Archer, L. The application of atmospheric pressure chemical ionization liquid chromatography-mass spectrometry in the chemotaxonomic study of flavonoids: Characterization of flavonoids from *Ocimum gratissimum* var. *gratissimum*. *Phytochem. Anal.* **2000**, *11*, 257–267. [CrossRef]
19. Youssef, D.; Ramadan, M.; Khalifa, A. Acetophenones, a chalcone, a chromone and flavonoids from *Pancratium maritimum*. *Phytochemistry* **1998**, *49*, 2579–2583. [CrossRef]
20. Iwashina, T.; Kitamjima, J.; Matsumoto, S. Flavonoids in the species of *Cyrtomium* (Dryopteridaceae) and related genera. *Biochem. Syst. Ecol.* **2006**, *34*, 14–24. [CrossRef]
21. Baracco, A.; Bertin, G.; Gnocco, E.; Legorati, M.; Sedocco, S.; Catinella, S.; Favretto, D.; Traldi, P. A comparison of the combination of fast-atom bombardment with tandem mass spectrometry and of gas chromatography with mass spectrometry in the analysis of a mixture of kaempferol, kaempferide, luteolin and oleuropein. *Rapid Commun. Mass Spectrom.* **1995**, *9*, 427–436. [CrossRef]
22. Saratha, V.; Pillai, I.; Subramanian, S. Isolation and characterization of lupeol, a triterpenoid from *Calotropis gigantea* latex. *Int. J. Pharm. Sci. Rev. Res.* **2011**, *10*, 54–57.

23. Adams, J. Alzheimer's disease, ceramide, visfatin and NAD. *CNS Neurol. Disord. Drug. Targets* **2008**, *7*, 492–498. [CrossRef]
24. Yan, B.; Pan, C.; Mao, X.; Yang, L.; Liu, Y.; Yan, L.; Mu, H.; Wang, C.; Sun, K.; Liao, F.; et al. Icariside II improves cerebral microcirculatory disturbance and alleviates hippocampal injury in gerbils after ischemia reperfusion. *Brain Res.* **2014**, *1573*, 63–73. [CrossRef] [PubMed]
25. Lee, T.; Juang, S.; Hsu, F.; Wu, S. Triterpene acids from the leaves of *Planchonella duclitan* (Blanco) Bakhuizan. *J. Chin. Chem. Soc.* **2005**, *52*, 1275–1280. [CrossRef]
26. Huang, L.; Guan, T.; Qian, Y.; Huang, M.; Tang, X.; Li, Y.; Sun, H. Anti-inflammatory effects of maslinic acid, a natural triterpene, in cultured cortical astrocytes via suppression of nuclear factor-kappa B. *Eur. J. Pharmacol.* **2011**, *672*, 169–174. [CrossRef] [PubMed]
27. Tak, P.; Taylor, P.; Breedveld, F.; Smeets, T.; Daha, M.; Kluin, P.; Meinders, A.; Maini, R. Decrease in cellularity and expression of adhesion molecules by anti-tumor necrosis factor α monoclonal antibody treatment in patients with rheumatoid arthritis. *Arthritis Rheum.* **1996**, *39*, 1077–1081. [CrossRef] [PubMed]
28. Mandel, S.; Youdim, M. Catechin polyphenols: Neurodegeneration and neuroprotection in neurodegenerative diseases. *Free Radic. Biol. Med.* **2004**, *37*, 304–317. [CrossRef] [PubMed]
29. Islam, N.; Ishita, I.; Jung, H.; Choi, J. Vicenin-2 isolated from Artemisia capillaris exhibited potent anti-glycation properties. *Food Chem. Toxicol.* **2014**, *69*, 55–62. [CrossRef] [PubMed]
30. Li, J.; Ge, R.; Tang, L.; Li, Q. Protective effects of farrerol against hydrogen-peroxide-induced apoptosis in human endothelium-derived EA.hy926 cells. *Can. J. Physiol. Pharmacol.* **2013**, *91*, 733–740. [CrossRef] [PubMed]
31. Kim, J.; Choi, S.; Cho, H.; Hwang, H.; Kim, Y.; Lim, S.; Kim, C.; Kim, H.; Peterson, S.; Shin, D. Protective effects of kaempferol (3,4′,5,7-tetrahydroxyflavone) against amyloid beta peptide (Abeta)-induced neurotoxicity in ICR mice. *Biosci. Biotechnol. Biochem.* **2010**, *74*, 397–401. [CrossRef] [PubMed]
32. Tang, J.; Li, J.; Qi, W.; Qiu, W.; Li, P.; Li, B.; Song, B. Inhibition of SREBP by a small molecule, betulin, improves hyperlipidemia and insulin resistance and reduces atherosclerotic plaques. *Cell Metab.* **2011**, *13*, 44–56. [CrossRef] [PubMed]
33. Lucetti, D.; Lucetti, E.; Bandeira, M.; Veras, H.; Silva, A.; Leal, L.; Lopes, A.; Alves, V.; Silva, G.; Brito, G.; et al. Anti-inflammatory effects and possible mechanism of action of lupeol acetate isolated from Himatanthus drasticus (Mart) Plumel. *J. Inflamm.* **2010**, *7*, 60. [CrossRef] [PubMed]

18

Fucoidan Inhibits Radiation-Induced Pneumonitis and Lung Fibrosis by Reducing Inflammatory Cytokine Expression in Lung Tissues

Hsin-Hsien Yu [1,2,†], Edward Chengchuan KO [3,4,5,†], Chia-Lun Chang [6,7], Kevin Sheng-Po Yuan [8], Alexander T. H. Wu [9], Yan-Shen Shan [1,10,*] and Szu-Yuan Wu [7,11,*]

1 Institute of Clinical Medicine, College of Medicine, National Cheng Kung University, Tainan 701, Taiwan; klaus610@gmail.com
2 Division of General Surgery, Department of Surgery, Wan Fang Hospital, Taipei Medical University, Taipei 116, Taiwan
3 School of Dentistry, College of Dental Medicine, Kaohsiung Medical University, Kaohsiung 807, Taiwan; ko.edward.kaseizen@gmail.com
4 Division of Oral and Maxillofacial Surgery, Kaohsiung Medical University Hospital, Kaohsiung 807, Taiwan
5 Department of FUJISOFT Cartilage and Bone Regeneration, Tissue Engineering, The University of Tokyo, Tokyo 113-0033, Japan
6 Department of Hemato-Oncology, Wan Fang Hospital, Taipei Medical University, Taipei 116, Taiwan; richardch9@hotmail.com
7 Department of Internal Medicine, School of Medicine, College of Medicine, Taipei Medical University, Taipei 11031, Taiwan
8 Department of Otorhinolaryngology, Wan Fang Hospital, Taipei Medical University, Taipei 116, Taiwan; dryuank@gmail.com
9 Ph.D. Program for Translational Medicine, Taipei Medical University, Taipei 11031, Taiwan; chaw1211@tmu.edu.tw
10 Department of Surgery, National Cheng Kung University Hospital, College of Medicine, National Cheng Kung University, Tainan 701, Taiwan
11 Department of Radiation Oncology, Wan Fang Hospital, Taipei Medical University, Taipei 116, Taiwan
* Correspondence: ysshan@mail.ncku.edu.tw (Y.-S.S.); szuyuanwu5399@gmail.com (S.-Y.W.)
† These authors have contributed equally to this study.

Abstract: Purpose: Radiotherapy is a crucial treatment approach for many types of cancer. Radiation pneumonitis (RP) is one of the major complications in chest irradiation. Fucoidan is a sulfated polysaccharide found mainly in various species of brown seaweed. Recent studies have demonstrated the anti-inflammatory effects of fucoidan. However, no study has reported a well-established prophylactic agent for RP. Therefore, we investigated the effects of fucoidan on RP and radiotherapy (RT)-induced lung fibrosis. **Materials and Methods**: We compared RP and RT-induced fibrosis in lung tissue specimens obtained from irradiated (10 Gy/shot) C57BL/6 mice with or without fucoidan administration (200 mg/kg/day, oral gavage for 14 days). The expression patterns of cytokines in the pleural fluid were determined using a cytokine array and confirmed through enzyme immunoassays. **Results**: Fucoidan administration attenuated RP and RT-induced fibrosis in lung tissues. Decreased neutrophil and macrophage accumulation was observed in irradiated lung tissues, and radiation-induced lung fibrosis, as demonstrated by Masson trichrome staining, was attenuated. We investigated the expression patterns of inflammatory cytokines in the irradiated lung pleural fluid through the protein array; results revealed that fucoidan administration changed the expression patterns of inflammatory cytokines in irradiated lung tissues. Furthermore, the expression levels of TIMP-1, CXCL1, MCP-1, MIP-2, and interleukin-1Ra were substantially enhanced in the pleural fluid, but fucoidan administration significantly reduced their expression. **Conclusions**: Fucoidan changes the expression patterns of inflammatory cytokines, which may consequently attenuate RP and RT-induced lung fibrosis.

Keywords: radiation pneumonitis; lung fibrosis; fucoidan; cytokine; macrophage; neutrophil

1. Introduction

Currently, radiotherapy (RT) is an important approach for treating tumors [1]. The treatment protocol can include curative, adjuvant, neoadjuvant, therapeutic, or palliative therapy, depending on the tumor type, location, and stage as well as the health status of patients [2,3]. Radiation pneumonitis (RP) is the acute manifestation of radiation-induced lung disease and is relatively common following RT for chest wall or intrathoracic malignancies [4]. The acute phase typically occurs between 4 and 12 weeks following the completion of the RT course; however, it may occur as early as 1 week after RT, particularly in patients receiving a high total dose or concurrent chemotherapy [5]. The late phase is characterized by lung fibrosis that occurs as early as 6 months following RT and can progressively continue for several years [6]. Typical symptoms include cough, dyspnea, low-grade fever, chest discomfort, and pleuritic pain. Moreover, the pathology of RP reflects an acute response of the lung to radiation and includes loss of type I pneumocytes and increased capillary permeability that result in interstitial and alveolar edema and the ingress of inflammatory cells into alveolar spaces. Immune-mediated lymphocytic alveolitis has been postulated as the underlying cause of changes in nonirradiated lung tissues [7,8]. Cytokines have been found to play crucial roles in RP and late RT-induced lung fibrosis [9–11].

Studies have indicated that preventing or treating RT-induced lung injury is difficult. Until now, no study has reported well-established prophylactic agents for RT-induced lung injury prevention or treatment. Patients who require chest RT have a risk of RP or lung fibrosis, which exerts acute or long-term effects. Therefore, it is necessary to identify an effective prophylactic agent that not only prevents RT-induced lung injury, but also guides the dose escalation of RT to achieve improved local control and overall survival.

A heparin-like molecule, referred to as fucoidan, containing high percentages of L-fucose and sulfated ester groups and small proportions of D-xylose, D-galactose, D-mannose, and glucuronic acid was found in the cell wall matrix of brown seaweed [12]. Various biological activities, such as antioxidant, anti-inflammatory, antiproliferative, anticancer, and proapoptotic activities, have been observed in brown seaweed [13–15]. Furthermore, radioprotective effects of fucoidan were observed in mice treated with total body irradiation [16]. The present study investigated the effects of fucoidan on RP and RT-induced lung fibrosis.

2. Material and Methods

2.1. Fucoidan Reagent

Fucoidan powder extracted from Sargassum hemiphyllum was obtained from Hi-Q Oligo-fucoidan, a commercial product provided by Hi-Q Marine Biotech International Ltd. (New Taipei City, Taiwan). Fucoidan powder or dextran powder (D9260; Sigma-Aldrich, St. Louis, MO, USA) was dissolved in double-distilled H2O and stirred at 25 °C for 30 min. The dissolved solution was filtered using 0.22-μm sterile filters (Millipore, Billerica, MA, USA). Fucoidan used in this study was obtained through the enzyme hydrolysis of original fucoidan. The average molecular weight, fucose content, and sulfate content of fucoidan used in this study were 0.8 KDa (92.1%), 210.9 ± 3.3 mmol/g, and 38.9% ± 0.4% (*w*/*w*), respectively [17].

2.2. Animals and Grouping

Eight-week-old male C57BL/6 mice, weighing approximately 25 g, were used as experimental subjects. These mice were divided into four study groups: sham (mice not treated with lung irradiation but were immobilized), RT (mice treated with lung irradiation and administered double-distilled

H_2O; 200 μL/day, oral gavage for 14 days), RT + fucoidan (mice treated with lung irradiation and administered fucoidan; 200 mg/kg/day in 200 μL, oral gavage for 14 days), and fucoidan (mice administered fucoidan; 200 mg/kg/day in 200 μL, oral gavage for 14 days). RT + dextran (mice treated with lung irradiation and administered dextran; 200 mg/kg/day in 200 μL, oral gavage for 14 days), and fucoidan (mice administered fucoidan; 200 mg/kg/day in 200 μL, oral gavage for 14 days). In the fucoidan or dextran-receiving groups, fucoidan or dextran was administered through oral gavage for 3 days before RT; we defined the first day of fucoidan or dextran administration as day 1. RT was administered on day 3, and fucoidan or dextran was administered for 14 days. To obtain the lung tissue for neutrophil and macrophage identification and the pleural fluid, some mice were sacrificed on day 15. To obtain the lung tissue for fibrosis determination, some mice were sacrificed on day 31. Mice were inhalationally anesthetized with 5% isoflurane (2-chloro-2-(difluoromethoxy)-1,1,1-trifluoro-ethane) for 5 min and then placed in a CO_2 chamber. A fill rate of approximately 10% to 30% of the chamber volume per minute with 100% CO_2 was used, and mice were unconscious within 2–3 min. We maintained CO_2 flow for a minimum of 1 min after their respiration ceased. This study protocol was approved by the Institutional Animal Care and Use Committee at Wan Fang Hospital, Taipei Medical University (No. LAC-2015-0167). All animal experiments were performed in accord with relevant guidelines and regulations.

2.3. *Mouse Lung Irradiation*

C57BL/6 mice were immobilized using a customized harness that allowed for the exposure of the trunk along with the whole lung. Fluoroscopy and computed tomography were conducted to determine the position of the lung, design the radiation field, and calculate the dose distribution. The whole lung was irradiated with a rectangular field. The remainder of the body was shielded 5 half-value layers of lead. A linear accelerator (Elekta, 6-MV photon beam, Crawley, UK) was used to perform whole lung irradiation at 10 Gy.

2.4. *Lung Tissue Dissection*

Irradiated or sham C57/B6 mice were sacrificed at the aforementioned time points. Mice were anesthetized with 5% isoflurane, and their pleural fluid was withdrawn 30 s after administering 0.5 mL of normal saline intrapleurally by using a 23-gauge needle. The pleural fluid was then centrifuged at 3000 rpm for 10 min, and the supernatant was collected to perform cytokine analysis, ELISA, or functional assays. To avoid the damage caused by intrapleural injection, lung tissue samples were collected from another group of mice and subsequently embedded in paraffin for sectioning. To determine the expression of collagen I in the lung tissue, the freshly excised whole left lung lobe tissue was homogenized in liquid nitrogen. The total protein content of this tissue was extracted using a cell lysis buffer (Thermo Fisher Scientific, Waltham, MA, USA) and quantified using the Bio-Rad protein assay (Hercules, CA, USA).

2.5. *Immunohistochemistry*

The paraffin-embedded tissue slides were rehydrated in PBS for 15 min, and endogenous peroxidase activity was inhibited by 3% H_2O_2 or methanol for 10 min at room temperature. For blocking, 5% nonfat milk or PBS was added for 30 min at room temperature. The slides were incubated with an anti-F4/80 antibody or anti-Ly6G antibody or control IgG at 1:100 dilution for 16 h at 4 °C (F4/80 [C-7] is a mouse monoclonal antibody raised against amino acids 335–634 mapped within an extracellular domain of F4/80 of mouse origin; sc-377009; Santa Cruz Biotechnology; anti-Ly6G antibody is a monoclonal antibody NIMP-R14 is highly specific for murine Ly-6G [NIMP-R14]; (ab2557); Abcam). A peroxidase-conjugated secondary antibody was incubated for 1 h at room temperature and detected by immersing the slides in 0.06% 3,3′-diaminobenzidine tetrahydrochloride, followed by counterstaining with Gill Hematoxylin V.

2.6. *Masson Trichrome Staining*

Masson trichrome staining is widely used to study muscular pathologies, including tissue fibrosis and myofibroblasts, and also to detect and analyze myofibroblasts in lung biopsies [18,19]. Lung sections were stained with Masson Trichrome (Sigma-Aldrich, Saint Louis, MO, USA).

2.7. *Real-Time Quantitative Reverse Transcription–Polymerase Chain Reaction*

The mRNA expressions of Ly6G and F4/80 in the lung tissue were measured using a fluorescein real-time quantitative reverse transcription–polymerase chain reaction (qRT-PCR) detection system (Light Cycler DNA Master SYBR Green I; Roche Molecular Biochemicals, Indianapolis, IN, USA). Primer pairs used were as follows: GAPDH: 5′-GGGAAGGTGAAGGTCGG-3′ and 5′-TGGACTCCACGACGTACTCAG-3′; Ly6G: 5′-TGGACTCTCACAGAAGCAAAG-3′ and 5′-GCAGAGGTCTTCCTTCCAACA-3′; and F4/80: 5′-CTCTGTGGTCCCACCTTCAT-3′ and 5′-GATGGCCAAGGATCTGAA AA-3′. The amplification program consisted of one cycle of initial incubation at 60 °C for 20 min, followed by 40 cycles of denaturation at 95 °C for 10 s, annealing at 55 °C for 10 s, and extension at 72 °C for 10 s. The relative mRNA level was calculated using the $2^{-\Delta\Delta Ct}$ method. The amount of indicated mRNA was normalized to that of GAPDH mRNA and presented in arbitrary units, with 1 U corresponding to the value of the sham group.

2.8. *Cytokine Array*

A mouse cytokine array (Ary006; Proteome Profiler, R&D Systems, Minneapolis, MN, USA) was used to analyze cytokine expression patterns in the pleural fluid. The pleural fluid was first mixed with a biotinylated detection antibody cocktail at room temperature for 1 h, and the array membrane was blocked with the blocking solution provided by the manufacturer. The membrane was then incubated with the samples overnight at 4 °C on a shaker. After washing, horseradish peroxidase-conjugated streptavidin was added to the membrane for 30 min at room temperature, and signal development was achieved by the addition of commercial chemiluminescence detection reagents. A digital imaging system (Bio Pioneer Tech Co., New Taipei City, Taiwan) was used to detect signals, which were further analyzed using the ImageJ program. The number of specimens, N, was 3 per experimental group, and a mean value was calculated.

2.9. *Determination of TIMP-1, CXCL1, MCP-1, MIP-2, and Interleukin-1Ra*

The protein lysate or serum levels of TIMP-1, CXCL1, MCP-1, MIP-2, and interleukin (IL)-1Ra were determined using enzyme immunoassay (EIA) kits (R&D Systems, Minneapolis, MN, USA). The protein levels of pro-collagen I alpha in the lung tissue lysate were determined using a mouse pro-collagen I alpha 1 ELISA kit (ab210579).

2.10. *Functional Test of the Pleural Fluid for Type I Collagen Expression in Fibroblasts*

NIH-3T3 cells were purchased from the American Type Culture Collection (Rockville, MD, USA). Cells are maintained in DMEM (Life Technologies, New York, NY, USA) supplemented with 10% (*vol*/*vol*) fetal bovine serum plus penicillin–streptomycin under sterile tissue culture conditions and cultured in a humidified atmosphere of 5% CO_2 and 95% air at 37 °C. NIH3T3 cells were cultured in 24-well plates until they reached a density of 1×10^5 cells/well. To prevent contamination of collagen in the pleural fluid, cells were treated with 100 μL of the pleural fluid obtained from different groups for 1 h. Subsequently, cells were washed, fresh medium was added, and the cell culture supernatant was collected after 24 h. The protein levels of type I collagen secreted into the cell culture supernatant were determined through ELISA.

2.11. Statistical Analysis

One-way ANOVA with Tukey's post hoc test was used to compare data among the groups. All statistical analyses were performed using SPSS for Windows, version 18.0 (SPSS Inc., Chicago, IL, USA). A p value of <0.05 was considered statistically significant.

3. Results

3.1. Fucoidan Attenuated RT-Induced Lung Fibrosis in Irradiated Mouse Lung Tissues

On the basis of the anti-inflammatory effect of fucoidan, we investigated its role in RT-induced lung fibrosis in a mouse model. Mice were divided into four groups, namely sham, RT, RT + fucoidan, and fucoidan, and sacrificed on day 31. We first determined pulmonary fibrosis in each group through Masson trichrome staining (Figure 1, left panel). Type I collagen, which is the major component of pulmonary fibrosis, is encoded by the COL1A1 gene. The COL1A1 gene produces a component of type I collagen, named pro-collagen 1 alpha. Thus, the whole left lobe of the lung was homogenized to determine the pro-collagen 1 alpha level through ELISA (Figure 1, right panel). The results of ELISA revealed increased collagen deposition in the RT group and attenuated collagen deposition in the RT + fucoidan group. The quantitative results of pro-collagen 1 alpha demonstrated that RT significantly enhanced collagen formation in the lung tissue (0.92 $\pm$ 0.05 mg/g in the sham group vs. 3.22 $\pm$ 0.39 mg/g in the RT group) and fucoidan administration significantly reduced the collagen level in the RT + fucoidan group (1.83 $\pm$ 0.23 mg/g). These results indicated that fucoidan attenuated RT-induced lung fibrosis in irradiated mouse lung tissues.

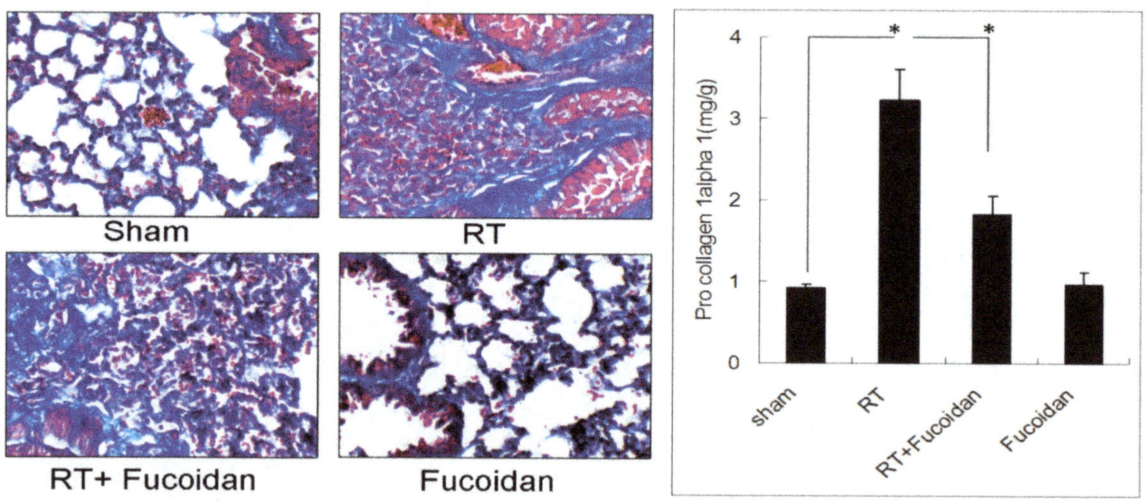

Figure 1. Effects of fucoidan on lung fibrosis in irradiated mouse lung tissues. (**Left** panel): mice from indicated groups were sacrificed on day 31. Representative images of Masson trichrome staining of mouse lung tissues (400×). (**Right** panel): the whole left lobe of the lung of each mouse in each group was homogenized to determine the pro-collagen 1 alpha level through ELISA. N = 5/group. * $p < 0.05$ by one-way ANOVA with Tukey's post hoc test.

3.2. Fucoidan Reduced Neutrophil and Macrophage Infiltration in Irradiated Lung Tissues

Lung fibrosis is a sequential effect of inflammation. To address the specific effect of Fucoidan, dextran, which is a complex branched glucan is used as polysaccharide control. To observe the phenomenon of neutrophil and macrophage infiltration in lung tissue specimens, mice were divided into four study groups, namely sham, RT, RT + fucoidan, and RT + dextran, and sacrificed on day 15. A part of the lung tissue of each mouse was dissected to prepare paraffin-embedded sections. Neutrophil infiltration was determined through Ly6G antibody staining, which is a specific marker for mouse neutrophils are shown in Figure 2 (left panels). Macrophage infiltration in paraffin-embedded lung tissues was identified through F4/80 antibody staining, which is a specific marker for mouse macrophages (Figure 3, left panels). The whole left lobe of the lung of each mouse in each group was homogenized for use in qRT-PCR performed to determine the expression levels of Ly6G and F4/80, which are specific markers for neutrophils (Figure 2, right panel) and macrophages (Figure 3, right panel), respectively. The quantitative results of Ly6G and F4/80 mRNA demonstrated increased neutrophil (1-fold in the sham group vs. 16.8 ± 4.8-fold in the RT group) and macrophage (1-fold in the sham group vs. 4.8 ± 1.6-fold in the RT group) infiltration in the lung tissues of the RT group. However, the infiltration of neutrophils (7.74 ± 4.01-fold) and macrophages (1.94 ± 0.54-fold) significantly decreased in the RT + fucoidan group but not in RT + dextran group. Meanwhile, Fucoidan administration alone did not change the levels of neutrophil and macrophage infiltration in lung tissues (data not show).

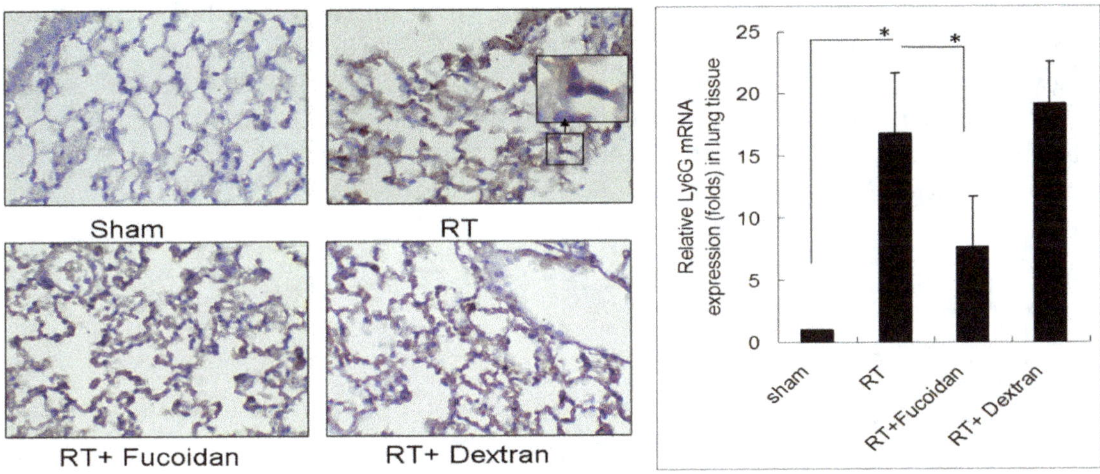

Figure 2. Effects of fucoidan on neutrophil infiltration in irradiated mouse lung tissues. (**Left** panel): mice from indicated groups were sacrificed on day 15. A representative image of neutrophil infiltration in lung tissues (400×). (**Right** panel): the whole left lobe of the lung of each mouse in each group was homogenized for use in qRT-PCR performed for determining the expression level of Ly6G. N = 5/group. * $p < 0.05$ by one-way ANOVA with Tukey's post hoc test.

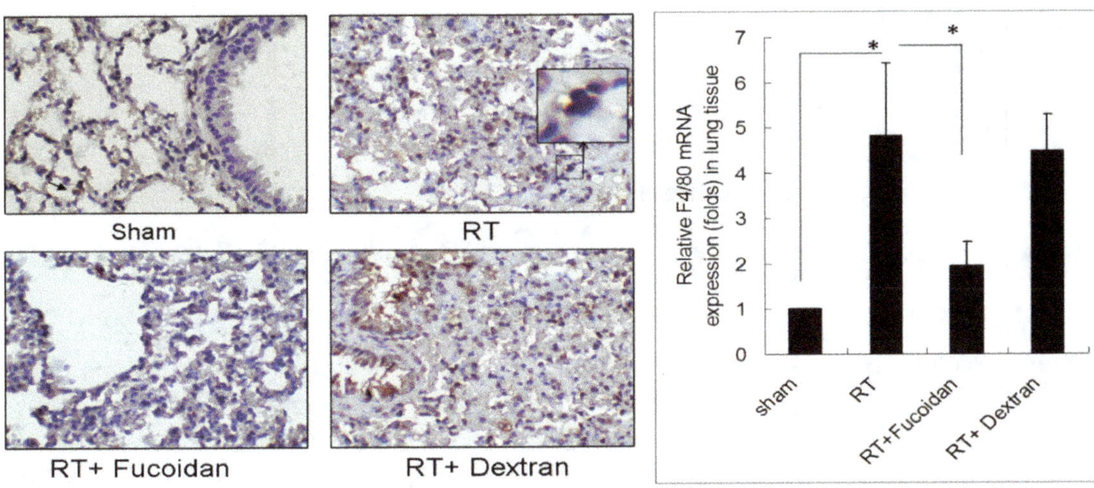

Figure 3. Effects of fucoidan on F4/80 macrophage infiltration in irradiated mouse lung tissues. (**Left** panel): mice from indicated groups were sacrificed on day 15. A representative image of F4/80 macrophage infiltration in lung tissues (400×). (**Right** panel): the whole left lobe of the lung of each mouse in each group was homogenized for use in qRT-PCR performed for determining the expression level of F4/80. N = 5/group. * $p < 0.05$ by one-way ANOVA with Tukey's post hoc test.

3.3. Fucoidan Reduced Cytokine Expression in the Pleural Fluid Obtained from Irradiated Mice

Cytokine expression may reflect the status of inflammation. To examine the expression of cytokines in the lung tissue, mice were divided into four study groups, namely sham, RT, RT + fucoidan, and fucoidan, and sacrificed on day 15. The pleural fluid was collected to analyze the expression patterns of inflammatory cytokines by using a cytokine array. The images of the cytokine array (Figure 4, upper panel) and their corresponding quantitative results demonstrated that fucoidan administration changed the expression patterns of inflammatory cytokines in the pleural fluid obtained from irradiated mice (Figure 4, lower panel). The top five cytokines that were significantly induced in the pleural fluid of the irradiated group than in that of the sham group are as follows: TIMP-1 (3.71 $\pm$ 0.11-fold), CXCL1 (4.32 $\pm$ 0.12-fold), MCP-1 (4.27 $\pm$ 0.13-fold), MIP-2 (13.71 $\pm$ 0.14-fold), and IL-1Ra (3.37 $\pm$ 0.1-fold). Furthermore, they were significantly reduced in RT + fucoidan group. Additionally, TREM-1 was also induced in the pleural fluid of the irradiated group than in that of the sham group (2.27 $\pm$ 0.11-fold) and it was reduced in RT + fucoidan group. On the other hand, by comparing with sham group, the quantitative result revealed that SDF-1/CXCL12 (2.57 $\pm$ 0.13-fold) and IL-16 (1.93 $\pm$ 0.1-fold) were induced in the pleural fluid of the fucoidan administration only group. However, the expression of SDF-1/CXCL12 (0.37 $\pm$ 0.12-fold) and IL-16 (0.68 $\pm$ 0.08-fold) in RT + fucoidan group were low.

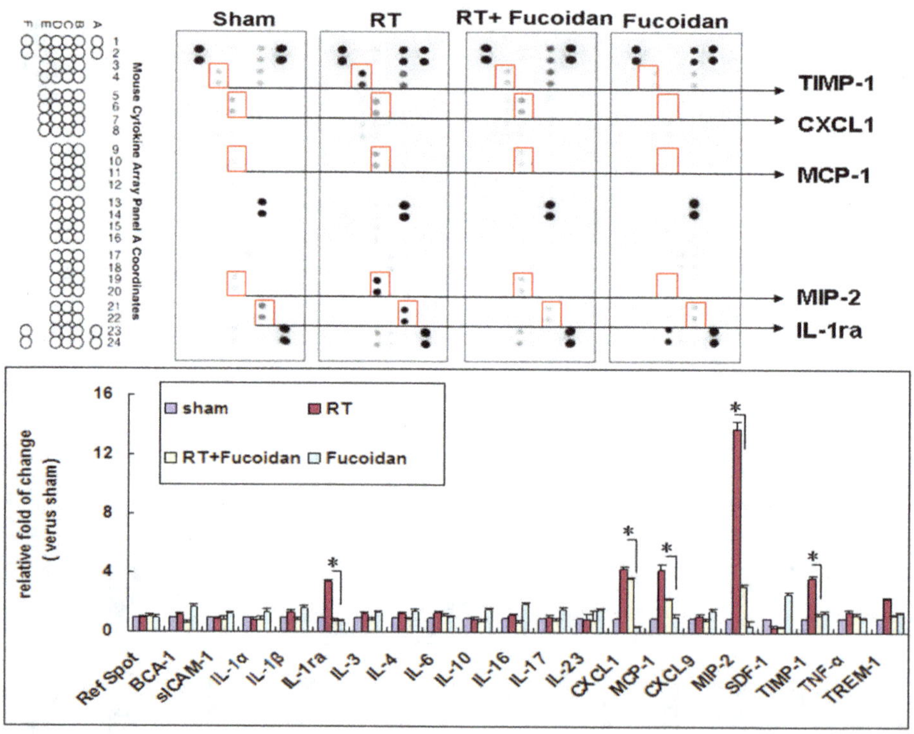

Figure 4. Effects of fucoidan on cytokine expression in the pleural fluid obtained from irradiated mice. (**Upper** panel): pleural fluid was collected from the mice of indicated groups on day 15. Representative image of the cytokine array of pleural fluids. Five spots with obvious changes are indicated. (**Lower** panel): quantitative results of cytokine spots. N = 3/group.

3.4. Fucoidan Reduced TIMP-1, CXCL1, MCP-1, MIP-2, and IL-1Ra Expression in the Pleural Fluid Obtained from Irradiated Mice

On the basis of the findings of the cytokine array described in Figure 4, we chose the following top five cytokines that were significantly induced in the sham group than in the RT groups: TIMP-1, CXCL1, MCP-1, MIP-2, and IL-1Ra. We determined the concentrations of these cytokines in the pleural fluid of mice in each group through EIA. The results revealed that the expression levels of TIMP-1 (203.1 $\pm$ 84.8 ng/mL in the sham group vs. 509.7 $\pm$ 151.1 ng/mL in the RT group; Figure 5A), CXCL1 (42.5 $\pm$ 17.9

pg/mL in the sham group vs. 145.8 ± 45 pg/mL in the RT group; Figure 5B), MCP-1 (28.6 ± 6.4 pg/mL in the sham group vs. 246.5 ± 80.4 pg/mL in the RT group; Figure 5C), MIP-2 (31.6 ± 16.8 pg/mL in the sham group vs. 143.2 ± 42.6 pg/mL in the RT group; Figure 5D), and IL-1Ra (98.4 ± 45.3 in the sham group vs. 1319.4 ± 203.4 µg/mL in the RT group; Figure 5E) were significantly enhanced in the collected pleural fluid. However, in the RT + fucoidan group, the levels of TIMP-1 (223.1 ± 30.7 ng/mL), CXCL1 (73.3 ± 26.4 pg/mL), MCP-1 (146.4 ± 30.8 pg/mL), MIP-2 (55 ± 27.3 pg/mL), and IL-1Ra (474.4 ± 146.7 µg/mL) were significantly decreased. In order to examine the effect of the cytokines induced by RT in the pleural fluid on fibroblasts and to assess fibrosis induction capability, NIH-3T3 cells, which is a well-known mouse fibroblast cell line, were treated with the pleural fluid obtained from mice in the sham, RT, RT + fucoidan, and fucoidan groups. The pro-collagen 1 alpha level in the cell culture supernatant was determined through ELISA (Figure 5F). The results revealed that, compared with the sham group, the pleural fluid obtained from mice in the RT group significantly increased the type I collagen level in the culture supernatant of NIH-3T3 cells (29.9 ± 6.9 ng/mL in the sham group vs. 70.6 ± 18.4 ng/mL in the RT group). However, compared with the RT group, the type I collagen level was decreased in the cell culture supernatant of NIH-3T3 cells treated with the pleural fluid obtained from mice in the RT + fucoidan group (42.8 ± 9.3 ng/mL).

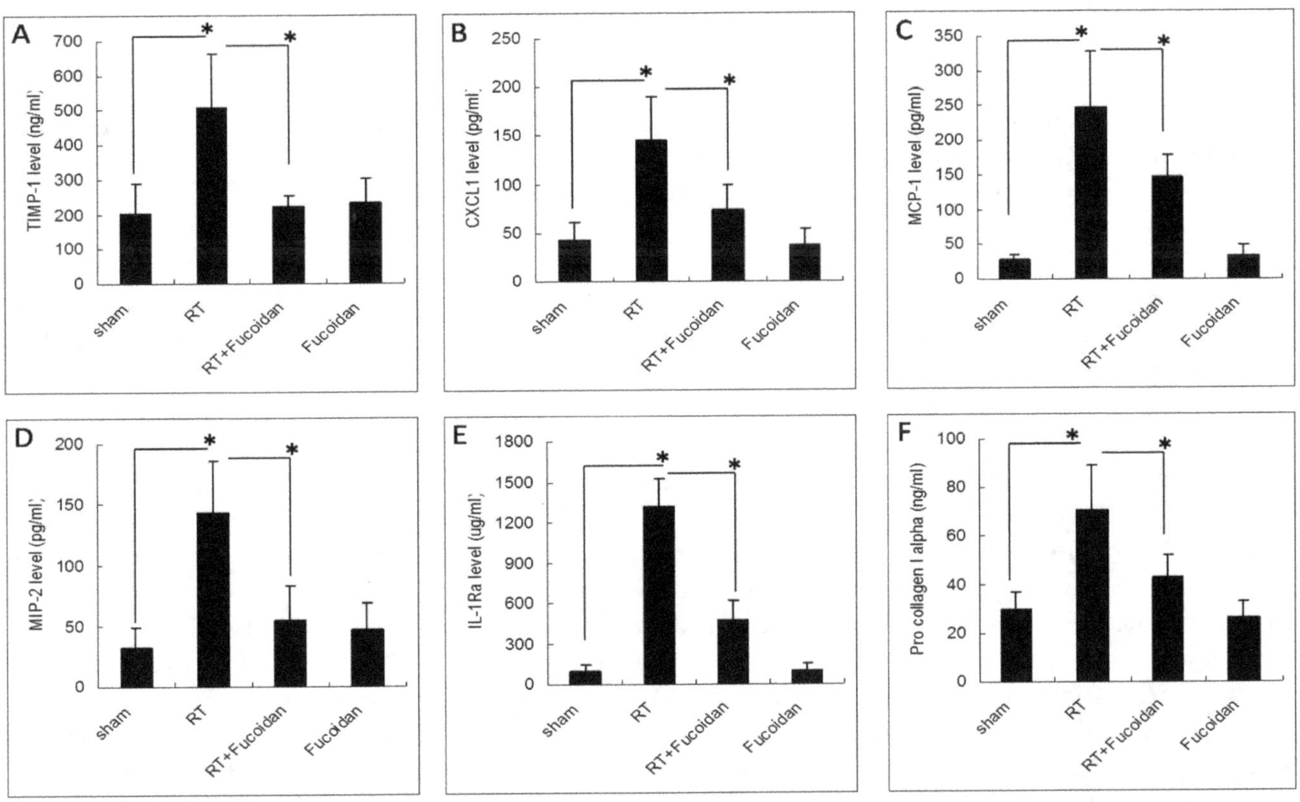

Figure 5. Effects of fucoidan on cytokine levels in the pleural fluid obtained from irradiated mice. The pleural fluid was collected from the mice of indicated groups on day 15. The expression levels of (**A**) TIMP-1, (**B**) CXCL1, (**C**) MCP-1, (**D**) MIP-2, and (**E**) IL-1ra were determined through enzyme immunoassays. Data are compared between indicated groups. * $p < 0.05$. N = 10/group. (**F**) NIH-3T3 cells were treated with the pleural fluid obtained from mice in the sham, RT, RT + fucoidan, and fucoidan groups for 1 h prior to the addition of fresh culture medium and then incubated for another 24 h. The cell culture supernatant was collected for determining the type I collagen level through ELISA. * $p < 0.05$. N = 6/group by one-way ANOVA with Tukey's post hoc test.

This study demonstrated that fucoidan administration in irradiated mice attenuated cytokine (TIMP-1, CXCL1, MCP-1, MIP-2, and IL-1Ra) expression in the collected pleural fluid and reduced pleural fluid-induced collagen expression in fibroblasts, which were correlated with the reduction of neutrophil and macrophage infiltration in lung tissues; macrophage and neutrophil infiltration may lead to RP and RT-induced lung fibrosis (Figure 6). This result may facilitate the design of fucoidan-based therapeutic approaches for preventing RP in clinical practice.

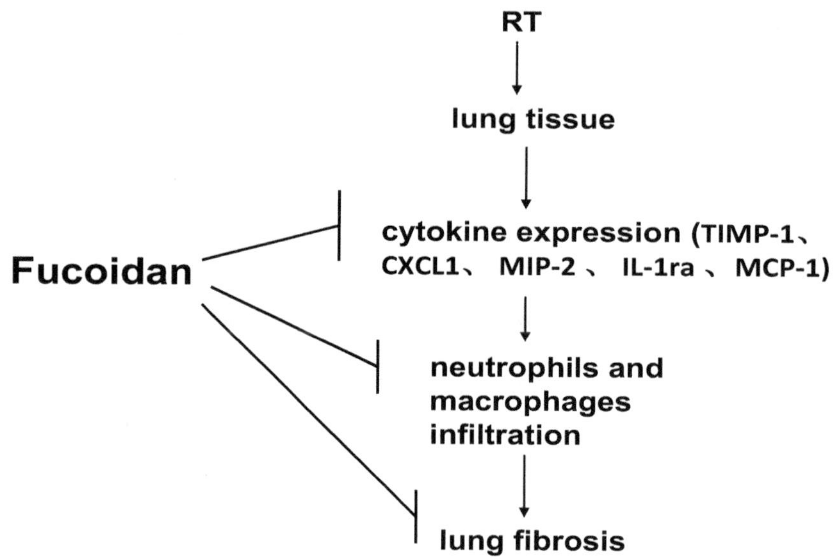

Figure 6. Schematic of possible molecular mechanisms underlying the preventive effects of fucoidan on radiotherapy (RT)-induced lung fibrosis mediated through the reduction of neutrophil and macrophage infiltration and alteration in cytokine expression patterns in lung tissues.

4. Discussion

According to a clinical description, RP occurs in the latent period. However, a molecular biology study revealed a cascade of events occurring immediately after injury and continuing up to the overall occurrence of clinical symptoms such as cough, dyspnea, low-grade fever, chest discomfort, and pleuritic pain [11]. Oxidative stress may cause DNA-damaging injuries; under such conditions, the immediate pulmonary response to radiation-induced injury is similar to many conventional wound healing responses. However, it remains unclear why radiation-induced lung injury is not completely repaired and resolved, with lung tissues consequently entering a progressive and dysregulated process that concludes in the late stage of RP and lung fibrosis. These injuries are now considered to be the result of a complex, structural interaction between multiple cell types, which is initiated and perpetuated through intercell and intracell signaling transduction pathways [20].

A previous study [21] investigated the tissue distribution of 100–200 mg/kg/day of fucoidan after intragastric administration in rats and reported considerable heterogeneity. Fucoidan preferentially accumulated in the kidneys (AUC0-t = 10.74 μg·h/g and Cmax = 1.23 μg/g after 5 h), spleen (AUC0-t = 6.89 μg·h/g and Cmax = 0.78 μg/g after 3 h), and liver (AUC0-t = 3.26 μg·h/g and Cmax = 0.53 μg/g after 2 h) and showed relatively long absorption time and extended circulation in the blood, with a mean residence time of 6.79 h. Although data regarding the fucoidan concentration in the lungs are not available, a study showed the anticancer effect of fucoidan on the lung tissue in vivo [22]. We did not perform a dose-dependent study before. The oral gavage dose administered in the current study was based on the dose suggested in previous studies (200 mg/kg) [23–25]. In addition, lung fibrosis is a sequential effect of inflammation. Because fucoidan may attenuate RT-induced inflammation and then reduce lung fibrosis, we examined the effects of fucoidan treatment only for 2 weeks, rather than for 3–4 weeks. We evaluated the phenomena of neutrophil and macrophage infiltration in lung tissue specimens.

RT techniques applied to patients with thorax-related malignancies have resulted in increased lung morbidity and mortality [26–30]. Such therapies involved the exposure of large areas of the heart or lungs to high radiation doses [2–4,29]. Although new treatment techniques have reduced both the dose of RT and the area of the heart or lungs exposed to the RT field, it is not clear whether the risk of late complications has been reduced in magnitude or has been merely delayed with regard to the onset time [27–30]. RT doses to the chest field, such as in breast, esophageal, or lung cancer, might be usually limited by lung or heart tolerance [26–29]. Furthermore, improved local control or overall survival through RT dose escalation is difficult because of the intolerance of normal tissues [26–29]. After a long-term follow-up, the grade of acute radiation-induced injury can often escalate to late radiation-induced injury, resulting in long-term RT-related complications [31]. In addition, similar to other organs, recovery from the acute effects of RT in the lungs does not always correlate with the prevention of late critical effects, including fibrosis, which contribute to organ failure [31]. An interventional agent, such as fucoidan, that can protect normal organ tissues from the acute and late effects of RT is crucial. The possibility of dose escalation for improved local control is important [32]. However, RT-induced toxicity in organs, such as the lungs, heart, or gastrointestinal tract, would be problematic in dose escalation because of the intolerance of normal tissues to RT [26–29]. Until now, no prospective controlled studies have evaluated the efficacy of any preventive drugs or therapies for RP in humans. This study is the first to evaluate the preventive effects of fucoidan on RP and RT-induced lung fibrosis.

In the present study, fucoidan attenuated RT-induced lung fibrosis in irradiated mouse lung tissues on day 31 (Figure 1). Radiation-induced lung injury results from the combination of direct cytotoxicity on normal lung tissues, and more importantly, from the development of fibrosis triggered by radiation-induced cellular signal transduction. The cytotoxic effects are mainly caused by DNA damage that leads to clonogenic death of normal lung epithelial cells, in addition to apoptotic pathways induced by radiation. Fucoidan significantly reduced neutrophil and macrophage infiltration in irradiated mouse lung tissues (Figures 2 and 3). A previous study reported that macrophages may also be present within the alveolar space; these macrophages are migratory cells from the bone marrow and act as a source of numerous cytokines, including IL-6 and TNF-α, to the lungs [33]. In our study, fucoidan attenuated RP and RT-induced lung fibrosis by reducing neutrophil and macrophage infiltration (Figure 6).

Several cytokines are upregulated following lung irradiation and together mediate the corresponding pathological changes. A previous clinical study demonstrated that RT induced the expression of transforming growth factor-beta 1 (TGF-β1), which induced fibroblast collagen deposition [34]. The plasma TGF-β1 level at the end of an RT course was observed to be a predictor of the risk of pneumonitis [34]. However, a subsequent clinical trial revealed no predictable pattern of TGF-β1 changes in individuals with and without radiation-induced lung injury [35]. The proinflammatory cytokines tumor necrosis factor-alpha (TNF-α) and IL-1α have been observed to be upregulated immediately following irradiation. The IL-6 concentration increases following RT, and an elevated pretreatment plasma IL-6 concentration has been shown to be correlated with an increased risk of radiation-induced lung injury [11,36]. However, in this study, we observed no significant differences in IL-1α, TNFα, or IL-6 levels between the sham and RT groups (Figure 4). The discrepancies in results might be due to different sites or the timing of sample collection in different studies. In our study, we collected the pleural fluid from mice of indicated groups on day 15, whereas in previous studies, samples were obtained from human plasma irradiated on day 1 [10,11,35,36]. In our study, the levels of TIMP-1, CXCL1, MCP-1, MIP-2, and IL-1ra were elevated in irradiated mice, which were reduced by fucoidan on day 15. The levels of TIMP-1, CXCL1, MCP-1, MIP-2, and IL-1ra were also determined through EIAs (Figure 5). Fucoidan reduced the expression of TIMP-1, CXCL1, MCP-1, MIP-2, and IL-1ra in the pleural fluid obtained from irradiated mice on day 15. The decreased expression of TIMP-1, CXCL1, MCP-1, MIP-2, and IL-1ra in the pleural fluid obtained from irradiated mice on day 15 was proportional to RT-induced lung fibrosis in mice from the indicated groups that were sacrificed on day 31 (Figure 1). In our study, the increased expression of TIMP-1, CXCL1, MCP-1, MIP-2, and IL-1ra was strongly associated with RT-induced lung fibrosis through the induction of alternatively activated macrophages and neutrophils [37–45]. In our current animal model, the pleural fluid was collected on day 15, and mice were sacrificed on day 31. These findings are consistent with late RT-induced lung injuries, such as lung fibrosis (Figure 1). The present results indicated that fucoidan might attenuate RT-induced lung fibrosis by reducing inflammatory cytokine expression and macrophage and neutrophil infiltration. In addition, the mechanism and role of fucoidan on the SDF-1/CXCL12 and IL-16 expression in normal lung tissue need to be further investigated.

Figure 6 presents a brief schematic of the possible molecular mechanism underlying the preventive effects of fucoidan on RT-induced lung fibrosis mediated through the reduction of inflammatory cytokine expression and neutrophil and macrophage infiltration in lung tissues. The strength of our study is that it is the first study to demonstrate the preventive effects of fucoidan on RP and RT-induced lung fibrosis. This finding can be considered in future clinical practice and randomized controlled studies. Therefore, to obtain crucial information on population specificity and disease occurrence, a large-scale randomized trial comparing the effects of fucoidan on carefully selected patients receiving chest irradiation is essential.

5. Conclusions

In our study, fucoidan changed the expression patterns of inflammatory cytokines, which may consequently attenuate RP and RT-induced lung fibrosis. Fucoidan can be a potential therapeutic agent for RP attenuation or prevention.

Author Contributions: Conception and design: S.-Y.W. Financial support: Taipei Medical University and Wan Fang Hospital (107-swf-08). Collection and assembly of data: E.C.K., C.-L.C., H.-H.Y., Y.-S.S., K.S.-P.Y., A.T.H.W. and S.-Y.W. Data analysis and interpretation: E.C.K., C.-L.C., H.-H.Y., Y.-S.S. and S.-Y.W. Administrative support: S.-Y.W. Manuscript writing: All authors. Final approval of manuscript: All authors.

Acknowledgments: Taipei Medical University and Wan Fang Hospital (107-swf-08).

Abbreviations

RT	Radiotherapy
RP	Radiation Pneumonitis
H&E	Hematoxylin and Eosin
EIAs	Enzyme Immunoassays
DAKO	Diaminobenzidine Tetrahydrochloride
ACEI	Angiotensin-Converting Enzyme Inhibitor
TGF-β1	Transforming Growth Factor-Beta 1
TNF-α	Tumor Necrosis Factor-Alpha
IL-1α	Interleukin 1-Alpha
IL-6	Interleukin 6

References

1. McDonald, S.; Rubin, P.; Phillips, T.L.; Marks, L.B. Injury to the lung from cancer therapy: Clinical syndromes, measurable endpoints, and potential scoring systems. *Int. J. Radiat. Oncol. Biol. Phys.* **1995**, *31*, 1187–1203. [CrossRef]
2. Morgan, G.W.; Breit, S.N. Radiation and the lung: A reevaluation of the mechanisms mediating pulmonary injury. *Int. J. Radiat. Oncol. Biol. Phys.* **1995**, *31*, 361–369. [CrossRef]
3. Marks, L.B.; Bentzen, S.M.; Deasy, J.O.; Kong, F.M.; Bradley, J.D.; Vogelius, I.S.; El Naqa, I.; Hubbs, J.L.; Lebesque, J.V.; Timmerman, R.D.; et al. Radiation dose-volume effects in the lung. *Int. J. Radiat. Oncol. Biol. Phys.* **2010**, *76*, S70–S76. [CrossRef] [PubMed]

4. Marks, L.B.; Yorke, E.D.; Jackson, A.; Ten Haken, R.K.; Constine, L.S.; Eisbruch, A.; Bentzen, S.M.; Nam, J.; Deasy, J.O. Use of normal tissue complication probability models in the clinic. *Int. J. Radiat. Oncol. Biol. Phys.* **2010**, *76*, S10–S19. [CrossRef] [PubMed]
5. Lingos, T.I.; Recht, A.; Vicini, F.; Abner, A.; Silver, B.; Harris, J.R. Radiation pneumonitis in breast cancer patients treated with conservative surgery and radiation therapy. *Int. J. Radiat. Oncol. Biol. Phys.* **1991**, *21*, 355–360. [CrossRef]
6. Rubin, P.; Casseratt, G.W.; Saunders, W. Respiratory system. In *Clinical Radiation Pathology*, 3rd ed.; W.B. Saunders: Philadelphia, PA, USA, 1968; pp. 423–470.
7. Kwa, S.L.; Lebesque, J.V.; Theuws, J.C.; Marks, L.B.; Munley, M.T.; Bentel, G.; Oetzel, D.; Spahn, U.; Graham, M.V.; Drzymala, R.E.; et al. Radiation pneumonitis as a function of mean lung dose: An analysis of pooled data of 540 patients. *Int. J. Radiat. Oncol. Biol. Phys.* **1998**, *42*, 1–9. [CrossRef]
8. Graham, M.V.; Purdy, J.A.; Emami, B.; Harms, W.; Bosch, W.; Lockett, M.A.; Perez, C.A. Clinical dose-volume histogram analysis for pneumonitis after 3D treatment for non-small cell lung cancer (NSCLC). *Int. J. Radiat. Oncol. Biol. Phys.* **1999**, *45*, 323–329. [CrossRef]
9. Rubin, P.; Johnston, C.J.; Williams, J.P.; McDonald, S.; Finkelstein, J.N. A perpetual cascade of cytokines postirradiation leads to pulmonary fibrosis. *Int. J. Radiat. Oncol. Biol. Phys.* **1995**, *33*, 99–109. [CrossRef]
10. Anscher, M.S.; Kong, F.M.; Marks, L.B.; Bentel, G.C.; Jirtle, R.L. Changes in plasma transforming growth factor beta during radiotherapy and the risk of symptomatic radiation-induced pneumonitis. *Int. J. Radiat. Oncol. Biol. Phys.* **1997**, *37*, 253–258. [CrossRef]
11. Chen, Y.; Williams, J.; Ding, I.; Hernady, E.; Liu, W.; Smudzin, T.; Finkelstein, J.N.; Rubin, P.; Okunieff, P. Radiation pneumonitis and early circulatory cytokine markers. *Semin. Radiat. Oncol.* **2002**, *12*, 26–33. [CrossRef] [PubMed]
12. Senthilkumar, K.; Manivasagan, P.; Venkatesan, J.; Kim, S.K. Brown seaweed fucoidan: Biological activity and apoptosis, growth signaling mechanism in cancer. *Int. J. Biol. Macromol.* **2013**, *60*, 366–374. [CrossRef] [PubMed]
13. Atashrazm, F.; Lowenthal, R.M.; Woods, G.M.; Holloway, A.F.; Dickinson, J.L. Fucoidan and cancer: A multifunctional molecule with anti-tumor potential. *Mar. Drugs* **2015**, *13*, 2327–2346. [CrossRef] [PubMed]
14. Kwak, J.Y. Fucoidan as a marine anticancer agent in preclinical development. *Mar. Drugs* **2014**, *12*, 851–870. [CrossRef] [PubMed]
15. Wu, S.Y.; Wu, A.T.; Yuan, K.S.; Liu, S.H. Brown seaweed fucoidan inhibits cancer progression by dual regulation of mir-29c/ADAM12 and miR-17-5p/PTEN axes in human breast cancer cells. *J. Cancer* **2016**, *7*, 2408–2419. [CrossRef] [PubMed]
16. Lee, J.; Kim, J.; Moon, C.; Kim, S.H.; Hyun, J.W.; Park, J.W.; Shin, T. Radioprotective effects of fucoidan in mice treated with total body irradiation. *Phytother. Res.* **2008**, *22*, 1677–1681. [CrossRef] [PubMed]
17. Hwang, P.A.; Phan, N.N.; Lu, W.J.; Ngoc Hieu, B.T.; Lin, Y.C. Low-molecular-weight fucoidan and high-stability fucoxanthin from brown seaweed exert prebiotics and anti-inflammatory activities in Caco-2 cells. *Food Nutr. Res.* **2016**, *60*, 32033. [CrossRef] [PubMed]
18. Szapiel, S.V.; Elson, N.A.; Fulmer, J.D.; Hunninghake, G.W.; Crystal, R.G. Bleomycin-induced interstitial pulmonary disease in the nude, athymic mouse. *Am. Rev. Respir. Dis.* **1979**, *120*, 893–899. [PubMed]
19. Moore, B.B.; Hogaboam, C.M. Murine models of pulmonary fibrosis. *Am. J. Physiol. Lung Cell Mol. Physiol.* **2008**, *294*, L152–L160. [CrossRef] [PubMed]
20. Folkman, J.; Camphausen, K. Cancer. What does radiotherapy do to endothelial cells? *Science* **2001**, *293*, 227–228. [CrossRef] [PubMed]
21. Pozharitskaya, O.N.; Shikov, A.N.; Faustova, N.M.; Obluchinskaya, E.D.; Kosman, V.M.; Vuorela, H.; Makarov, V.G. Pharmacokinetic and tissue distribution of fucoidan from fucus vesiculosus after oral administration to rats. *Mar. Drugs* **2018**, *16*, 132. [CrossRef] [PubMed]
22. Hsu, H.Y.; Lin, T.Y.; Wu, Y.C.; Tsao, S.M.; Hwang, P.A.; Shih, Y.W.; Hsu, J. Fucoidan inhibition of lung cancer in vivo and in vitro: Role of the Smurf2-dependent ubiquitin proteasome pathway in TGFbeta receptor degradation. *Oncotarget* **2014**, *5*, 7870–7885. [CrossRef] [PubMed]
23. Chen, L.M.; Liu, P.Y.; Chen, Y.A.; Tseng, H.Y.; Shen, P.C.; Hwang, P.A.; Hsu, H.L. Oligo-fucoidan prevents IL-6 and CCL2 production and cooperates with p53 to suppress ATM signaling and tumor progression. *Sci. Rep.* **2017**, *7*, 11864. [CrossRef] [PubMed]

24. Chen, C.H.; Sue, Y.M.; Cheng, C.Y.; Chen, Y.C.; Liu, C.T.; Hsu, Y.H.; Hwang, P.A.; Huang, N.J.; Chen, T.H. Oligo-fucoidan prevents renal tubulointerstitial fibrosis by inhibiting the CD44 signal pathway. *Sci. Rep.* **2017**, *7*, 40183. [CrossRef] [PubMed]
25. Tsai, H.L.; Tai, C.J.; Huang, C.W.; Chang, F.R.; Wang, J.Y. Efficacy of low-molecular-weight fucoidan as a supplemental therapy in metastatic colorectal cancer patients: A double-blind randomized controlled trial. *Mar. Drugs* **2017**, *15*, 122. [CrossRef] [PubMed]
26. Bradley, J.D.; Paulus, R.; Komaki, R.; Masters, G.; Blumenschein, G.; Schild, S.; Bogart, J.; Hu, C.; Forster, K.; Magliocco, A.; et al. Standard-dose versus high-dose conformal radiotherapy with concurrent and consolidation carboplatin plus paclitaxel with or without cetuximab for patients with stage IIIA or IIIB non-small-cell lung cancer (RTOG 0617): A randomised, two-by-two factorial phase 3 study. *Lancet Oncol.* **2015**, *16*, 187–199. [PubMed]
27. Wang, K.; Eblan, M.J.; Deal, A.M.; Lipner, M.; Zagar, T.M.; Wang, Y.; Mavroidis, P.; Lee, C.B.; Jensen, B.C.; Rosenman, J.G.; et al. Cardiac toxicity after radiotherapy for stage III non-small-cell lung cancer: Pooled analysis of dose-escalation trials delivering 70 to 90 Gy. *J. Clin. Oncol.* **2017**, *35*, 1387–1394. [CrossRef] [PubMed]
28. Speirs, C.K.; DeWees, T.A.; Rehman, S.; Molotievschi, A.; Velez, M.A.; Mullen, D.; Fergus, S.; Trovo, M.; Bradley, J.D.; Robinson, C.G. Heart dose is an independent dosimetric predictor of overall survival in locally advanced non-small cell lung cancer. *J. Thorac. Oncol.* **2017**, *12*, 293–301. [CrossRef] [PubMed]
29. Dess, R.T.; Sun, Y.; Matuszak, M.M.; Sun, G.; Soni, P.D.; Bazzi, L.; Murthy, V.L.; Hearn, J.W.D.; Kong, F.M.; Kalemkerian, G.P.; et al. Cardiac events after radiation therapy: Combined analysis of prospective multicenter trials for locally advanced non-small-cell lung cancer. *J. Clin. Oncol.* **2017**, *35*, 1395–1402. [CrossRef] [PubMed]
30. Jones, J.M.; Ribeiro, G.G. Mortality patterns over 34 years of breast cancer patients in a clinical trial of post-operative radiotherapy. *Clin. Radiol.* **1989**, *40*, 204–208. [CrossRef]
31. Epperly, M.; Bray, J.; Kraeger, S.; Zwacka, R.; Engelhardt, J.; Travis, E.; Greenberger, J. Prevention of late effects of irradiation lung damage by manganese superoxide dismutase gene therapy. *Gene Ther.* **1998**, *5*, 196–208. [CrossRef] [PubMed]
32. Morganti, A. Higher-dose radiotherapy ups survival in pancreatic cancer. In Proceedings of the European Society for Radiotherapy & Oncology, Vienna, Austria, 15 May 2017.
33. Chen, G.; Lin, S.C.; Chen, J.; He, L.; Dong, F.; Xu, J.; Han, S.; Du, J.; Entman, M.L.; Wang, Y. CXCL16 recruits bone marrow-derived fibroblast precursors in renal fibrosis. *J. Am. Soc. Nephrol.* **2011**, *22*, 1876–1886. [CrossRef] [PubMed]
34. Anscher, M.S.; Kong, F.M.; Andrews, K.; Clough, R.; Marks, L.B.; Bentel, G.; Jirtle, R.L. Plasma transforming growth factor beta1 as a predictor of radiation pneumonitis. *Int. J. Radiat. Oncol. Biol. Phys.* **1998**, *41*, 1029–1035. [CrossRef]
35. Mazeron, R.; Etienne-Mastroianni, B.; Perol, D.; Arpin, D.; Vincent, M.; Falchero, L.; Martel-Lafay, I.; Carrie, C.; Claude, L. Predictive factors of late radiation fibrosis: A prospective study in non-small cell lung cancer. *Int. J. Radiat. Oncol. Biol. Phys.* **2010**, *77*, 38–43. [CrossRef] [PubMed]
36. Chen, Y.; Rubin, P.; Williams, J.; Hernady, E.; Smudzin, T.; Okunieff, P. Circulating IL-6 as a predictor of radiation pneumonitis. *Int. J. Radiat. Oncol. Biol. Phys.* **2001**, *49*, 641–648. [CrossRef]
37. Selman, M.; Ruiz, V.; Cabrera, S.; Segura, L.; Ramirez, R.; Barrios, R.; Pardo, A. TIMP-1, -2, -3, and -4 in idiopathic pulmonary fibrosis. A prevailing nondegradative lung microenvironment? *Am. J. Physiol. Lung Cell Mol. Physiol.* **2000**, *279*, L562–L574. [CrossRef] [PubMed]
38. Ruiz, V.; Ordonez, R.M.; Berumen, J.; Ramirez, R.; Uhal, B.; Becerril, C.; Pardo, A.; Selman, M. Unbalanced collagenases/TIMP-1 expression and epithelial apoptosis in experimental lung fibrosis. *Am. J. Physiol. Lung Cell Mol. Physiol.* **2003**, *285*, L1026–L1036. [CrossRef] [PubMed]
39. Wynn, T.A. Integrating mechanisms of pulmonary fibrosis. *J. Exp. Med.* **2011**, *208*, 1339–1350. [CrossRef] [PubMed]
40. Li, D.; Guabiraba, R.; Besnard, A.G.; Komai-Koma, M.; Jabir, M.S.; Zhang, L.; Graham, G.J.; Kurowska-Stolarska, M.; Liew, F.Y.; McSharry, C.; et al. IL-33 promotes ST2-dependent lung fibrosis by the induction of alternatively activated macrophages and innate lymphoid cells in mice. *J. Allergy Clin. Immunol.* **2014**, *134*, 1422–1432. [CrossRef] [PubMed]

41. Hasegawa, M.; Sato, S.; Takehara, K. Augmented production of chemokines (monocyte chemotactic protein-1 (MCP-1), macrophage inflammatory protein-1alpha (MIP-1alpha) and (MIP-1beta) in patients with systemic sclerosis: MCP-1 and MIP-1alpha may be involved in the development of pulmonary fibrosis. *Clin. Exp. Immunol.* **1999**, *117*, 159–165. [PubMed]
42. Car, B.D.; Meloni, F.; Luisetti, M.; Semenzato, G.; Gialdroni-Grassi, G.; Walz, A. Elevated IL-8 and MCP-1 in the bronchoalveolar lavage fluid of patients with idiopathic pulmonary fibrosis and pulmonary sarcoidosis. *Am. J. Respir. Crit. Care Med.* **1994**, *149*, 655–659. [CrossRef] [PubMed]
43. Piguet, P.F.; Vesin, C.; Grau, G.E.; Thompson, R.C. Interleukin 1 receptor antagonist (IL-1ra) prevents or cures pulmonary fibrosis elicited in mice by bleomycin or silica. *Cytokine* **1993**, *5*, 57–61. [CrossRef]
44. Mall, M.; Grubb, B.R.; Harkema, J.R.; O'Neal, W.K.; Boucher, R.C. Increased airway epithelial Na^+ absorption produces cystic fibrosis-like lung disease in mice. *Nat. Med.* **2004**, *10*, 487–493. [CrossRef] [PubMed]
45. Hagiwara, S.I.; Ishii, Y.; Kitamura, S. Aerosolized administration of N-acetylcysteine attenuates lung fibrosis induced by bleomycin in mice. *Am. J. Respir. Crit. Care Med.* **2000**, *162*, 225–231. [CrossRef] [PubMed]

19

A Reassessment of the *Marrubium Vulgare* L. Herb's Potential Role in Diabetes Mellitus Type 2: First Results Guide the Investigation toward New Horizons

Javier Rodríguez Villanueva [1,*], Jorge Martín Esteban [2] and Laura Rodríguez Villanueva [3]

1 Biomedical Sciences Department, Pharmacy and Pharmaceutical Technology Unit, Faculty of Pharmacy, University of Alcalá, Ctra. de Madrid-Barcelona (Autovía A2) Km. 33,600, 28805 Alcalá de Henares, Madrid, Spain

2 Phytotherapy Faculty, University of Barcelona, Gran Via de les Corts Catalanes, 585, 08007 Barcelona, Spain; jorgemartinesteban@gmail.com

3 Faculty of Pharmacy, University of Alcalá, Ctra. de Madrid-Barcelona (Autovía A2) Km. 33,600 28805 Alcalá de Henares, Madrid, Spain; lau95.rv@gmail.com

* Correspondence: therealworldvsme@hotmail.com

Abstract: Despite the wide variety of pharmacological activities described for the *Marrubium vulgare* L. herb, amazingly, only one clinical trial can be found in scientific literature. It was designed for the evaluation of its antidiabetic activity. Worse, the outcomes of this trial were contradictory to what previous in vivo mice assays had concluded. Therefore, should *Marrubium vulgare* be ruled out due to its lack of therapeutic potential in diabetes? The authors suggest a reevaluation of the clinical trial methodology to establish valid and final results.

Keywords: *Marrubium vulgare* L. herb; diabetes mellitus type 2; clinical trial; methodology

1. Introduction

Marrubium L. (Lamiaceae) has about forty species, generally distributed in temperate regions of Central and Western Asia, North Africa, Europe, and South America. Generally, these plants are large annual or perennial shrubs [1]. The furane labdane diterpene marrubiin is assumed to be the chemotaxonomic marker among the various species of the *Marrubium* genus. Generally, marrubiin is isolated from dried whole plants of *Marrubium vulgare* Linn (white/common horehound, hoarhound, marriout, maromba, marroio-branco, or marrubio) in a proportion of 0.3–0.7% [2]. *M. vulgare* L., commonly known as "white horehound" can be identified as a robust perennial herb, with densely cottony stems and white flowers [3].

Researchers have tried to support the biological activities described for the *M. vulgare* L. herb (for an extended analysis, see Reference [4] and Figure 1) by the isolation and identification of biologically active phytochemicals such as diterpenes (marrubiin and related compounds), flavonoids (luteolin, apigenin, ladanein, quercetin, isoquercitrin, chrysoeriol, or vitexin), phenylpropanoid esters (including acteoside (or verbascoside), forsythoside B, arenarioside, ballotetroside, alyssonoide, marruboside, and acethyl marruboside), tannins (such as proanthocyanidins, catechin and epicatechin, condensed tannins), and sterols [5].

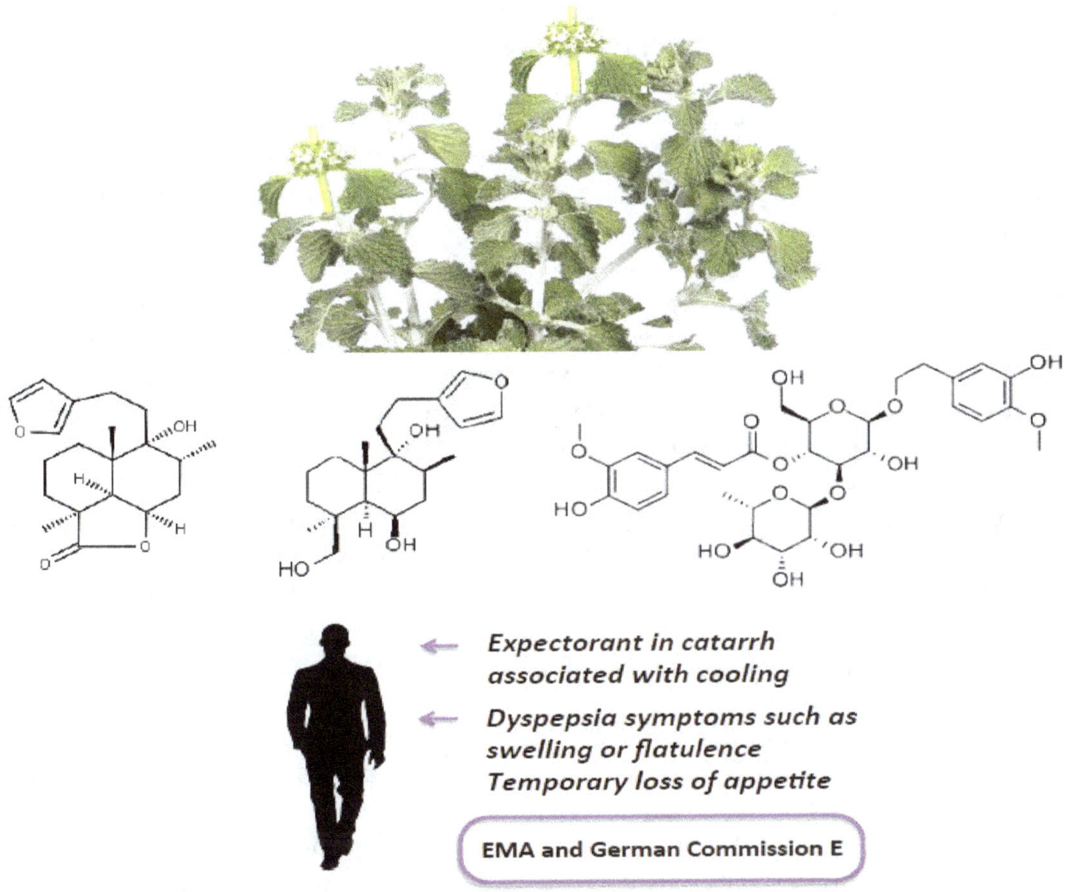

Figure 1. Top, photograph of the aerial part of *Marrubium vulgare* L.; Middle, marrubiin, marrubiol (both diterpenes), and martinoside (a phenylpropanoid), three of the plant's active compounds; Bottom, the European Medicine Agency (EMA) and German Commission E approved indications for the aerial part of *Marrubium vulgare* L.

Diabetes mellitus is a metabolic disease characterized by chronic hyperglycemia resulting from defects in insulin secretion, insulin action, or both. Diabetes mellitus type 2 (DM2), known as adult type or non-insulin-dependent diabetes mellitus, is treated by controlling the diet and oral hypoglycemic drugs [6]. In 2004, more than 120 million people in the world had diabetes. In 2015, there were approximately 415 million people with diabetes, and this is projected to increase to 642 million by 2040 (International Diabetes Federation atlas, 2015). In Mexico, DM2 affects 8.2% of the population between 20 and 69 years old and has the highest mortality rate of chronic degenerative diseases, representing 16.7% of deaths [7].

M. Vulgare L. has been reported to be used in the treatment of diabetes in traditional medicine in Mexico [8] and central Morocco [6], and scientific studies have revealed through in vivo research the hypoglycemic effect of this plant, supporting its traditional use in diabetes mellitus control [9].

2. Preclinical In Vivo Observations: The Starting Point

Initial studies showed that horehound infusion (132 g of the dried plant/1 L water, in a dose of 4 mL/kg body weight) decreased the glucose curve significantly when a 50% dextrose solution (4 mL/kg of weight) was administered [10].

Years later, the methanolic extract of the top parts of *M. vulgare* L. was also evaluated for the same purpose [11], and 500 g of the aerial part was homogenized with methanol for 15 min, three times each with 1000 mL (500 g/1 × 3 L), followed by distillation of the solvent under reduced pressure. The percentage yield was calculated as 12%. In this case, diabetes was induced in rats through streptozotocin (in 0.1 M sodium citrate buffer, pH 4.5) injected intraperitoneally at a dose of 55 mg/kg, as a single dose. The diabetic rats orally received the extract of *M. vulgare* in a dose of 500 mg dry extract/kg of weight in a 1% CMC-Na vehicle once a day, starting on the 11th day. The oral administration of the *M. vulgare* extract significantly reduced the plasma glucose level after three days by more than 7% (curiously, glibenclamide has no effect here). After 14 days, the reduction was marked, reaching 42% compared to the control values of the diabetic group. The plasma glucose level was reduced in the glibenclamide group by 31% compared to the control values of the diabetic group on the 28th day.

In 2012, Boudjelal et al. [9] proved through preclinical in vivo trials the hypoglycemic and hypolipidemic effects in diabetic albino rats (180–200 g) fed ad libitum with a pellet diet and water, kept and maintained under laboratory conditions of temperature and light (24 ± 1 °C and a 12 h light/dark cycle). Rats were randomly divided into six groups and injected intraperitoneally with a single injection of alloxan monohydrate (150 mg/kg) to cause hyperglycemia and fasting blood glucose levels greater than 300 mg/dL.

The extract of *M. Vulgare* administered was prepared by boiling 6 g of the aerial parts of the plant, dried at room temperature in the dark and ground to a powder, in 25 mL of distilled water for 15 min, the mixture of which was then left to reach room temperature and filtrated. Extracts in a dose of 100, 200, or 300 mg/kg of body weight were orally administered twice daily for 15 days. The positive control was glibenclamide (5 mg/kg of body weight); a normal control and a diabetic control were also included. A sharp decline in blood glucose levels was observed from the third day after the treatment with three doses of *M. vulgare* extracts and glibenclamide (more than 5% for 300 mg/kg of body weight, and up to 12% for glibenclamide). In particular, the highest percentage decrease of glycaemia levels was observed after 28 days for the treatments with 300 mg/kg of body weight of *Marrubium* infusion (−62.55%) and the positive control glibenclamide (−65.90%). Serum glucose, total lipids, triglycerides, and total cholesterol decreased after the administration of *M. vulgare* extract in all doses without attaining the values of the normal control. The effect was similar to that observed with the positive control, glibenclamide. The authors attribute these results to a stimulation of insulin secretion from beta cells of islets and/or inhibition of insulin degradation processes due to the high content of flavonoids in the drug (15.53 mg quercetin equivalent/g of dry plant material).

In both studies, there were no physical signs of toxicity, such as writhing, gasping, palpitation and respiratory rate, or mortality in the rats. The rats treated with different doses of *M. vulgare* did not show any drug-induced behavioral disorders.

3. From Animals to Humans: The Clinical Trial Issue for Herbal Medicine

More than 10 years ago, Wolsko and coworkers [12] stated that poor quality control in the United States was not surprising, given the US regulatory environment as dictated by the Dietary Supplement Health and Education Act of 1994. The same could be applied nowadays, for the United States as well as for the European Union. There is still currently no minimum standard of practice for manufacturing dietary supplements, no premarket safety or efficacy studies are needed, and dietary supplements do not need approval from the Food and Drug Administration (FDA) or the European Medicine Agency (EMA) before they are marketed. It continues to be purely the manufacturers' responsibility to ensure that supplements are safe and labeled properly before marketing. The FDA or the EMA (coordinated with the agency of each member state) can take action to restrict a product's use only after it has been shown that a dietary supplement is unsafe, sometimes years later, when it has taken the lives or has cost the health of innocent people. In the absence of evidence to the contrary, herbal supplements used in clinical trials have the same poor quality as demonstrated in the marketplace as a whole. This fact, linked with the number of pharmacognosy drugs of the same species and the different treatments being undergone, makes it very difficult if not impossible to establish valid conclusions that are not contradictory to what has been reported before in animals.

For the *Marrubium vulgare* L. herb, while some articles describe and sustain the ethnopharmacological use [13], only one clinical trial can be found in the scientific literature up to date [7]. This is striking given that, in 2015, preparations of this species were the best-selling herbal dietary supplements, reaching approximately $106 million in retail sales [14]. This randomized, double-blind, and controlled clinical trial was conducted to evaluate the clinical effect produced by its aqueous extract on type 2 non-controlled diabetes mellitus. The verum product consisted of fresh *M. vulgare* L. leaves that were dried under environmental temperatures and protected from direct light and then milled. Ethylene oxide was used for sterilization. Patients had to prepare the treatment immediately before administration. A 1-g filter-paper envelope was placed in a cup of boiling water for 5 min. *M. vulgare* L. extract was administered three times a day, before every meal. The infusion was analyzed through HPLC with UV detection at 255 nm only for chlorogenic acid determination. This compound was not found in the extract.

Outpatients of either sex, between 30 and 60 years old, who had been diagnosed with type 2 diabetes no more than five years earlier, were selected. All patients were under medical treatment but showing a fasting blood glucose >140 mg/dL. As usual, patients affected with diabetes complications or nephropathy, pregnant women, patients with gestational diabetes, and hospitalized patients were not selected. In this study, insulin-dependent or type I diabetics were excluded, and, for comfort and to assure results, people who needed to travel frequently were also not selected. A total of 43 patients were recruited, and 21 received an *M. vulgare* L. infusion. The other 22 received a *Cecropia obtusifolia* extract. All patients showed treatment adherence, evaluated by counting the used dosages.

The study was carried out for 21 days. Prior to infusion administration, every seven days and after the clinical trial, the fasting determination of glucose, cholesterol, triglycerides, urea, creatinine, and uric acid in blood was carried out using automatic equipment (Autolab) with standardized techniques by a certified external laboratory.

In this study, effectiveness was considered a decrease in the basal concentration of glucose, cholesterol, or triglycerides by at least 25%. *M. vulgare* L. caused that effect in only two of the 21 patients (9.52%). The mean of plasma glucose level was reduced by 0.64%, and that of cholesterol and triglycerides by 4.16% and 5.78%, respectively. These results were disappointing.

4. Some Result Considerations Must Be Kept in Mind: Paving the Way for Future Actions

Nevertheless, some considerations must be taken into account. First of all, as the authors state, a crude extract was evaluated, with a similar preparation to that used in traditional medicine. As previously described, effective results on animal models were obtained after the administration of specific extracts, available after processing crude plant material with different methods. The effect of preparation methods on composition or content (as well as on undesired ingredients) is not fully understood. The same applies for therapeutic activity. Also, the administration route influences the bioavailability, pharmacological activity, and clinical effectiveness of a phytotherapeutic preparation. Previously, clinical studies could only demonstrate observations if the botanic drug material and the study design were rationally based on that basis.

What is important here is that 6-octadecynoic acid, a fatty acid with a triple bond found in *Marrubium vulgare* L., exhibits PPARγ agonist activity by directly binding to helix 12 through the conformational change of the Ω loop. Compounds with PPARγ agonist activity have been clinically used for treatment of type 2 diabetes by improving insulin resistance [15]. However, it is only found in the organic (methanolic) extract of the aerial parts (tops, leaves, and flowers), as fatty acids are not soluble in water infusion. It is not difficult to propose that, between others, there may be a presumable relation between the efficacy of the methanolic extract in mice models/lack of efficacy as an aqueous extraction and the presence/absence of 6-octadecynoic acid.

Despite this, as we previously stated [16], a characterized compound with a perfectly defined mechanism of action at a particular dose fulfills the negative requirements (such as toxicity) inherited from classical pharmacology. However, new trends suggest an integrative approach in which a wide variety of compounds act on multiple targets together to produce a final action through a balance resulting from minor changes (synergy); something different is not expected here. Diterpenes, flavonoids, and phenylpropanoid esters may also play a role in the antidiabetic activity or in the diabetes concomitant effects as on animal models.

No less important is a diligent analysis of the dose translation from animals to humans, if possible with recognized recommendations (i.e., FDA, EMA, or Commission E if available). Elberry and colleagues [11] administered to rats 500 mg of dried extract (as previously described) per kg of weight. For an average person (weighing 60 kg), this dosage correlates with a dose of 81 mg/kg of weight. Taking into account the drug/extraction ratio, almost 39 g of the herbal substance (crude drug) is needed, which is impossible to achieve for an individual administration (the EMA recommends a 1–2 g dose of the cut drug, and the German Commission E recommends a 4–5 g dose of the fresh/dried plant material per day). Considering the hypothesis that 6-octadecynoic acid is the compound primarily involved in the antidiabetic activity and available in sufficient amounts of raw material, these results reveal that a more efficient extraction method should be developed (ethyl acetate showed good results in the study by Ohtera et al. [15], but possible toxicity risks must be abolished before achieving clinical trials with EtOAc extracts).

For example, we proposed that the extract prepared by El Bardai et al. [17,18] was obtained by aqueous infusion (5 g air parts/100 mL of water, yield after lyophilization) with a drug: extract ratio (DER) 6.2:1 and performance 13%. This extract minimizes possible toxicity due to organic solvents, allows oral administration, and makes feasible the fulfilment of the recommended therapeutic range, which allows a maximum amount of 6 g per drug per day.

Finally, it is important to notice the slighter side effects (described by one in every four patients) in the clinical trial, including nausea, oral dryness, sialorrhea, dizziness, and anorexia, although they were not adverse enough to necessarily cause a withdrawal from the study [7]. These results and the acquired experience in the traditional intake of the water infusion of *Marrubium vulgare* L. can be considered safe. In spite of this, the number of patients, as is usual in clinical trials of herb preparations, was reduced, and the establishment of general conclusions is therefore almost impossible.

References

1. Kahkeshani, N.; Gharedaghi, M.; Hadjiakhoondi, A.; Sharifzadeh, M. Antinociceptive effect of extracts of Marrubium astracanicum Jacq. aerial parts. *Avicenna J. Phytomed.* **2017**, *7*, 73–79. [PubMed]
2. Mittal, V.; Nanda, A. Intensification of marrubiin concentration by optimization of microwave-assisted (low CO_2 yielding) extraction process for *Marrubium vulgare* using central composite design and antioxidant evaluation. *Pharm. Biol.* **2017**, *55*, 1337–1347. [CrossRef] [PubMed]
3. Aouni, R.; Attia, M.B.; Jaafoura, M.H.; Bibi-Derbel, A. Effects of the hydro-ethanolic extract of *Marrubium vulgare* in female rats. *Asian Pac. J. Trop. Med.* **2017**, *10*, 160–164. [CrossRef] [PubMed]
4. Villanueva, R.J.; Esteban, M.J. An Insight into a Blockbuster Phytomedicine; *Marrubium vulgare* L. Herb. More of a Myth than a Reality? *Phytother. Res.* **2016**, *30*, 1551–1558. [CrossRef] [PubMed]
5. Garjani, A.; Tila, D.; Hamedeyazdan, S.; Vaez, H. An investigation on cardioprotective potential of *Marrubium vulgare* aqueous fraction against ischemia-reperfusion injury in isolated rat heart. *Folia Morphol. (Warsz)* **2015**. [CrossRef] [PubMed]
6. Barkaoui, M.; Katiri, A.; Boubaker, H.; Msanda, F. Ethnobotanical survey of medicinal plants used in the traditional treatment of diabetes in Chtouka Ait Baha and Tiznit (Western Anti-Atlas), Morocco. *J. Ethnopharmacol.* **2017**, *198*, 338–350. [CrossRef] [PubMed]
7. Herrera-Arellano, A.; Aguilar-Santamaria, L.; Garcia-Hernandez, B.; Nicasio-Torres, P. Clinical trial of Cecropia obtusifolia and *Marrubium vulgare* leaf extracts on blood glucose and serum lipids in type 2 diabetics. *Phytomedicine* **2004**, *11*, 561–566. [CrossRef] [PubMed]

8. Argueta, V.A.; Cano, L.M.; Rodarte, M.E. (Eds.) *Atlas de las Plantas de la Medicina Tradicional Mexicana*; Instituto Nacional Indigenista: Mexico DF, República de Mexico, 1994; Volume 3. Available online: www.medicinatradicionalmexicana.unam.mx/monografia.php?=3&t=Marrubio&id=76201 (accessed on 29 July 2017).
9. Boudjelal, A.; Henchiri, C.; Siracusa, L.; Sari, M. Compositional analysis and in vivo anti-diabetic activity of wild Algerian *Marrubium vulgare* L. infusion. *Fitoterapia* **2012**, *83*, 286–292. [CrossRef] [PubMed]
10. Roman Ramos, R.; Alarcon-Aguilar, F.; Lara-Lemus, A.; Flores-Saenz, J.L. Hypoglycemic effect of plants used in Mexico as antidiabetics. *Arch. Med. Res.* **1992**, *23*, 59–64. [PubMed]
11. Elberry, A.A.; Harraz, F.M.; Ghareib, S.A.; Gabr, S.A. Methanolic extract of *Marrubium vulgare* ameliorates hyperglycemia and dyslipidemia in streptozotocin-induced diabetic rats. *Int. J. Diabetes Mellit.* **2015**, *3*, 37–44. [CrossRef]
12. Wolsko, P.M.; Solondz, D.K.; Phillips, R.S.; Schachter, S.C. Lack of herbal supplement characterization in published randomized controlled trials. *Am. J. Med.* **2005**, *118*, 1087–1093. [CrossRef] [PubMed]
13. Ballero, M.; Sotgiu, A.M.; Piu, G. Empirical administration of preparations of *Marrubium vulgare* in the asthmatic syndrome. *Biomed. Lett.* **1998**, *57*, 31–36.
14. Izzo, A.A.; Hoon-Kim, S.; Radhakrishnan, R.; Williamson, E.M. A Critical Approach to Evaluating Clinical Efficacy, Adverse Events and Drug Interactions of Herbal Remedies. *Phytother. Res.* **2016**, *30*, 691–700. [CrossRef] [PubMed]
15. Ohtera, A.; Miyamae, Y.; Nakai, N.; Kawachi, A. Identification of 6-octadecynoic acid from a methanol extract of *Marrubium vulgare* L. as a peroxisome proliferator-activated receptor gamma agonist. *Biochem. Biophys. Res. Commun.* **2013**, *440*, 204–209. [CrossRef] [PubMed]
16. Villanueva, J.R.; Esteban, J.M.; Villanueva, R.L. Solving the puzzle: What is behind our forefathers' anti-inflammatory remedies? *J. Int. Ethnopharmacol.* **2017**, *6*, 128–143. [CrossRef] [PubMed]
17. El Bardai, S.; Hamaide, M.C.; Lyoussi, B.; Quetin-Leclercq, J.; Morel, N.; Wibo, M. Marrubenol interacts with the phenylalkylamine binding site of the L-type calcium channel. *Eur. J. Pharmacol.* **2004**, *492*, 269–272. [CrossRef] [PubMed]
18. El Bardai, S.; Lyoussi, B.; Wibo, M.; Morel, N. Comparative study of the antihypertensive activity of *Marrubium vulgare* and of the dihydropyridine calciumantagonistamlodipine in spontaneously hypertensive rat. *Clin. Exp. Hypertens.* **2004**, *26*, 465–474. [CrossRef] [PubMed]

20

Components from the Leaves and Twigs of Mangrove *Lumnitzera racemosa* with Anti-Angiogenic and Anti-Inflammatory Effects

Szu-Yin Yu [1,†], Shih-Wei Wang [1,2,†], Tsong-Long Hwang [3,4,5], Bai-Luh Wei [6], Chien-Jung Su [1], Fang-Rong Chang [1,7,*] and Yuan-Bin Cheng [1,8,*]

1 Graduate Institute of Natural Products, College of Pharmacy, Kaohsiung Medical University, Kaohsiung 807, Taiwan; s91412232@gmail.com (S.-Y.Y.); shihwei@mmc.edu.tw (S.-W.W.); scj820826@gmail.com (C.-J.S.)
2 Department of Medicine, Mackay Medical College, New Taipei City 252, Taiwan
3 Graduate Institute of Natural Products, College of Medicine, and Chinese Herbal Medicine Research Team, Healthy Aging Research Center, Chang Gung University, Taoyuan 333, Taiwan; htl@mail.cgu.edu.tw
4 Research Center for Chinese Herbal Medicine, Research Center for Food and Cosmetic Safety, and Graduate Institute of Health Industry Technology, College of Human Ecology, Chang Gung University of Science and Technology, Taoyuan 333, Taiwan
5 Department of Anesthesiology, Chang Gung Memorial Hospital, Taoyuan 333, Taiwan
6 Department of Life Science, National Taitung University, Taitung 950, Taiwan; blwei@nttu.edu.tw
7 National Research Institute of Chinese Medicine, Ministry of Health and Welfare, Taipei 112, Taiwan
8 Department of Medical Research, Kaohsiung Medical University Hospital, Kaohsiung 807, Taiwan
* Correspondence: aaronfrc@kmu.edu.tw (F.-R.C.); jmb@kmu.edu.tw (Y.-B.C.)

† These authors contributed equally to this work.

Abstract: One new neolignan, racelactone A (**1**), together with seven known compounds (**2**−**8**) were isolated from the methanolic extract of the leaves and twigs of *Lumnitzera racemosa*. The structure of racelactone A (**1**) was determined on the basis of the mass and NMR spectroscopic data interpretation. With respect to bioactivity, compound 1 displayed an anti-angiogenic effect by suppressing tube formation. Furthermore, compounds **1**, **4**, and **5** showed significant anti-inflammatory effects with IC_{50} values of 4.95 ± 0.89, 1.95 ± 0.40, and 2.57 ± 0.23 μM, respectively. The plausible biosynthesis pathway of racelactone A (**1**) was proposed.

Keywords: neolignan; *Lumnitzera racemosa*; anti-angiogenesis; anti-inflammation

1. Introduction

Mangroves are unique plants growing in the intertidal zone of the tropical and subtropical climates; these species are salt-tolerant and have mechanisms which affect a variety of cellular metabolic processes [1]. Plants of the mangrove genus *Lumnitzera* (Combretaceae) comprise more than 600 species in Asia, Austria, and Africa. Among them, *Lumnitzera racemosa* Willd. is native to the seashore of southern Taiwan. *L. racemosa* can grow up to a five-meter height; its bark is dark brown and rough, the leaves are slightly concave top round, and the fruits are drupe and with an ellipsoid shape [2]. The woods of *L. racemosa* are hard and have a long shelf life; they can be used as building materials, equipment, or fuels. *L. racemosa* is also fantabulous nectar plant, while the leaves are edible to date [3]. Traditionally, the sap of this plant is used to treat cutaneous pruritus, herpes, scabies, and thrush [4]. The chemical constituents of *L. racemosa* are fatty acids, flavonoids, polyisoprenoid alcohols, tannins, and triterpenoids [5]. Pharmacological studies of the extracts from *L. racemosa* demonstrated antibacterial, antifungal, antihypertensive, antioxidant, cytotoxic, and hepatoprotective activities [6–9].

Inflammation is tightly associated with carcinogenesis and the disease progression of cancer [10]. Angiogenesis has been reported to facilitate the growth and dissemination of cancer cells in tumor microenvironments [11]. Plentiful studies reveal that inhibition of inflammation and angiogenesis is an effective therapeutic strategy to suppress cancer development and metastasis [12,13]. Our preliminary pharmacological investigation indicated that methanolic extract of the leaves and twigs of *L. racemosa* exerted promising anti-angiogenic and anti-inflammatory responses. Herein, we describe the isolation, structural elucidation, and bioactivities of one new neolignan, racelactone A (**1**), along with seven known compounds (**2**–**8**).

2. Results

In the present study, the methanolic extracted from *L. racemosa* was partitioned with ethyl acetate (EtOAc) and water (H_2O). The EtOAc layer was further partitioned with *n*-hexane and 75% methanol (MeOH) in H_2O to give a 75% $MeOH_{(aq)}$ layer. One new compound, racelactone A (**1**), and seven known compounds: Botulin (**2**) [14,15], 3,4,3′-tri-*O*-methyl ellagic acid (**3**) [16], methyl gallate (**4**) [17], myricitrin (**5**) [18], stigmasterol (**6**) [19], kaempferol (**7**) [20], and isoguaiacin (**8**) [21] were identified from the 75% $MeOH_{(aq)}$ layer. The structures of compounds (**1**–**8**) are shown in Figure 1.

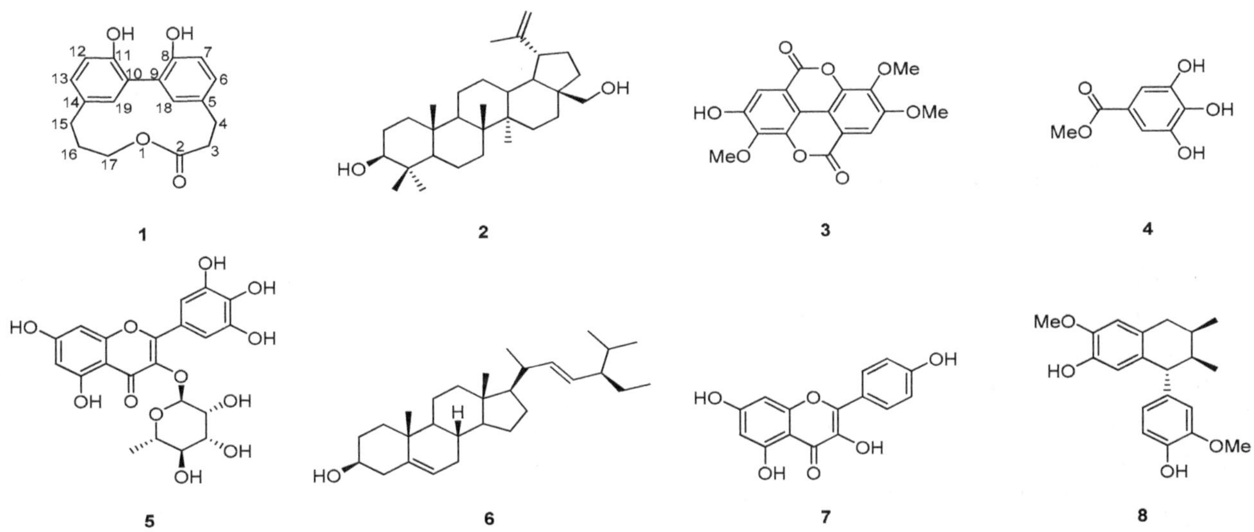

Figure 1. Structures of compounds **1**–**8**.

Racelactone A (**1**) was isolated as an amorphous powder, light yellow, having a molecular formula determined as $C_{18}H_{18}O_4$. Ten indices of hydrogen deficiency were calculated, in accord with the high-resolution electrospray ionisation mass spectrometry (HRESIMS) data (m/z 321.10955 $[M + Na]^+$) (Figure S1) and NMR spectrum. The IR spectrum (Figure S2) of **1** suggested the presence of hydroxy (3364 cm^{-1}), carbonyl (1709 cm^{-1}) and aromatic (1503, 1586 cm^{-1}) functionalities. In ^1H NMR (Figure S3), data revealed six olefinic methines (δ_H 6.81, 6.87, 7.01, 7.03, 7.06, and 7.18), and five methylenes (δ_H 2.25, 2.58, 2.82, 2.98, and 4.29) (Table 1). The ^{13}C (Figure S4) and DEPT NMR spectrum (Table 1) of **1** noted eighteen carbon signals, including one carbonyl (δc 175.0), six olefinic methines (δc 113.3, 115.9, 116.4, 128.3, 129.2, and 133.1), six nonprotonated carbons (δc 126.6, 127.2, 131.4, 132.7, 151.9, and 152.7), and five methylenes (δc 25.2, 29.7, 30.7, 35.7, and 65.7). Analyses on a set of signals and coupling constants at δ_H 6.87 (d, 1H, J = 8.2 Hz, H-12), 7.03 (dd, 1H, J = 8.2, 2.4 Hz, H-13), and 7.06 (d, 1H, J = 2.5 Hz, H-18) as well as another set at δ_H 7.01 (dd, 1H, J = 8.2, 2.5 Hz, H-6), 6.81 (d, 1H, J = 8.1 Hz, H-7), and 7.19 (d, 1H, J = 2.5 Hz, H-19) led to the identification of two 1,3,4-trisubstituted phenyl moieties. From analyses of the NMR, UV (Figure S5), and IR data, compound **1** was determined to be a neolignan. Compound **1** showed similar ^1H and ^{13}C NMR signals (Table 1), partially similar to those of corniculatolide A, which has an ether bridge between two propylphenyl moieties [22,23]—except for the presence of two unusual quaternary carbon signals at δc 126.6 and δc 127.2 instead of two signals at δc 149.0 and δc 154.2 in corniculatolide A. This indicated a new carbon–carbon linkage formation in the target molecule.

Table 1. ^{1}H and ^{13}C NMR data of **1**[a] in acetone-d_6.

Position	δ_H, mult (J in Hz)	δ_C, Type	HMBC (^{1}H-^{13}C)
2	-	175.0, C	-
3	2.58, m	35.7, CH_2	2, 4, 5
4	2.98, m	29.7, CH_2	2, 3, 5, 6, 18
5	-	132.7, C	-
6	7.01, dd (8.1, 2.5)	128.3, CH	7, 8, 18
7	6.81, d (8.1)	115.9, CH	5, 6, 8, 9
8	-	152.7, C	-
9	-	127.2, C	-
10	-	126.6, C	-
11	-	151.9, C	-
12	6.87, d (8.2)	116.4, CH	10, 11, 14
13	7.03, dd (8.2, 2.5)	129.2, CH	11, 12, 15, 19
14	-	131.4, C	-
15	2.82, m	30.7, CH_2	13, 14, 16, 17, 19
16	2.25, m	25.2, CH_2	14, 15, 17
17	4.29, t (5.0)	65.7, CH_2	2, 15, 16
18	7.06, d (2.5)	133.1, CH	4, 6, 8, 10
19	7.19, d (2.5)	133.3, CH	9, 11, 13

[a] ^{1}H and ^{13}C NMR data (δ) were measured at 400 and 100 MHz, respectively; chemical shifts are in ppm.

The planar structure of **1** was established by the correlation spectroscopy (COSY) (Figure S6) and heter onuclear multiple bond correlation (HMBC) (Figure S7) correlations (Figure 2). The COSY correlations established the fragments of H-3/H-4, H-6/H-7, H-12/H-13, and H-15/H-16/H-17 of compound **1**. The HMBC correlations of H-4/C-5, C-6, and C-18 and the correlations of H-15/C-13, C-14, and C-19 determined the linkages of two sets of propyl and phenyl functions, respectively. The macroring connection system of two phenylpropanoid moieties was completed on the basis of a key HMBC correlation between H-17/C-2, H-18/C-10, and H-19/C-9. As mentioned above, compound **1** was categorized as a macrolactone, and named racelactone A. The biosynthesis of racelactone A is proposed to be initiated by a PAL enzyme of phenylalanine to form dihydrocaffeic acid. The precursor was resonated to form intermediates A and B. Phenoxy radicals of intermediates A and B were linked to generate the intermediate C, which was structured as racelactone A during a cyclization (Figure 3).

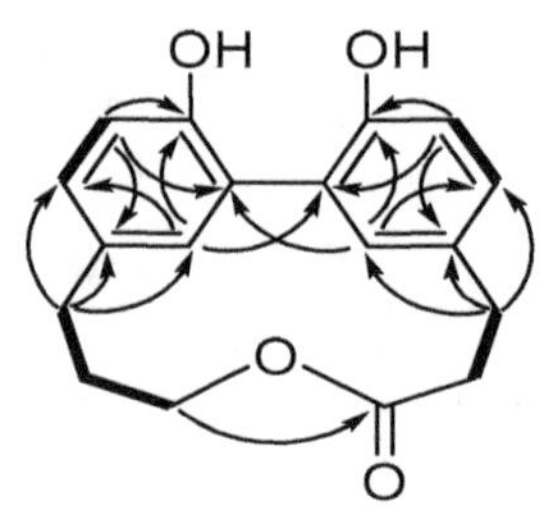

Figure 2. COSY (bold bond) and selected HMBC (arrow) correlations of **1**.

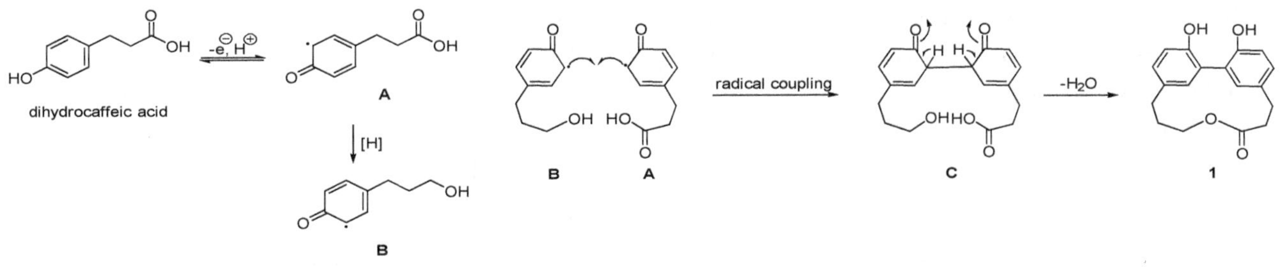

Figure 3. Plausible biosynthesis pathway of racelactone A (**1**).

Circulating endothelial progenitor cells (EPCs) have been reported to promote tumor angiogenesis and metastasis [24,25]. Tumors can secrete a variety of angiogenic factors to induce the recruitment of EPCs from bone marrow to the tumor site. Recruited EPCs enter the circulation system from their niche in bone marrow and extravasate with the chemotactic stimuli. After reaching the tumor site, EPCs differentiate into the structural part of the tumor vasculature, which contributes to tumor progression. Furthermore, EPCs have the ability to release pro-inflammatory cytokines that facilitate the growth and metastatic spread of tumors. Compelling evidence suggests that selective targeting of EPCs represents a novel therapeutic strategy for cancer treatment [26]. The differentiation and formation of capillary vessels is the most critical process during EPCs angiogenesis. Therefore, we performed tube formation assay to evaluate the anti-angiogenic activity of racelactone A in EPCs. As shown in Figure 4, the capillary tube-like structure was suppressed by racelactone A in a concentration-dependent manner. Sorafenib, a well-known angiogenesis inhibitor, was used as the positive control. To confirm this anti-angiogenic effect was not caused by the potential cytotoxicity of racelactone A, the release of lactate dehydrogenase (LDH) was measured in racelactone A-treated EPCs. We found that no statistical difference was observed between the control EPCs and EPCs treated with racelactone A. Collectively, these results reveal that the anti-angiogenic effect of racelactone A is not due to the cytotoxic action in human EPCs.

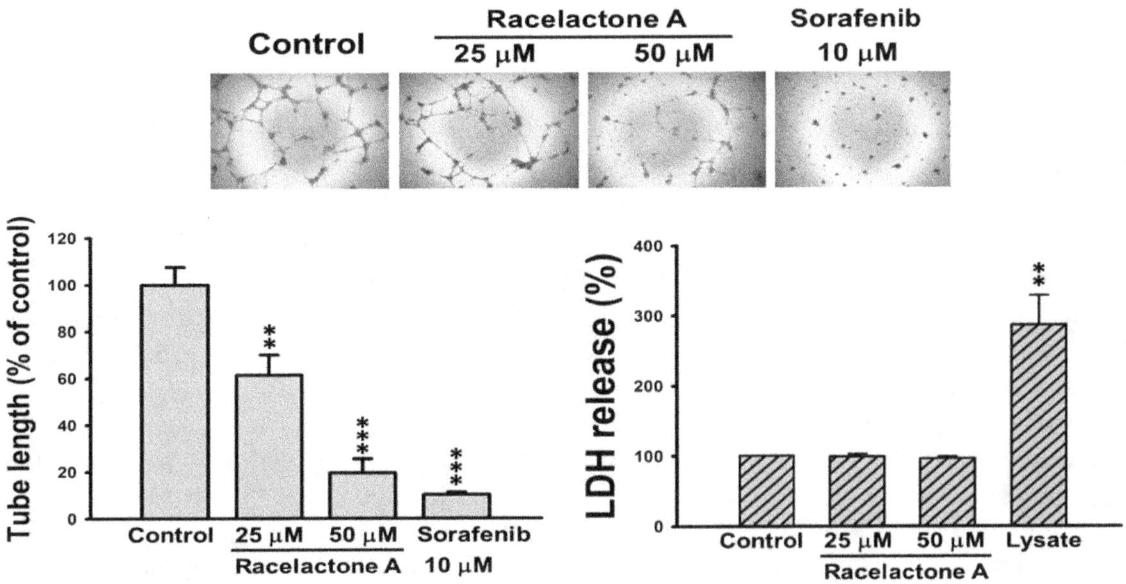

Figure 4. Effect of racelactone A (**1**) on tube formation and cytotoxicity of human endothelial progenitor cells (EPCs). EPCs were with the indicated concentrations of racelactone A and sorafenib for 24 h. The capillary-like structure formation and lactate dehydrogenase (LDH) release were determined by tube formation and cytotoxicity assay, respectively. Representative images of EPCs' tube formation were shown (phase contrast, 40×). Data represent the mean ± SEM of five independent experiments. ** $p < 0.01$, *** $p < 0.001$ compared with the control group.

All compounds were subjected to anti-inflammatory assays on superoxide anion generation and elastase release in fMLF/CB-induced human neutrophils inhibitory effects. Fortunately, the new compound **1** selectively displayed significant inhibitory activity on superoxide anion generation (IC_{50} = 4.95 ± 0.89 μM). The known compounds **4** and **5** also showed strong activity (Table 2).

Table 2. Inhibitory effects of isolates on superoxide anion generation and elastase release in fMLF/CB-induced human neutrophils.

Compound	Percentage of IC_{50} (μM) [a]			
	Superoxide Anion		Elastase Release	
1	4.95 ± 0.89	**	>10	
4	1.95 ± 0.40	***	>10	
5	2.57 ± 0.23	***	>10	
genistein [b]	1.54 ± 0.37	***	17.47 ± 2.80	***

Percentage of inhibition (Inh %) at 10 μM concentration. Results are presented as mean ± SEM (n = 3~5). ** $p < 0.01$, *** $p < 0.001$ compared with the control. [a] Concentration necessary for 50% inhibition (IC_{50}). [b] positive control.

3. Materials and Methods

3.1. General Experimental Procedures

Optical rotation was measured on a JASCO P-1020 digital polarimeter (Tokyo, Japan). UV data were recorded on a JASCO V-530 UV/VIS Spectrophotometer (Tokyo, Japan). High-resolution ESIMS data were obtained on a Bruker APEX II spectrometer (Billerica, MA, USA)). The IR spectrum was measured on a Perkin Elmer system 2000 FT-IR spectrophotometer (Waltham, MA, USA). The NMR spectra were obtained by JEOL JNM-ECS 400 MHz NMR (Akishima, Japan). Merck (Darmstadt, Germany) silica gel 60 and GE Healthcare (Chicago, IL, USA) Sephadex LH-20 were used for column chromatography. The instrumentation for HPLC was composed of a Shimadzu LC-10AD pump (Kyoto, Japan) and a Shimadzu SPD-M10A PDA detector.

3.2. Material

Specimens of *Lumnitzera racemosa* were collected in south Taiwan, in August 2015. The research samples were identified by Yuan-Bin Cheng. A voucher specimen (no. KMU-LR01) was deposited in the Graduate Institute of Natural Products, College of Pharmacy, Kaohsiung Medical University.

3.3. Extraction and Isolation

The air-dry twigs and leaves (15.0 kg) of *L. racemosa* were ground and extracted thrice with MeOH (40 L) at room temperature. The solvent was concentrated under reducing pressure to yield crude extracts. The MeOH crude extracts were partitioned between H_2O/EtOAc (1:1) to afford two portions. The EtOAc part was partitioned with *n*-hexane and 75% MeOH in water (1:1). The 75% $MeOH_{(aq)}$ layer (88.5 g) was subjected to a silica gel column stepwise eluted with *n*-hexane/EtOAc to yield botulin (221.1 mg), 3,4,3′-Tri-*O*-methyl ellagic acid (3330.0 mg), methyl gallate (4730.0 mg), myricitrin (5599.5 mg), and six fractions (A−J). Fraction C (830 mg) was isolated by silica gel column to give stigmasterol (63.4 mg). Fraction E (2.4 g) was chromatographed over a silica gel column to afford six subfractions (E.1−E.6). Subfraction E.4 (196.9 mg) was further separated by an LH-20 column, eluted with 100% MeOH to yield kaempferol (712.8 mg). Racelactone A (111.0 mg) and isoguaiacin (83.7 mg) were obtained from subfraction D.1 (144.7 mg) by LH-20 column, eluted with 100% MeOH and Phenyl-hexyl column (Luna phenyl-hexyl, 100 Å, 250 × 10 mm, Phenomenex®) stepwise from 70% to 100% $MeOH_{(aq)}$.

Racelactone A (1): Light yellow amorphous powder; $[\alpha]^{26}_{D}$ -0.6 (*c* 0.05, MeOH); UV (MeOH) λ_{max} (log ε) 299 (2.85), 252 (2.95), 215 (3.34) nm; IR (neat) υ_{max}: 3364, 1709, 1503, 1411 cm^{-1}; ^1H NMR and ^{13}C NMR data, see Table 1; HRESIMS *m/z* 321.10955 $[M + Na]^+$ (calcd for $C_{18}H_{18}O_4Na^+$: 321.10973).

3.4. Preparation of Human EPCs

The ethical approval for the collection of human EPCs was granted by the Institutional Review Board of Mackay Medical College, New Taipei City, Taiwan (P1000002). Prior to collecting the peripheral blood from healthy donors, informed consent was acquired. After density centrifugation Ficoll-Paque plus (Amersham Biosciences, Uppala, Sweden), peripheral blood mononuclear cells (PBMCs) were isolated from the fractionated blood components. CD34-positive progenitor cells were isolated from PMBCs with CD34 MicroBead kit and MACS Cell Separation System (Miltenyi Biotec, Bergisch Gladbach, Germany). Further isolation and preservation of CD34-positive EPCs were performed as described previously [27,28]. In the present study, all experiments were carried out on EPCs between passages 10 and 18. EPCs were cultured with 1% gelatin-coated plasticware and MV2 complete medium (PromoCell, Heidelberg, Germany) with 20% defined fetal bovine serum (FBS) (HyClone, Logan, UT, USA) in humidified incubator containing 5% CO_2 at 37 °C.

3.5. Tube Formation Assay

The capillary tube formation assay was carried out on Matrigel-coated 96-well plates. EPCs were seeded with the density of 1.25×10^4 cells per well and incubated in an MV2 complete medium with 2% FBS and the indicated concentration of tested compounds for 24 h at 37 °C. Quantifications of EPCs differentiation and capillary-like tube formation were done with photomicrographs taken by an inverted phase contrast microscope. The long axis of each tube was measured with Image J software in 3 randomly chosen fields per well.

3.6. Cytotoxicity Assay

5×10^3 of EPCs per well were seeded onto 96-well plates and incubated with an MV2 complete medium containing 2% FBS in the presence of vehicle (DMSO) or racelactone A. The quantification of LDH release in the medium was done with a cytotoxicity assay kit (Promega, Madison, WI, USA).

3.7. Superoxide Anion and Elastase Release Assays

The assay on superoxide anion generation and elastase release in response to fMLF stimulation of neutrophils were assayed by the same method as those of the reference published by co-author Professor Tsong-Long Hwang [29].

4. Conclusions

In summary, eight compounds, including one unusual macrolactone neolignan, were isolated and identified during a phytochemical investigation of the Taiwanese mangrove, *L. racemosa*. The new compound shows promising activities to anti-angiogenic and anti-inflammatory effects. Our findings suggest that racelactone A (**1**) may serve as a lead compound worthy of further development against angiogenesis-related diseases or inflammation-facilitated disorders, especially for the treatment of cancer.

Supplementary Materials:
Figure S1: HRESIMS of racelactone A (**1**). Figure S2: IR spectrum of racelactone A (**1**). Figure S3: ^{1}H NMR Spectrum of racelactone A (**1**) in acetone-d_6. Figure S4: ^{13}C NMR Spectrum of racelactone A (**1**) in acetone-d_6. Figure S5: UV spectrum of racelactone A (**1**). Figure S6: COSY Spectrum of racelactone A (**1**) in acetone-d_6. Figure S7: HMBC Spectrum of racelactone A (**1**) in acetone-d_6.

Author Contributions: S.-Y.Y., S.-W.W., B.-L.W., F.-R.C., and Y.-B.C. contributed to manuscript preparation; Y.-B.C. designed the whole experiment; S.-W.W., T.-L.H., and C.-J.S. analyzed the data and performed data acquisition.

Acknowledgments: We appreciated the Ministry of Science and Technology, Taiwan (MOST 105-2628-B-037-001-MY3 and MOST 106-2320-B-037-008-MY2 award to F.-R. Chang; MOST106-2320-B-037-016 and MOST 107-2628-B-037-001 award to Y.-B. Cheng).

References

1. Parida, A.L.; Jha, B. Salt tolerance mechanisms in mangroves: A review. *Trees* **2010**, *24*, 199–217. [CrossRef]
2. Chen, J. *Flora of China*; Missouri Botanical Garden: St. Louis, MO, USA; Harvard University Herbaria: Cambridge, MA, USA, 2007; Volume 13, p. 310.
3. Tomlinson, P.B. *The Botany of Mangroves*; Cambridge University Press: Cambridge, UK, 2016; p. 236, ISBN 9781107080676.
4. Chong, K.Y.; Tan, H.T.W.; Corlett, R.T. *A Checklist of the Total Vascular Plant Flora of Singapore Native, Naturalized and Cultivated Species*; National University of Singapore: Singpore, 2009; p. 273.
5. Anjaneyulu, A.S.R.; Murthy, Y.L.N.; Rao, V.L.; Sreedhar, K. A new aromatic ester from the mangrove plant *Lumnitzera racemosa* willd$^+$. *ARKIVOC* **2003**, *3*, 25–30. [CrossRef]
6. Lin, T.C.; Hsu, F.L.; Cheng, J.T. Antihypertensive activity of corilagin and chebulinic acid, tannins from *Lumnitzera racemosa*. *J. Nat. Prod.* **1993**, *56*, 629–632. [CrossRef]
7. D'Souza, L.; Wahidulla, S.; Devi, P. Antibacterial phenolics from the mangrove *Lumnitzera racemosa*. *Indian J. Mar. Sci.* **2010**, *39*, 294–298.
8. Ravikumar, S.; Gnanadesigan, M. Hepatoprotective and antioxidant activity of a mangrove plant *Lumnitzera racemosa*. *Asian Pac. J. Trop. Biomed.* **2011**, *1*, 348–352. [CrossRef]
9. Thao, N.P.; Luyen, B.T.T.; Diep, C.N.; Tai, B.H.; Kim, E.J.; Kang, H.K.; Lee, S.H.; Jang, H.D.; Cuong, N.T.; Thanh, N.V.; et al. In vitro evaluation of the antioxidant and cytotoxic activities of constituents of the mangrove *Lumnitzera racemosa* Willd. *Arch. Pharm. Res.* **2015**, *38*, 446–455. [CrossRef] [PubMed]
10. Clevers, H. At the crossroads of inflammation and cancer. *Cell* **2004**, *118*, 671–674. [CrossRef] [PubMed]
11. Chung, A.S.; Lee, J.; Ferrara, N. Targeting the tumour vasculature: Insights from physiological angiogenesis. *Nat. Rev. Cancer* **2010**, *10*, 505–514. [CrossRef] [PubMed]
12. Weis, S.M.; Cheresh, D.A. Tumor angiogenesis: Molecular pathways and therapeutic targets. *Nat. Med.* **2011**, *17*, 1359–1370. [CrossRef] [PubMed]
13. Zha, S.; Yegnasubramanian, V.; Nelson, W.G.; Isaacs, W.B.; Marzo, A.M.D. Cyclooxygenases in cancer: Progress and perspective. *Cancer Lett.* **2004**, *215*, 1–20. [CrossRef] [PubMed]
14. Liao, C.-R.; Kuo, Y.-H.; Ho, Y.-L.; Wang, C.-Y.; Yang, C.-S.; Lin, C.-W.; Chang, Y.-S. Studies on cytotoxic constituents from the leaves of *Elaeagnus oldhamii* Maxim. in non-small cell lung cancer A549 Cells. *Molecules* **2014**, *19*, 9515–9534. [CrossRef] [PubMed]
15. Schmidt, J.; Himmelreich, U.; Adam, G. Brassinosteroids, sterols and lup-20(29)-en-2α,3β,28-triol from *Rheum Rhabarbarum*. *Phytochemistry* **1995**, *40*, 527–531. [CrossRef]
16. Begum, S.S.; Tauseef, S.; Siddiqui, B.S.; Nizami, S.S.; Ghulam, H.; Ahmad, A. In vitro antibacterial and antifungal activity of flower buds (clove) of *Syzygium aromaticum*. *J. Chem. Soc. Pak.* **2014**, *36*, 723–728.
17. Madikizela, B.; Aderogba, M.A.; Finnie, J.F.; Staden, J.V. Isolation and characterization of antimicrobial compounds from *Terminalia phanerophlebia* Engl. & Diels leaf extracts. *J. Ethnopharmacol.* **2014**, *156*, 228–234. [CrossRef] [PubMed]
18. Saldanha, L.L.; Vilegas, W.; Dokkedal, A.L. Characterization of flavonoids and phenolic acids in *Myrcia bella* Cambess. using FIA-ESI-IT-MS^n and HPLC-PAD-ESI-IT-MS combined with NMR. *Molecules* **2013**, *18*, 8402–8416. [CrossRef] [PubMed]
19. Forgo, P.; Kövér, K.E. Gradient enhanced selective experiments in the ^{1}H NMR chemical shift assignment of the skeleton and side-chain resonances of stigmasterol, a phytosterol derivative. *Steroids* **2004**, *69*, 43–50. [CrossRef] [PubMed]
20. Moraes, L.S.; Donza, M.R.H.; Rodrigues, A.P.D.; Silva, B.J.M.; Brasil, A.S.B.; Zoghbi, M.G.B.; Andrade, E.H.A.; Guilhon, G.M.S.P.; Silva, E.O. Leishmanicidal activity of (+)-phyllanthidine and the phytochemical profile of *Margaritaria nobilis* (Phyllanthaceae). *Molecules* **2015**, *20*, 22157–22169. [CrossRef] [PubMed]
21. Wang, B.-G.; Hong, X.; Li, L.; Zhou, J.; Hao, Z.-J. Chemical constituents of two Chinese Magnoliaceae plants, *Tsoongiodendron odorum* and *Manglietiastrum sinicum*, and their inhibition of platelet aggregation. *Planta Med.* **2000** *66*, 511–515. [CrossRef] [PubMed]

22. Vongvanich, N.; Kittakoop, P.; Charoenchai, P.; Intamas, S.; Danwisetkanjana, K.; Thebtaranonth, Y. Combretastatins D-3 and D-4, new macrocyclic lactones from *Getonia floribunda*. *Planta Med.* **2005**, *71* 191–193. [CrossRef] [PubMed]
23. Pettit, G.R.; Quistorf, P.D.; Fry, J.A.; Herald, D.L.; Hamel, E.; Chapuis, J.-C. Antineoplastic agents. 565. synthesis of combretastatin D-2 phosphate and dihydro-combretastatin D-2[1]. *J. Nat. Prod.* **2009**, *72*, 876–883. [CrossRef] [PubMed]
24. Carmeliet, P. Angiogenesis in life, disease and medicine. *Nature* **2005**, *438*, 932–936. [CrossRef] [PubMed]
25. Urbich, C.; Dimmeler, S. Endothelial progenitor cells: Characterization and role in vascular biology. *Circ. Res.* **2004**, *95*, 343–353. [CrossRef] [PubMed]
26. Moschetta, M.; Mishima, Y.; Sahin, I.; Manier, S.; Glavey, S.; Vacca, A.; Roccaro, A.M.; Ghobrial, I.M. Role of endothelial progenitor cells in cancer progression. *BBA-Rev. Cancer* **2014**, *1846*, 26–39. [CrossRef] [PubMed
27. Chung, C.-H.; Chang, C.-H.; Chen, S.-S.; Wang, H.-H.; Yen, J.-Y.; Hsiao, C.-J.; Wu, N.-L.; Chen, Y.-L.; Huang, T.-F.; Wang, P.-C.; et al. Butein inhibits angiogenesis of human endothelial progenitor cells via the translation dependent signaling pathway. *Evid.-Based Complement. Altern. Med.* **2013**, *2013*, e943187. [CrossRef] [PubMed]
28. Lee, M.-S.; Wang, S.-W.; Wang, G.-J.; Pang, K.-L.; Lee, C.-K.; Kuo, Y.-H.; Cha, H.-J.; Lin, R.-K.; Lee, T.-H. Angiogenesis inhibitors and anti-inflammatory agents from *Phoma* sp. NTOU4195. *J. Nat. Prod.* **2016**, *79* 2983–2990. [CrossRef] [PubMed]
29. Yang, S.-C.; Chung, P.-J.; Ho, C.-M.; Kuo, C.-Y.; Hung, M.-F.; Huang, Y.-T.; Chang, W.-Y.; Chang, Y.-W.; Chan, K.-H.; Hwang, T.-L. Propofol inhibits superoxide production, elastase release, and chemotaxis in formyl peptide–activated human neutrophils by blocking formyl peptide receptor 1. *J. Immunol.* **2013**, *190* 6511–6519. [CrossRef] [PubMed]

21

A Review on Ethno-Medicinal and Pharmacological Activities of *Sphenocentrum jollyanum* Pierre

Olubukola Sinbad Olorunnisola, Olumide Samuel Fadahunsi * and Peter Adegbola

Department of Biochemistry, Faculty of Basic Medical Sciences, Ladoke Akintola University of Technology, Ogbomoso, PMB 4000, Oyo State, Nigeria; osolorunnisola@lautech.edu.ng (O.S.O.); useablevesselofgod@gmail.com (P.A.)

* Correspondence: fadahunsiolumide5@gmail.com

Academic Editor: James D. Adams

Abstract: *Sphenocentrum jollyanum* Pierre is a member of a diverse family of plants known as Menispermaceae. They are famous for a plethora of important biological functions. *S. jollyanum* is a shrub native to the tropical forest zones of West Africa and thrives in deep shade. It is widely cultivated in Cameroun, Sierra Leone, Nigeria, Ghana, and Côte d'Ivoire. *S. jollyanum* is employed in folk medicine as a cure for wounds, fever, coughs, high blood pressure, breast tumor, constipation, and as an aphrodisiac. Phytochemical investigations revealed that the plant is a rich source of secondary metabolites such as annin, alkaloids, saponins, and flavonoids. Pharmacological activities include anti-diabetic, anti-inflammatory, anti-bacterial, anti-viral, anti-malarial, angiogenic, and anxiogenic. Thus, this present review summarizes the phytochemical and nutritional constituents and important biological studies on various crude extracts, fractions, and isolated principles of all morphological organs of *S. jollyanum*.

Keywords: ethno-medicinal uses; pharmacological activities; phytochemical profile; *Sphenocentrum jollyanum* Pierre

---

1. Introduction

Globally, the employment of medicinal plants as a substitute for orthodox drugs in the management of various diseases has been increasing due to the unavailability of modern health facilities, relative availability of medicinal herbs, poverty, and recent revelations that they possess active compounds that may be responsible for different biological and pharmacological actions [1]. According to Newman and Cragg [2], natural materials are the source of about two -third of all drugs developed in the past three decades. According to a World Health Organization (WHO) report, it is estimated that close to 80% of the people living in the third world nations of the world depend on traditional and complementary medicines for their basic health care [3]. Thus, this review is aimed at elucidating the traditional and biological importance of *Sphenocentrum jollyanum*.

S. jollyanum Pierre is a member of the plant family Menispermaceae (Table 1). These are diverse group of plants which are popular for important biological activities. *S. jollyanum* is a shrub native to the tropical forest zones of West Africa and is widely distributed in Sierra Leone, Nigeria, Ghana, Ivory Coast, and Cameroun [4]. It is extensively employed in folkloric medicine in the management of various ailments. *S. jollyanum* is commonly known locally as *"Aduro kokoo"* (red medicine), *"Okramankote"* (dog's penis), and *"Krakoo"* among the Akan and Asante tribes of Ghana. In South-Western Nigeria, the plant is traditionally known as Akerejupon or Ajo, Oban abe in Republic of Benin, and Ouse-abe in Côte d'Ivoire [5].

2. Plant Description

Sphenocentrum jollyanum (Figure 1) is a perennial under growth of dense forest, which thrives in deep shade, from sea-level up to 400 m altitude. It is mostly found in regions withmean annual rainfall of 1800 mm or more, mean minimum temperature of 20 °C, and mean maximum of 29 °C. It grows to an average height of about 1.5 m, with few scanty branches. *S. jollyanum* leaves are wedge-shaped, about 5–12 cm wide, smooth onboth sides, and can grow up to about 20 cm long with a small-arrowed apex [6,7]. The fruit (Figure 2) occurs as clusters, ovoid-ellipsoid, with a single large oval-shaped seed. It is fleshy, edible, and bright yellow or orange when ripe [8,9]. The roots are visibly bright yellow and are characterized by a sour acidic taste that causes things eaten thereafter to taste sweet [8].

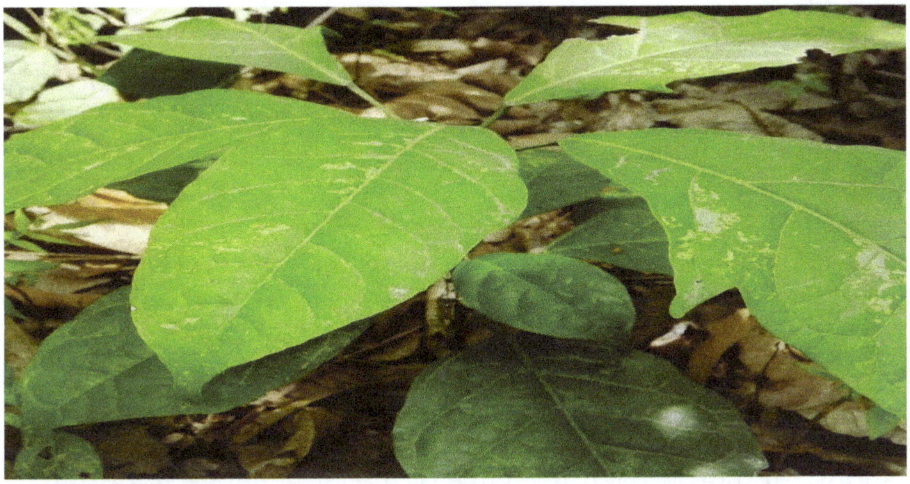

Figure 1. *Sphenocentrum jollyanum* in its natural habitat.

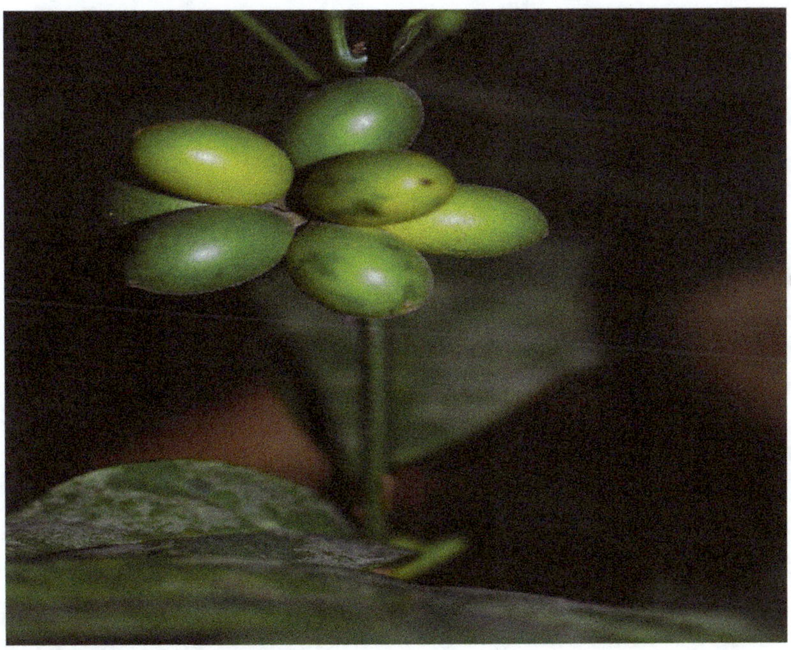

Figure 2. *Sphenocentrum jollyanum* fruits.

Table 1. Taxonomical classification of *Sphenocentrum jollyanum* [5].

Kingdom	Plantae
Division	Magnoliophyta (Cronquist)
Subdivision	Magnoliophytina (Frohne and Jensen)
Class	Ranunculopsida (Brongn)
Subclass	Ranunculidae (Takht)
Suborder	Ranunculanae (Takht)
Order	Menispermales (Bromhead)
Family	Menispermaceae (Juss.)
Genus	Sphenocentrum (Pierre)
Species	Jollyanum

3. Ethno-Medicinal Uses

Different parts of *S. jollyanum* are traditionally employed in folkloric medicine. In Ghana, the root of the plant is widely used by the men as an aphrodisiac. It is steeped in alcohol for few days to allow extraction of some constituents, which is thereafter drank as bitters to strengthen penile erection, and this effect is known to be long-lasting [10,11].

It has been documented in several literature studies that the root is employed for its effectiveness in stimulating the central nervous system (CNS), the management of mental and inflammatory disorders, pain and depression [12]. The dried, powdered root is used in combination with some anti-malarial plant as panacea for fever and muscular pains. Aerial parts of the plant (leafy twigs and fruits) are vastly employed in the treatment of chronic wounds, feverish conditions, and coughs when combined with *Piper guineense* (West African pepper) and lime juice [8,9].

In Nigeria, the roots are chewed in traditional medicine to relieve constipation, promote appetite, and increase digestion. All morphological organs of *S. jollyanum* are important ingredients in the management of sickle cell disease (SCD) [8]. Traditional healers in Ghana and Côte d'Ivoire have also reported the roots to possess medicinal properties against high blood pressure, breast tumor, irregular menstrual cycle, and diabetes mellitus [7,13–16]. Furthermore, the powdered roots are eaten in combination with *Aframomum melegueta* (alligator pepper) seeds, salt, and *Elaeis guineensis* (African oil palm) in the management of abdominal discomfort [17]. The charred fruits are used in the treatment of fibroids and as edible anti-fatigue snack [9,18]. It is also reported that the leaves decoctions are used in expelling intestinal parasites and to stop spitting of blood [15].

4. Phytochemical and Proximate Analysis

The majority of the reported biological and pharmacological activity of *S. jollyanum* extracts (Table 2) has been attributed to their bioactive principles and constituent phytochemicals. A detailed phytochemical analysis of the ethanol root extract of *S. jollyanum* revealed that it contains compounds such as terpenoids and flavonoids, while alkaloids are reported to be the most dominant chemical constituents [19]. Phytochemical investigation by Nia et al. [4] revealed the presence of tannins, saponins, terpenes, and alkaloids in the different fractions of methanol extracts of the stem bark. The chloroform fraction was found to be the most active of all fractions, and it tested positive to the test of flavonoids and alkaloids. In the submission of Aboabaand Ekundayo [20], detailed analysis of the essential oil of *S. jollyanum* root using gas chromatography-mass spectrometry analysis (GC-MS) revealed a total of 19 compounds (α-pinene, α-ylangene, guaia-6,9-diene-4α-ol, globulol, guaiene-11-ol, α-eudesmol, isocaryophyllene, aromadendrene, selina-4(15),6-dien *E*-β-isocaryophyllene, γ-terpinene, γ-humulene, epi-zonarene, δ-amorphene, 1,8-cineol,camphene, B-pinene, p-cymene, d3-carene, Figure 3) consisting of monoterpenoids (33.5%) and sesquiterpenoids (56.3%), while (10.2%) of the total oil constituents remain unidentified. Phytochemistry of the seed extracts by Ibironke et al. [21] revealed the bio-availability of flavonoids, alkaloids, and saponins, while phylobatannin and free anthraquinone were not present. Proximate analysis of the seed extract showed the crude fat, moisture, crude protein, carbohydrate, ash, and fiber contents to be 9.65%, 16.70% 48.09%, 16.79%, 3.26%, and 5.51%, respectively, while the energy value was 1460 kcal/100 kg. This suggests that the fruits are an important source of nutrients and energy [21]. Interestingly, the flame photometric and atomic absorption spectrophotometric (AAS) analysis of the mineral element composition of the seeds showed an appreciable amount of macro and micro elements that are required for the growth in humans and animals [21]. Minerals such as calcium (8.92 mg/L), magnesium (0.44 mg/L), potassium (4.26 mg/L), iron (0.22 mg/L), manganese (0.19 mg/L), zinc (1.38 mg/L), and sodium (4.70 mg/L) were present in appreciable quantity. This indicates the importance of the plant in building strong bones, the production of energy, and carrying out some metabolic reactions in the body [21]. Previous scholarly articles documented the isolation of three furanoditerpenes (columbin, isocolumbine, and fibeucin) (Figure 4) and alkaloids (protoberberine) from the fruit [22].

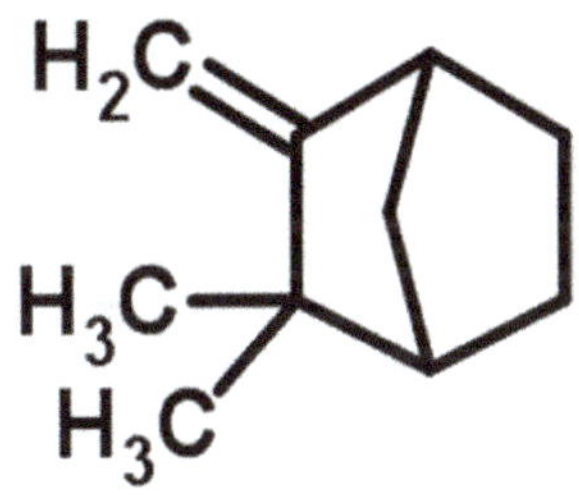

Camphene

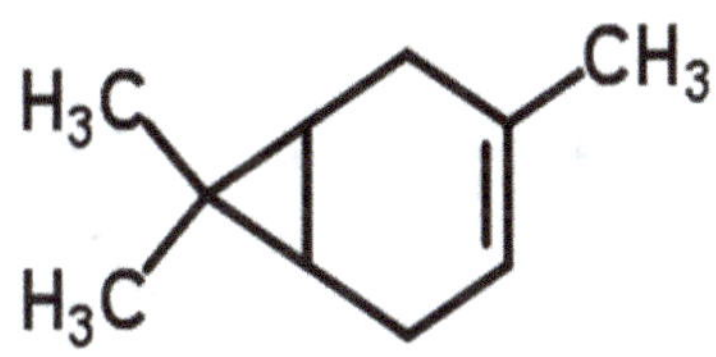

d3-Carene

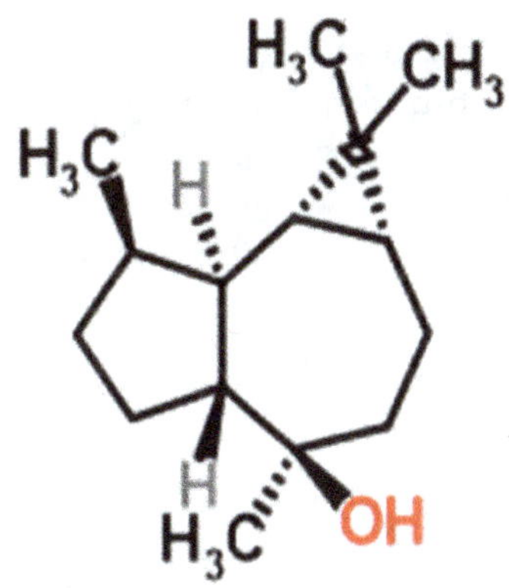

Globulol

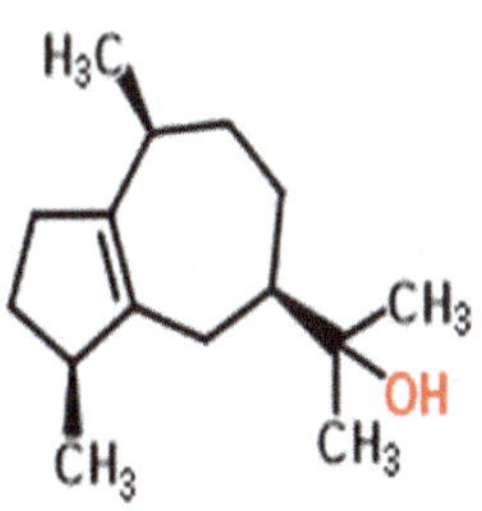

Guaiene-11-ol

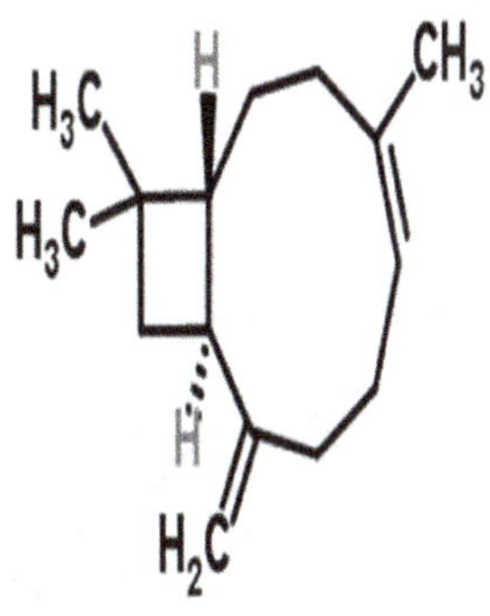

Isocaryophyllene

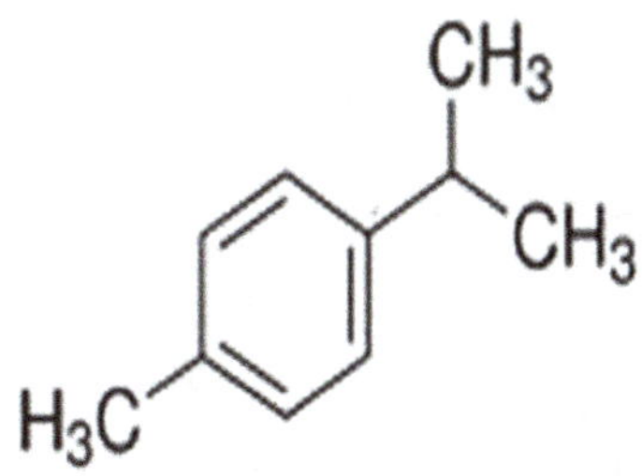

p-Cymene

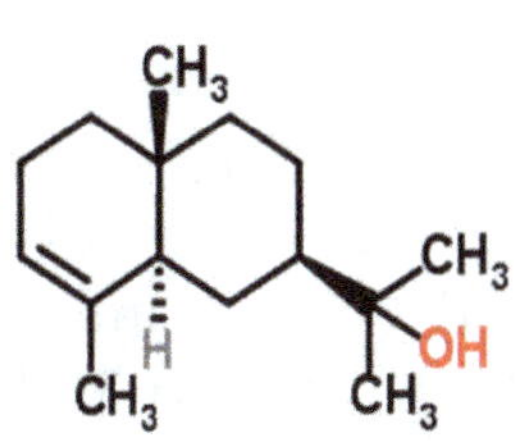

α-Eudesmol

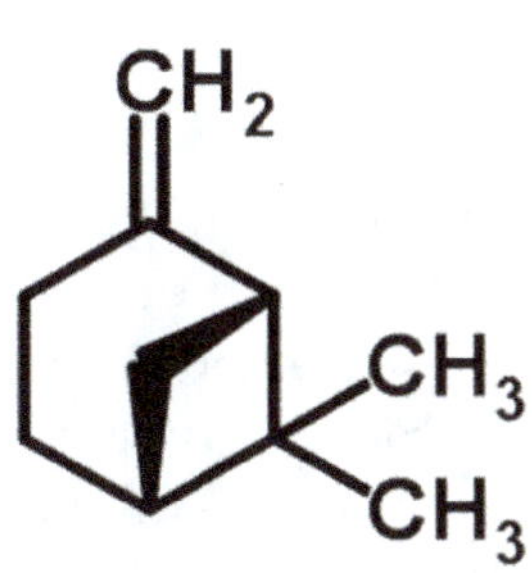

β-Pinene

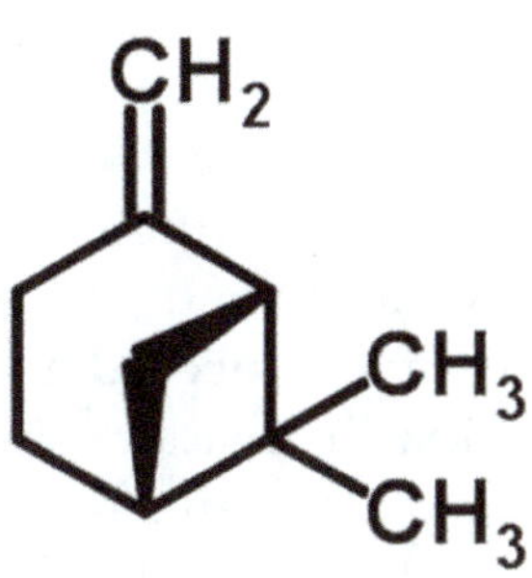

γ-Terpinene

Figure 3. Some identified compounds from the root oil of *S. jollyanum.*

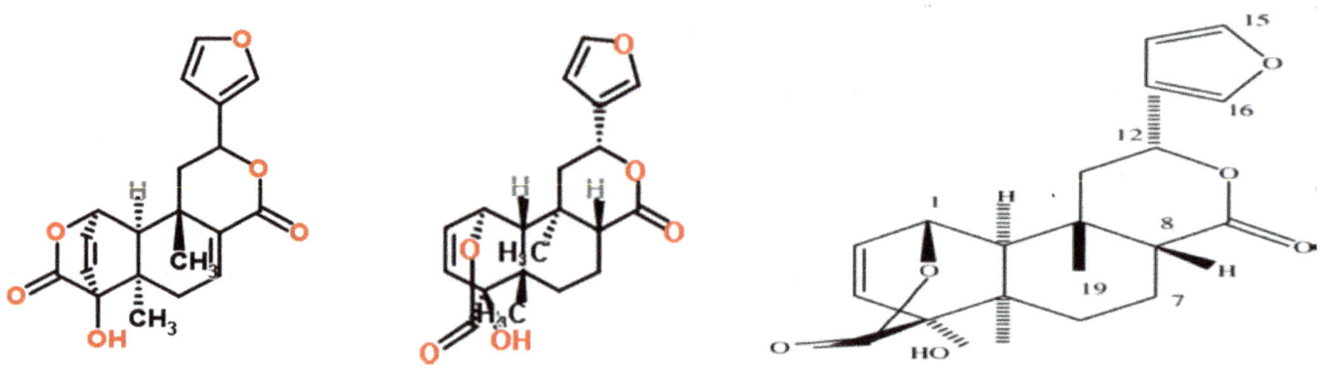

(a) (b) (c)

Figure 4. Isolated compounds from fruits of *S. jollyanum*. Structure of isolated fibleucin (**a**) and isocolumbin (**b**) [22], Structure of isolated columbine (**c**) [22].

Table 2. Summary of pharmacological activities *of S. jollyanum.*

Pharmacological Activities	Part Used	Extracts	References
Angiogenic	Stem bark,	Methanol, Chloroform	[4]
Anti-Oxidant	Stem bark, Root, Leaf	Methanol, Hexane, Chloroform, Ethanol, Butanol, Aqueous	[4,23,24]
Anti-Bacteria	Root	Essential oil, Ethanol	[20,25]
Haematological	Leaf , Root	Methanol	[22,23,26]
Anti-Inflammatory	Fruit, Root,	Methanol, Ethanol, Aqueous	[22,27,28]
Anti-Diabetic	Root, Stem, Fruit, Leaf	Aqueous, Ethanol, Methanol	[29–32]
Hypolipidemic	Root	Ethanol	[32]
Hepatoprotective,Toxicological	Stem bark, Leaf, Root,	Methanol, Ethanol, Essential oil	[23,26,33]
Anti-Malaria	Leaf, Root	Methanol	[24,34]
Weight Loss Prevention	Leaf , Root, Seed	Ethanol, Essential oil	[24,26,33,35]
Anti-Allergy	Fruit	Ethanol	[36]
Anti-viral	Stem, Root, Leaf	Hexane, Methanol	[37,38]
Anti-depressant	Root	Ethanol	[39]
Anxiogenic	Root	Ethanol	[40,41]
Analgesic, Antipyretic	Leaf	Methanol	[42]
Sexual, Reproductive	Root	Ethanol, Methanol	[43,44]

5. Pharmacological and Biological Activities

5.1. Anti-Diabetic Activity

Investigation of the different extracts of morphological organs of *S. jollyanum* indicated its blood glucose lowering potential. The effect of petroleum ether seed extract on oral glucose tolerant test (OGTT) and alloxan-induced diabetic rabbits revealed that 1 g/kg of the extract administered 30 min before glucose load considerably reduced blood glycemic level by 20% relative to the untreated group. The study also reported the anti-hyperglycemic activity of the extract on alloxan-induced diabetic rabbits [29]. In another study, a 9-day treatment regimen revealed that the extract caused a significant ($p < 0.05$) dose-dependent decrease in the plasma glucose level from the 3rd to the 9th day. The three-dosage group showed a peak percentage decrease of 12.3%, 29.2%, and 32.7%, which compared favorably with glinbenclamide at 51.9%. Furthermore, the aqueous root extract demonstrated a dose-dependent reduction in blood glycemic level of alloxan-induced diabetic rabbits [30]. Ethanol extracts of *S. jollyanum* leaf at concentrations of 50, 100, 200 mg/kg significantly

($p < 0.05$) lowered the blood glycemic index of alloxan-induced diabetic rabbits in a dose-dependent manner, with plasma glucose level of 200.2 mg/100 mL (42.8%) at 200 mg/kg [31]. Alese et al. [32] reported that the methanol root extract demonstrated hypoglycemic effects on streptozotocin-induced diabetic Wistar rats. Oral dosage of 200 mg/kg extracts for 2 weeks caused a significant decrease in blood glucose to 6.62 mmol/L relatively to the uncontrolled group with blood glucose level of 16.3 mmol/L. The results of these studies validate the traditional claim of the blood glucose lowering activity of the plant, and thus may serve as a potential source of potent anti-diabetic compounds.

5.2. Antioxidant Activity

Studies on superoxide radical and hydrogen peroxide scavenging ability of the methanolic stem extract revealed a dose-dependent anti-oxidant activity with IC_{50} value of 13.11 μg/mL and 30.04 μg/mL when compared to ascorbic acid 15.34 μg/mL and 35.44 μg/mL respectively [23]. In a separate study, Olorunnisola and Afolayan[24] reported that the plant significantly ($p < 0.05$) ameliorated the oxidative stress related with *P. berghei* infection in mice, which was evident in the reduced levels of total protein and liver MDA (malondialdehyde). In addition, there was increased activity of serum and liver catalase (CAT), superoxide dismutase (SOD) and glutathione (GSH) levels. Alternatively, Nia et al. [4] point to the anti-oxidant activity of extracts of all morphological organs on 2,2-diphenyl-1-picrylhydrazyl hydrate (DPPH). The stem bark was observed to be the most active with IC_{50} of 1.80 μg/mL, when compared with ascorbic acid 0.80 μg/mL. The leaf had the weakest activity, IC_{50} of 4.35 μg/mL, while IC_{50} of the root bark was 3.50 μg/mL. Fractions of the stem bark were screened, and the chloroform fraction exhibited the most potent activity with an IC_{50} of 1.54 μg/mL. The findings emanating from these studies indicate the potential of *S. jollyanum* as an anti-oxidant (Table 2), and thus could be explored in the development of new pharmaceuticals.

5.3. Anti-Inflammatory

Studies on the in vivo anti-inflammatory activity of *S. jollyanum* crude extracts and isolated compounds were investigated in healthy adult rats inoculated with carrageenan [22]. It was reported that the methanol fruit extract at a concentration of 200 mg/kg showed the stronger inhibition (79.58%) of oedema formation on hind paws, while root extract demonstrated a 53.75% inhibition. The same study also revealed that three furanoditerpenes (namely columbin, isocolumbine, and fibleucin) isolated from the methanolic fruit extract demonstrated considerable anti-inflammatory potentials. Columbin and flavonoids-rich fraction at 200 mg/kg exhibited 67.08% and 76.25% anti-inflammatory activities that were in a comparable range with acetylsalicylic acid. Olorunnisola et al. [27,28] evaluated the in vitro inflammatory potential and possible modes of action of crude extracts and secondary metabolites of *S. jollyanum* organs. The results also provided some vindication for the traditional usage of *S. jollyanum* in managing inflammatory-related diseases in the West African sub-region.

5.4. Anti-Allergy Activities

The anti-allergic study was performed on milk-induced leukocytosis and oesinophilia in mice. The ethanolic fruit extracts demonstrated a considerable dose-dependent decrease in the absolute eosinophil and lymphocyte counts. The results suggested the anti-allergy property of the fruit extract, and the mode of activity may involve multiple mechanisms due to phytochemical interactions [36].

5.5. Anti-Malarial Activities

Anti-malarial studies on the leaf and root extracts of *S. jollyanum* were reported by Olorunnisola in [24,34] respectively. The in vivo anti-plasmodial activity of methanol extracts was evaluated using chloroquine-resistant *Plasmodium berghei* NK67 strain-inoculated Swiss albino mice. The leaf and root extracts demonstrated statistically significant concentration-dependent activities of (74.4%) and (54.1%), respectively. However, the standard drug arthemether-lumefartrin had a better antimalaria activity (81.4%). Further research is necessary to identify and characterize the active components and determine the possible mode of activity.

5.6. Anti-Bacterial Activities

Aboaba and Ekundayo [20] studied the essential oil composition of the root extract of *S. jollyanum* against *Bacillus subtilis*, *Salmonellatyphi*, *Staphylococcus aureus*, *Bacillus cereus*, *Proteus mirabilis*, and *Pseudomonas aeruginosa*. It was observed that the essential oil was effective against *Bacillus subtilis* and *Pseudomonas aeruginosa* strains with inhibition zones of 10 mm and 9.0 mm, respectively, at 1000 μg/mL. In a separate study, Koleosho et al. [25] showed the plant extract to be a potent inhibitor of *S. typhi*. The moderate antimicrobial activity displayed supports the traditional use of the root as a laxative which aids proper bowel movements and digestion.

5.7. Anti-Viral Activities

Moody et al. [37,38] revealed that the methanol extracts of the different morphological parts were assessed for their antiviral activities on polio virus Types 1, 2, and 3. It was observed from the study that the leaf and root extracts were active against polio virus Type 2. Additionally, hexane and methanol extracts were investigated and reported for their mosaic virus inhibitory potentials in cowpea.

5.8. Haematological Activities

Methanol root and leaf extracts of *S. jollyanum* were investigated for possible hematopoietic activity in Wistar mice infected with chloroquine-resistant *Plasmodium berghei* NK67. Methanol extracts of leaf and root were administered orally for 7 days. The study revealed that there was a significant increase in the pack cell volume (PCV), mean corpuscular volume (MCV), mean corpuscular hemoglobin concentration (MCHC), and hemoglobin (Hb). There was also an observable elevation in red and white blood cell levels, with the exception of monocytes and neutrophils. The study is suggestive of the ability of the extract to stimulate hematopoietic stem cells [22,23,26].

5.9. Effect on Weight

The effect of leaf and root extracts on weight change was investigated in malaria and diabetic rat. It was observed that there was a significant ($p < 0.05$) increase in weight gain in Wistar mice treated with the extracts. Comparative analysis suggested that the extracts significantly prevented loss of weight in a concentration-dependent pattern in the extract-administered group when compared to the negative control [24,26,33,35]. Consequently, the physical status of the extract-treated animals was improved. This may be related to the ameliorative effect of the extracts to prevent the acute fluid loss, fat catabolism, and protein catabolism which are evident in weight loss.

5.10. Hepatoprotective and Toxicological Studies

Scientific examination of the hepatoprotective potential of stem bark extract revealed that the extract significantly ameliorated/prevented liver damage in carbon tetrachloride (CCl_4)-induced rats. The study showed that the extract considerably ($p < 0.05$) reversed the elevated aspartate aminotransferase (AST), alkaline phosphatase (ALP), alanine amino transferase (ALT), and total bilirubin, and decreased the level of total serum protein in a concentration-dependent pattern [23]. In the submission of Mbaka et al. [26,33], no mortality or morbidity was recorded in the 120-days administration of ethanol leaf extract during the toxicity studies. Detailed assessment also indicated that there was no obvious inflammation of the internal organs. In addition, there were no appreciable increases in serum AST and ALT in the extract-administered animals. This observation denotes that the extract poses no damaging effect on the liver. The result of the histological study on the liver tissue morphology confirmed that no toxic effects of the extract were visible. Furthermore, minimum cytotoxic dose (MCD50) of the methanol leaf extract was also investigated on Hep-2 (Human epithelia cell line) and it was found to range within 3.9×10^{-3} mg/mL [37]. The Ames microbial mutagenicity test of the root ethanol extract showed no statistically observable increase in the number of revertant colonies in the four strains of *S. typhimurium* TA_{97}, TA_{98}, TA_{100}, and TA_{102} at any concentration. This indicates that *S. jollyanum* has no ability to cause mutation in relation to the in vitro assay [19]. According to Aboaba and Ekundayo [20], the toxicity of the essential oil of *S. jollyanum* to brine shrimp lethality test showed a lethal concentration LC_{50} of 84.87 ppm. Therefore, the observed safety level of the plant extracts vindicates its age-long ethno-pharmacological usage.

5.11. Hypolipidemic Activity

Effect of the ethanol root extract on serum lipid profile was investigated on streptozotocin-induced diabetic albino rats. It was noticed that there was no observable difference in total cholesterol (TC) amount of the extract- and glinbenclamide-administered animals. Additionally, there was a significant ($p < 0.02$) difference in antiartherogenic index (AAI) and high-density lipoprotein level in extract-treated group (0.77 $\pm$ 0.02 mmol/L) when compared to untreated infected group (0.85 $\pm$ 0.02 mmol/L) [32].

5.12. Antidepressant Activity

The anti-depressant effect of the ethanol extract of the root was evaluated on mice using forced swimming and tail suspension examination. The plant extract (100–1000 mg/kg) increased the duration of mobility in both models in a concentration-dependent manner. However, it was observed that the standard drugs imipramine and fluoxetine were 20–50 times more potent than the extracts. This implied that the antidepressant activity of the extract might be as a result of its modifying activity on monoamine transport and metabolism [39].

5.13. Anxiogenic Activity

Anxiogenic activity was carried out by administration of 100–1000 mg/kg of the ethanol extract. The animals exhibited anxiety-like effects dose-dependently in a similar way to those induced by caffeine (10–100 mg/kg), and this was in contrast to the anxiolytic effect of diazepam (0.1–1 mg/kg) [40,41]. The result validates the conventional use of the plant for its stimulatory effect on the central nervous system and as mood enhancer.

5.14. Anti-Angiogenic Activity

Angiogenesis has been reported as a fundamental process in the transition of benign tumors to malignant ones, and therefore Nia et al. [4] evaluated the anti-angiogenic activities of the methanol extract of morphological organs using in vivo chick chorioallantoic membrane (CAM) angiogenesis assay. It was revealed that the stem bark had the most potent activity, with an IC_{50} value of 1.00 μg/mL. In addition, the chloroform fraction of the stem bark exhibited the strongest inhibitory IC_{50} (1.54 μg/mL) activity against the formation of new endothelial cells [4], thus validating the ethno-botanical usage of *S. jollyanum* as an important anti-tumor agent.

5.15. Antipyretic and Analgesic Activities

Muko et al. [42] disclosed that the petroleum ether and methanol extracts of *S. jollyanum* leaves possess significant in vitro analgesic and antipyretic activities.

5.16. Reproductive and Sexual Activity

Investigation on the potential of the plant extracts to affect sexual activities and hormonal levels in laboratory animals was carried out by Owiredu et al. [43]. It was observed that there was an increased urge by the male animals to mount on the female for the first time, increased duration of ejaculation, and shortened refractory period. Furthermore, a decrease in post-ejaculatory, climbing and intromission latency was observed in the extract-treated animals. These are relevant perceptions of sexual performance and satisfaction. In addition, testosterone level was increased by four-fold and about there was a one-third increment in follicle stimulating hormone (FSH) activity. However, there was a contradictory report by Raji et al. [44] that pointed to a considerable reduction in the total sperm count, fertilization ability of the sperm cells, movement and swimming (asthenozoospermia) abilities. There was also a considerable increase in superoxide dismutase activity in relation to the testes and degeneration of seminiferous tubules. However, it was suggested that *S. jollyanum* could produce deleterious effects on reproductive ability, which can be measured as a function of poor sperm quantity (epididymal sperm count), quality (sperm movement, viability, structure), and gradual impairment, loss of function of the tissues and cells of the testes.

6. Conclusions

The importance of *S. jollyanum* in the traditional medicinal system of Africa cannot be over-emphasized. The medicinal value of the plant is owed to it richness in alkaloids, tannins, saponins, flavonoids, and essential oils. These bioactive principles have been reported to be responsible for the various pharmacological efficacies reported in this review. Hence, all morphological organs of the plant stand an important chance as a major source of potent therapeutic compounds useful in the management of several human diseases.

Author Contributions: O.S.O. conceived the idea and outlined the content, O.S.F. and P.A. searched the internet and wrote the manuscript. All authors read and approved the final manuscript for submission.

References

1. Tiwari, A.K.; Mehta, R. Medicinal plants used by traditional healers in Jashpur district of Chhattisgarh India. *Life Sci. Leafl.* **2013**, *1*, 31–41.
2. Newman, D.J.; Cragg, G.M. Natural products as sources of new drugs over the 30 years from 1981 to 2010. *J. Nat. Prod.* **2012**, *75*, 311–335. [CrossRef] [PubMed]
3. Farnsworth, N.R.; Akerele, O.; Bingel, A. Medicinal plants in therapy. *Bull. World Health Organ.* **1985**, *63*, 965–981.
4. Nia, R.; Paper, D.H.; Essien, E.E. Evaluation of the anti-oxidant and anti-angiogenic effects of *Sphenocentrum jollyanum* Pierre. *Afr. J. Biomed. Res.* **2004**, *7*, 129–132.
5. Amidu, N. An Evaluation of the Central and Sexual Behavioral Effects and Toxicity of the Root Extract of *Sphenocentrum jollyanum* Pierre (Menispermaceae). Ph.D. Thesis, Department of Molecular Medicine, Kwame Nkrumah University of Science & Technology, Kumasi, Ghana, 2008.
6. Dalziel, J.M. *The Useful Plants of West Tropical Africa*; Crown Agents: London, UK, 1985.
7. Iwu, M.M. *Handbook of African Medicinal Plants*; CRC Press: Boca Raton, FL, USA, 1993; p. 239.
8. Abbiw, D.K. *Useful Plants of Ghana*; Intermediate Technology Publications and Royal Botanic Gardens: Kew, UK, 1990.
9. Neuwinger, H.D. *African Ethno Botany: Poisons and Drugs*; Chapman and Hall: London, UK, 1996.
10. Irvine, F.R. *Woody Plants of Ghana: With Special Reference to the Uses*; Oxford University Press: London, UK, 1961.
11. Burkill, H.M. *Volume 1: The Useful Plants of West Tropical Africa*; Royal Botanical Gardens: Kew, UK, 1985.
12. Oke, J.M.; Hamburger, M.O. Screening of some Nigeria medicinal plant Antioxidant Acitivity Using 22-Diphenyl-picryl-hydrazyl radical. *Afr. J. Biomed. Res.* **2002**, *5*, 77–79.
13. Odugbemi, T. *Medicinal Plants by Species Names: Outlines and Pictures of Medicinal Plants from Nigeria*; Lagos University Press: Ojo, Lagos State, Nigeria, 2006.
14. Oliver-Bever, B. *Medicinal Plants in Tropical West Africa*; Cambridge University Press: Cambridge, UK, 1986.
15. Kayode, J.; Ige, O.E.; Adetogo, T.A.; Igbakin, A.P. Conservation and Bio derversity in Ondo State, Nigeria. Survey of plant barks used in native pharmaceutical extraction in Akoko region. *EthnoBot. Leafl.* **2009**, *13*, 665–667.

16. Fasola, T.R.; Egunyomi, A. Bark extraction and uses of some medicinal plants. *Niger. J. Biotechnol.* **2002**, *15*, 23–36.
17. Ghana Herbal Pharmacopoeia. *Ghana Herbal Pharmacopoeia*; Advent Press: Accra, Ghana, 1992.
18. Egunyomi, A.; Fasola, T.R.; Oladunjoye, O. Charring Medicinal Plants: A Traditional Method of Preparing Phytomedicines in Southwestern Nigeria. *EthnoBot. J.* **2005**, *3*, 261–265. [CrossRef]
19. Amidu, N.; Woode, E.; Owiredu, K.B.; William, A.; George-Boateng, A.K.; Opoku-Okrah, C. An Evaluation of Toxicity and Mutagenicity of *Sphenocentrum jollyanum*. *Int. J. Pharm.* **2008**, *4*, 67–77.
20. Aboaba, S.A.; Ekundayo, O. Constituents, antibacterial activities and toxicological assay of essential oils of *Artocarpus communis* Forst (Moraceae) and *Sphenocentrum jollyanum* (Menispermaceae). *Int. J. Biol. Chem. Sci.* **2010**, *4*, 1455–1461. [CrossRef]
21. Ibironke, A.A.; Olusola, O.O. Phytochemical analysis and mineral element composition of ten medicinal plant seeds from South-west Nigeria. *N. Y. Sci. J.* **2013**, *6*, 2–28.
22. Moody, J.O.; Robert, V.A.; Connolly, J.D.; Houghton, P.J. Anti-inflammatory activities of the methanol extracts and an isolated furanoditerpene constituent of *Sphenocentrum jollyanum* Pierre (Menispermaceae). *J. Ethnopharmacol.* **2006**, *104*, 87–91. [CrossRef] [PubMed]
23. Olorunnisola, O.S.; Akintola, A.A.; Afolayan, A.J. Hepatoprotective and antioxidant effect of *Sphenocentrum jollyanum* (Menispermaceae) stem bark extract against CCl4-induced oxidative stress in rats. *Afr. J. Pharm. Pharmacol.* **2011**, *5*, 1241–1246. [CrossRef]
24. Olorunnisola, O.S.; Afolayan, A.J. In Vivo antioxidant and biochemical evaluation of *Sphenocentrum jollyanum* leaf extract in *P. berghei* infected mice. *Pak. J. Pharm. Sci.* **2013**, *26*, 445–450. [PubMed]
25. Koleosho, A.T.; Jose, A.R.; Oyibo, P.G.; Roland-Ayodele, M.A.; Uloko, M.E. Antimicrobial Activity of *Sphenocentrum jollyanum* and *Mangifera indica*Linn On *Salmonella Typhi*. *Pak. J. Pharm. Sci.* **2013**, *5*, 50–54.
26. Mbaka, G.O.; Adeyemi, O.O.; Oremosu, A.A. Acute and sub-chronic toxicity studies of the ethanol extract of the leaves of *Sphenocentrum jollyanum* (Menispermaceae). *Agric. Biol. J. N. Am.* **2010**, *1*, 265–272. [CrossRef]
27. Olorunnisola, O.S.; Fadahunsi, O.; Adetutu, A.; Olasunkanmi, A. Evaluation of Membrane Stabilizing, Proteinase and Lipoxygenase Inhibitory Activities of Ethanol Extract of Root and Stem of *Sphenocentrum jollyanum* Pierre. *J. Adv. Biol. Biotechnol.* **2017**, *13*, 1–8.
28. Olorunnisola, O.S.; Fadahunsi, O.S.; Owoade, O.A. In Vitro anti-inflammatory activities of extracts of the leaves of *Sphenocentrum jollyanum* Pierre. *J. Appl. Life Sci. Int.* **2017**, accepted.
29. Mbaka, G.O.; Adeyemi, O.O.; Adesina, S.A. Anti-diabetic activity of the seed extract of *Sphenocentrum jollyanum* and morphological changes on pancreatic beta cells in alloxan-induced diabetic rabbits. *J. Med. Med. Sci.* **2010**, *1*, 550–556.
30. Mbaka, G.; Adeyemi, O.; Osinubi, A.; Noronha, C.; Okanlawon, A. The effect of aqueous root extract of *Sphenocentrum jollyanum* on blood glucose level of rabbits. *J. Med. Plants Res.* **2009**, *3*, 870–874.
31. Mbaka, G.O.; Adeyemi, O.O.; Anunobi, C.C. Anti-hyperglycemic effects of ethanol leaf extract of *Sphenocentrum jollyanum* in normal and alloxan-induced diabetic rabbits. *Glob. J. Pharmacol.* **2008**, *2*, 46–51.
32. Alese, M.O.; Adewale, O.S.; Ijomone, O.M.; Ajayi, S.A.; Alese, O.O. Hypolipidemic and hypoglycemic activities of methanol extract of *Sphenocentrum jollyanum* on stretozocin induced diabetic Wistar rats. *Eur. J. Med. Plants* **2014**, *4*, 353–364. [CrossRef]
33. Mbaka, G.O.; Owolabi, M.A. Evaluation of Haematinic Activity and Sub chronic Toxicity of *Sphenocentrum jollyanum* (Menispermaceae) Seed Oil. *Eur. J. Med. Plants* **2011**, *1*, 140–152. [CrossRef]
34. Olorunnisola, O.S.; Afolayan, A.J. In Vivo antimalaria of methanol leaf and root extracts *Sphenocentrum jollyanum*. *Afr. J. Pharm. Pharmacol.* **2011**, *5*, 1669–1673. [CrossRef]
35. Mbaka, G.O.; Adeyemi, O.O.; Ogbonnia., S.O.; Noronha, C.C.; Okanlawon, O.A. The protective effect of ethanol root extract of *Sphenocentrum jollyanum* on the morphology of pancreatic beta cells of alloxan challenged rabbits. *J. Morphol.* **2011**, *28*, 37–45.
36. Olorunnisola, O.S.; Adetutu, A.; Fadahunsi, O.S. Anti-allergy potential and possible modes of action of *Sphenocentrum jollyanum* Pierre fruit extracts. *J. Phytopharm.* **2017**, *6*, 20–26.
37. Moody, J.O.; Robert, V.A.; Adeniji, J.A. Anti-viral effect of selected medicinal plants: *Diospyros bateri, D. monbutensis* and *Sphenocentrum jollyanum* on polio viruses. *Niger. J. Nat. Prod. Med.* **2002**, *6*, 4–6.

38. Moody, J.O.; Robert, V.A.; Hughes, J.A. Anti-viral activities of selected medicinal plantsand effect of extracts of Diospyrosmon butensis and *Sphenocentrum jollyanum* on cowpea mosaic viruses. *Pharm. Biol.* **2002**, *40*, 342–345. [CrossRef]
39. Woode, E.; Amidu, N.; Owiredu, K.; Boakye, G.; Ansah, C.; Duweijua, M. Antidepressant–Like effects of an ethanol extract of *Sphenocentrum jollyanum* Pierre Roots in Mice. *Int. J. Pharmacol.* **2009**, *5*, 22–29. [CrossRef]
40. Woode, E.; Duwiejua, M.; Ansah, C.; Kuffour, G.A.; Obiri, D.D.; Amidu, N. Effect of *Sphenocentrum jollyanum* in experimental mouse models of anxiety. In Proceedings of the 2nd Western Africa Network of Natural Products Research Scientists (WANNPRES), Elmina 32, Ghana, 1–4 August 2006; p. 32.
41. Woode, E.; Amidu, N.; Owiredu, K.; Boakye, G.; Laing, E.F.; Ansah, C.; Duweijua, M. Anxiogenic—Like effect of a root extract of *Sphenocentrum jollyanum* Pierre in Murine behaviour models. *J.Pharmacol. Toxicol.* **2009**, *4*, 91–108. [CrossRef]
42. Muko, K.N.; Ohiri, P.C.; Ezugwu, C.O. Antipyretic and analgesic activities of *Sphenocentrum jollyanum*. *Niger. J. Nat. Prod. Med.* **1998**, *2*, 52–53.
43. Owiredu, W.A.; Amidu, N.; Amissah, F.; Woode, E. The effects of ethanol extract of root of *Sphenocentrum jollyanum* Pierre on sexual behavior and hormonal levels in rodents. *J. Sci. Technol.* **2007**, *27*, 9–21.
44. Raji, Y.; Fadare, O.O.; Adisa, R.A.; Salami, S.A. Comprehensive assessment of the effect of *Sphenocentrum jollyanum* root extract on male albino rats. *Reprod. Med. Biol.* **2006**, *5*, 283–292. [CrossRef]

22

Antimicrobial, Cytotoxic, Phytotoxic and Antioxidant Potential of *Heliotropium strigosum* Willd.

Muhammad Khurm [1,*], Bashir A. Chaudhry [1], Muhammad Uzair [1] and Khalid H. Janbaz [2]

[1] Faculty of Pharmacy, Natural Product Chemistry Unit, Bahauddin Zakariya University, Multan 60800, Pakistan; drbashirahmadch@bzu.edu.pk (B.A.C.); muhammaduzair@bzu.edu.pk (M.U.)

[2] Akson College of Pharmacy, Mirpur University of Science and Technology, Mirpur 10250, Pakistan; KHjanbaz@hotmail.com

* Correspondence: khuram.ghori19@gmail.com

Academic Editor: James D. Adams

Abstract: Background: *Heliotropium strigosum* Willd. (Chitiphal) is a medicinally important herb that belongs to the *Boraginaceae* family. Traditionally, this plant was used in the medication therapy of various ailments in different populations of the world. The aim of the study is to probe the therapeutic aspects of *H. strigosum* described in the traditional folklore history of medicines. **Methods:** In the present study, the dichloromethane crude extract of this plant was screened to explore the antimicrobial, cytotoxic, phytotoxic and antioxidant potential of *H. strigosum*. For antibacterial, antifungal and antioxidant activities, microplate alamar blue assay (MABA), agar tube dilution method and diphenyl picryl hydrazine (DPPH) radical-scavenging assay were used, respectively. The cytotoxic and phytotoxic potential were demonstrated by using brine shrimp lethality bioassay and *Lemna minor* assay. **Results:** The crude extract displayed positive cytotoxic activity in the brine shrimp lethality assay, with 23 of 30 shrimps dying at the concentration of 1000 µg/mL. It also showed moderate phytotoxic potential with percent inhibition of 50% at the concentration of 1000 µg/mL. The crude extract exhibited no significant antibacterial activity against *Staphylococcus aureus*, *Shigella flexneri*, *Escherichia coli* and *Pseudomonas aeruginosa*. Non-significant antifungal and radical scavenging activity was also shown by the dichloromethane crude extract. **Conclusion:** It is recommended that scientists focus on the identification and isolation of beneficial bioactive constituents with the help of advanced scientific methodologies that seems to be helpful in the synthesis of new therapeutic agents of desired interest.

Keywords: *Heliotropium strigosum*; antimicrobial activity; cytotoxicity; phytotoxicity; antioxidant activity; *Boraginaceae* family

1. Introduction

For the past few decades, the importance of medicinal plants for treating various infections has been tremendously increased because of the fact that a large number of people belonging to different populations depend upon the usage of phytomedicines due to the unavailability of primary healthcare facilities [1]. According to World Health Organization reports on phytomedicines, more than 25% of drugs which have been prescribed in recent years are obtained from different plant sources [2]. The family *Boraginaceae* is comprised of 100 genera and about 2000 species. The plants of this family are widely distributed in temperate, especially Mediterranean and tropical, regions. In Pakistan, this family is represented by 32 genera and 135 species. Moreover, some species, namely *Cordia*, *Echium* and *Anchusa* are cultivated [3]. *Heliotropium*, *Cordia*, *Arnebia*, *Martensia* and *Trichodesma* are the important genera of the *Boraginaceae* family. Fruits of *Cordia* are used as diaphoretic and sometimes as astringent [4]. The leaves and roots of *Trichodesma indicum* are effective against snake bites and urinary diseases and are used as a diuretic. The roots of this plant are also applied as a paste on swellings and joints and are used in dysentery in children [5]. Today, *Alkanna* (*Alkanna tinctoria*) root is used almost exclusively as a cosmetic dye. Orally, it has been used for diarrhea and gastric ulcers. Traditionally, *Alkanna* root has been used topically to treat skin wounds and diseases [6].

Heliotropium is one of the most complex and largest genera of the family *Boraginaceae*. In tropical and temperate regions, it was represented by 270–275 species while in Pakistan 23 species of this genus are present [3]. In folk medicinal history, species of genus *Heliotropium* have attained noticeable pharmacological importance. In Somalia, the pulp of roots of *H. aegyptiacum* was considered to be effective against scorpion stings and snake bites [7]. In India, the paste of the leaves of *H. indicum* was used for rheumatism [8]. In Mauritius, the decoction of whole plant of *H. amplexicaule* was used in the therapeutic management of coughs and fevers [9]. The variety of traditional medicinal uses of *H. strigosum* made it distinguishable among other species of genus *Heliotropium*. The powder and decoction of the whole plant material of *H. strigosum* has been used in the medication therapy of rheumatic arthritis and jaundice and it is also used as a blood purifier [10]. The paste of roots of this plant is used for healing wounds [11]. For the curing of snake bites, gum boils, eye sores and nettle stings, the juice of this whole plant is administered [12]. This juice has also been used as diuretic and demonstrated some laxative effect [13]. In the current study, the dichloromethane crude extract of *H. strigosum* was examined for different biological activities, which could be related to the potential therapeutic value of this plant as prescribed in traditional medicine.

2. Experimental Section

2.1. Materials and Methods

The current study was conducted in the natural product chemistry laboratory, Faculty of Pharmacy, Bahauddin Zakariya University, new campus Multan and International Centre for Chemical and Biological Sciences, Hussain Ebrahim Jamal Research Institute of Chemistry, University of Karachi, Karachi, Pakistan, from August 2014 to August 2015.

2.2. Collection and Identification of Plant Material

The plant *Heliotropium strigosum* was collected in September 2014 from the surroundings of the railway ground district Khanewal (Pakistan) and identified by Dr. Muhammad Zafarullah, Assistant professor of Institute of Pure and Applied Biology, Bahauddin Zakariya University, Multan, Pakistan. A voucher no. "Stewart 591" was assigned to the specimen and preserved in the University herbarium.

2.3. Preparation of Dichloromethane Extract

Drying of the whole plant material was achieved by placing it under shade on old newspapers for 25 days to accomplish the process of effective extraction. When the plant material was completely dried, it was made into a coarse powder by crushing in the grinding mill. The extraction of this powdered plant material was carried out by the process of simple maceration. About 600 g of measured powdered material was put into the extraction bottle and a known volume of dichloromethane (3×1.5 L) was added into the bottle. For the purpose of maximum possible extraction, the mixture was continuously shaken after every 15 min for 3 to 4 h and then make it homogenized by the method of ultra-sonication. After 24 h, this mixture was filtered off. Repeated the same procedure thrice with dichloromethane. After the third collection, the dichloromethane extract was concentrated separately with the help of a rotary evaporator. This was done under reduced pressure. Then the dichloromethane extract was collected in the separated sample bottle and assigned the code as HSWPD (Heliotropium strigosum whole plant dichloromethane extract). The powdered plant material yielded 5.15 g of crude dichloromethane extract which is approximately 0.85% of total dry weight.

2.4. Antimicrobial Assays

2.4.1. Antibacterial Assay—Microplate Alamar Blue Assay (MABA)

The dichloromethane extract of *H. strigosum* was tested for significant antibacterial activity by using microplate alamar blue assay (MABA) (Invitrogen Corporation, San Diego, CA, USA). Strains of four pathogenic bacteria such as *Staphylococcus aureus* (NCTC 6571), *Shigella flexneri*, *Pseudomonas aeruginosa* (ATCC 10145) and *Escherichia coli* (NCTC 10418) were used in this assay. Mueller Hinton medium was prepared in a separate petri dish by following the specifications and guidelines given by the manufacturer (Sigma-Aldrich, St. Louis, MO, USA) and adjusted the pH to 6.6–7.3 normally at 25 °C. In this method, the tested micro-organisms were cultured in Mueller Hinton medium. Then the adjustment of turbidity index of inoculums up to 0.5 McFarland was done. We prepared the standard solution of 1g dichloromethane crude extract in 1 mL sterile dimethyl sulfoxide (DMSO) and distributed the above prepared media into the wells. This work was repeated thrice. All the tested micro-organisms were also placed into the wells. We made sure that the control wells did not contain any testing organism. The volume of well plate 96 was settled up to the level of 200 μL. At the end, added 5×10^6 cells into all the control and testing wells. Sealed all the plates with the help of paraffin. We placed these plates into the incubator at 37 °C for at least 18–20 h without shaking. After 20 h, we added 5 μL alamar blue dye into every well and shook gently at the speed of 80 revolutions per minute for 2–3 h by using the shaking incubator at 37 °C. Plates were covered with foil in shaking incubator. If the color of alamar blue dye was changed from blue to pink, it confirmed the growth of bacteria. Finally, the absorbance at the wavelength of 570 nm–600 nm was recorded with the help of Elisa reader [14].

2.4.2. Antifungal Assay—Agar Tube Dilution Method

The dichloromethane extract of whole plant of *H. strigosum* was tested for certain antifungal activity against six fungal strains such as *Trychophyton rubrum*, *Aspergillus niger*, *Fusarium solani*, *Candida albicans* and *Microsporum canis* by using agar tube dilution assay. We took 24 mg of dichloromethane crude extract and mixed in 1 mL sterile dimethyl sulfoxide (DMSO) to prepare its stock solution. For the preparation of Sabouraud dextrose agar (SDA) medium, we dissolved 32.5 g of Sabouraud glucose (2%) or maltose agar in 500 mL of distilled water. Adjusted the pH of this medium up to 5.5–5.6. Steaming of this media was done to dissolve all the suitable contents and added an appropriate volume (4 mL) into the test tubes having screw caps. These tubes were placed into the autoclave for 15 min at the temperature of 121 °C. After this, these tubes were placed at the temperature of 50 °C to achieve the effective cooling. Then, we loaded the non-solidified agar media by using pipette with 66.6 μL of tested sample taken from the stock solution. At room temperature, these tubes were placed for solidification in a slanting position. In every tube, a piece of fungus obtained from the seven day old fungus culture with the diameter of 4 mm was inoculated. All these tubes containing culture of fungus were placed in the incubator at the optimum temperature of 27 °C–29 °C. These culture containing tubes were allowed to grow for 3–7 days. This culture was observed twice a week during the period of incubation. When the incubation for 3–7 days was completed, the tube in which the growth of fungus culture was not visible was taken for the measurement of MIC value of the tested sample which is expressed in μg/mL [15].

2.5. Cytotoxic Assay—Brine Shrimp Lethality Bioassay

We stored the brine shrimp (*Artemia salina* Leach) eggs usually at the very low temperature of 4 °C. When filtration of brine solution was achieved, the hatching tray was filled half with this solution. Then we sprinkled eggs (50 mg) on the hatching try and incubated at the temperature of 37 °C. Then, we prepared the stock solution by taking 20 mg of crude dichloromethane extract and dissolved it in 2 mL of sterile dimethyl sulfoxide. From this stock solution, we transferred 5 μL, 50 μL and 500 μL into three separate glass vials at the concentrations of (10, 100 and 1000) μg/mL by using micro-pipette.

We placed these solvent containing vials over night for the evaporation of solvent. After two days of hatching process, we placed 10 larvae individually in the vials by using Pasteur pipette. We made the final volume of solvent up to 5 mL with the addition of sea water. These vials were placed into the incubator at the temperature of 25–27 °C for 24 h beneath the illumination. We took an extra two vials, one of which had the standard cytotoxic drug (Etoposide) served as positive control and the other vials in which respective solvent was added and served as negative control. Larvae were observed in each vial after 24 h. The number of survivors should be determined. Finney computerized system (Probit analysis) was used to analyze the data for the determination of LD_{50} values with 95% confidence intervals. Shrimps can be used 48–72 h after the initiation of hatching. After 72 h they should be discarded [15–17].

2.6. *Phytotoxic Assay—Lemna Bioassay for Phytotoxicity*

We prepared the inorganic E-medium (stock solution) by mixing appropriate inorganic constituents [15] into 1 liter of distilled water. The pH of E-medium was adjusted by adding potassium hydroxide pellets up to 6–7. To prepare the working E-medium, 100 mL of this stock solution was taken and dissolved it in 900 mL of distilled water. Then, we prepared the solution of tested crude extract by dissolving 30 mg of crude extract in 1.5 mL of ethyl alcohol. Three flasks were taken and pipetted 10 µL, 100 µL and 1000 µL into these flasks from concentration solutions of (10, 100 and 1000) µg/mL. Placed these solvent containing flasks over night for the evaporation of solvent. In each flask, added 20 mL stock solution of working E-medium along with the addition of 2 to 3 fronds (total fronds used 20) from the rosette of the plant *Lemna minor*. Two supplemented flasks, one with the standard drug (Paraquat) and other with the E-medium were served as positive and negative control respectively. We placed all these flasks into the growth chamber for 7 days by maintaining the temperature at 28 °C along with the light intensity of 9000 lux and relative humidity of 56% ± 10%. When the incubation period was completed, counted and verified the number of fronds of each flask on the 7th day [18,19]. The results which were analyzed as growth inhibition (%), compared with reference drug to negative control were given as shown below.

$$\%\,\text{inhibition of growth} = 100 - (\text{No. of fronds in tested sample/No. of fronds in negative control}) \times 100$$

2.7. *Antioxidant Assay—DPPH (2,2-Diphenyl-1-Picrylhydrazl) Radical Scavenging Assay*

We dissolved the weighed amount of tested sample in a suitable volume of pure dimethyl sulfoxide. Then we prepared the 300 µL solution of DPPH (2,2-diphenyl-1-picrylhydrazl) by using appropriate volume of pure ethyl alcohol. About 5 µL of the tested sample solution was added into the 96-well plate and measured the absorbance at the wavelength of 515 nm. After this, to each well was added 95 µL solution of DPPH. We then incubated the 96 well plate at the temperature of 37 °C for the period of 30 min. We covered this plate with paraffin so that the solvent evaporation must be avoided. The pure dimethyl sulfoxide was served as control. By using a micro-plate reader, final absorbance at the wavelength of 515 nm was recorded. Percentage of radical scavenging activity (%RSA) can be determined by the following equation [20].

$$\%\,\text{RSA} = 100 - (\text{Original dose of tested sample/Original dose of control}) \times 100$$

3. Results

3.1. *Antibacterial Activity*

In the present study, antibacterial potential of crude dichloromethane extract was examined. The percent (%) inhibition showed by sample extract against various tested bacteria are specified in the Table 1. The results of preliminary antibacterial activity demonstrated that the dichloromethane crude extract of *H. strigosum* showed inhibition up to 16% against *S. aureus* while against *S. flexneri*, and showed an inhibition of 3% respectively at the concentration used, which is 150 μg/mL. The pathogens *E. coli* and *P. aeruginosa* showed no inhibition against the tested sample. Thus, crude dichloromethane extract showed non-significant antibacterial activity against all the four tested bacterial strains when compared with the reference drug used, which was Ofloxacin (0.25 μg/mL).

Table 1. Results of preliminary antibacterial assay of *H. strigosum*.

Name of Bacteria	Percent (%) Inhibition of Tested Sample	Percent (%) Inhibition of Standard Drug (Ofloxacin)
S. aureus	16	92.35
E. coli	0	90.20
P. aeruginosa	0	89.35
S. flexneri	3	91.40

Concentration of tested sample used = 150 μg/mL; Concentration of standard drug used = 0.25 μg/mL; Positive control = Ofloxacin (standard antibiotic); Negative control = DMSO (Dimethyl sulfoxide); Percent inhibition activity, 0–39 = Low (non-significant); 40–59 = moderate; 60–69 = Good; above 70 = Significant.

3.2. *Antifungal Activity*

The dichloromethane extract of the whole plant of *H. strigosum* was tested for significant antifungal activity. The results shown by tested crude extract against different fungal strains are given in Table 2. The results revealed that none of the tested fungal strains showed any kind of inhibition against the tested sample. So, the dichloromethane extract was found to be inactive against all the tested fungus species at the concentration of the sample used (400 μg/mL).

Table 2. Results of antifungal assay of *H. strigosum*.

Name of Fungus	Linear Growth (mm)		% Inhibition (Tested Sample)	Standard Drug	MIC (μg/mL)
	Sample	Control			
T. rubrum	100	100	0	Miconazole	97.8
A. niger	100	100	0	Amphotericin B	20.70
F. solani	100	100	0	Miconazole	73.50
C. albicans	100	100	0	Miconazole	113.1
M. canis	100	100	0	Miconazole	98.1

MIC = Minimum inhibitory concentration; Concentration of tested sample used = 400 μg/mL; Percent inhibition activity, 0–39 = Low (non-significant); 40–59 = moderate; 60–69 = Good; above 70 = Significant; Positive control = Miconazole and Amphotericin B (*A. niger*); Negative control = DMSO (Dimethyl sulfoxide).

3.3. *Cytotoxic Activity*

Brine shrimp lethality bioassay was used for cytotoxic screening of dichloromethane extract of the whole plant of *H. strigosum*. The consequences of dichloromethane screening are expressed in Table 3. The results showed that, at the concentration of 10 μg/mL and 100 μg/mL, the number of dead shrimps was only one. However, when the concentration of the tested sample increased up to 1000 μg/mL, the number of dead shrimps was 23 and only 7 shrimps survived. Thus, from the above revealed data, an LD_{50} of 462 μg/mL was calculated as compared with the reference agent (etoposide) that resulted in an LD_{50} of 7.46 μg/mL.

Table 3. Results of brine shrimp lethality bioassay of *H. strigosum*.

Dose of Tested Sample (μg/mL)	No. of Shrimps	No. of Survivors	LD_{50} (μg/mL)	Standard Drug	LD_{50} (μg/mL)
10	30	29	462	Etoposide	7.46
100	30	29			
1000	30	7			

Positive control = Etoposide; Negative control = DMSO (Dimethyl sulfoxide); No. of replicates = 3; Incubation conditions = 28 ± 1 °C.

3.4. Phytotoxic Activity

The phytotoxic potential of dichloromethane extract of whole plant of *H. strigosum* was studied by using *Lemna minor* phytotoxicity bioassay. The growth inhibition (%) shown by the tested crude extract is given in Table 4. The results revealed that the tested sample showed percent growth inhibition up to 35% and 40% at the concentration of 10 and 100 μg/mL but at the concentration of 1000 μg/mL, it showed 50% growth inhibition. So, the dichloromethane extract exhibited low phytotoxic activity at the concentrations of 10 and 100 μg/mL but showed moderate activity at the highest tested concentration that was 1000 μg/mL when compared with the standard drug (Paraquat) which inhibited the growth of *L. minor* at the concentration of 0.015 μg/mL.

Table 4. Results of phytotoxicity assay of *H. strigosum*.

Name of Plant	Concentration of Tested Sample (μg/mL)	No. of Fronds		% Growth Inhibition	Concentration of Standard Drug (Paraquat) (μg/mL)
		Sample	Control		
Lemna minor	10	13	20	35	0.015
	100	12		40	
	1000	10		50	

Positive control = Paraquat; Negative control = Volatile solvent (ethanol); Incubation conditions = 28 ± 1 °C.

3.5. Antioxidant Activity

DPPH radical scavenging assay was used to determine the significant antioxidant activity of dichloromethane extract of the whole plant of *H. strigosum*. The radical scavenging activity exhibited by the tested dichloromethane extract is shown in Table 5. The results demonstrated that the crude extract showed non-significant antioxidant potential with very low radical scavenging activity up to 13% at the tested concentration that was 500 μM when compared with N-acetyl cysteine (standard drug) which exhibited significant radical scavenging activity up to 96% with IC_{50} of 111.44 ± 0.7 μM respectively at the same concentration.

Table 5. Results of diphenyl picryl hydrazine (DPPH) radical scavenging assay of *H. strigosum*.

Concentration of Tested Sample (μM)	% RSA (Radical Scavenging Activity)	IC_{50} ± SEM (μM)
500 [a]	13	>500
500 [b]	96	111.44 ± 0.7

[a] = Dichloromethane extract; [b] = N-acetyl cysteine (Standard drug & Positive control); Negative control = DMSO (Dimethyl sulfoxide); μM = Micro-molar (10^{-3} mol/m^3); SEM = Standard error mean; Data is expressed as mean ± SEM of three independent readings.

4. Discussion

The history of human beings has revealed that, for the past 60,000 years, plants have been used as a source of treating various ailments in different civilizations of the world [21]. Due to the increased resistance of microbes worldwide, scientists are always looking for the development of newer antibacterial agents [22]. Medicinal plants are considered as a source in the discovery and advancement of new pharmaceuticals which are effective in the management of different diseases [23,24]. In our study, the dichloromethane extract of whole plant material of *H. strigosum* showed non-significant antibacterial activity against *S. aureus*, *S. flexneri*, *E. coli* and *P. aeruginosa*. The results of our studies are quite comparable with the antibacterial activity revealed by other species of genus *Heliotropium* and some other plant species of different families. The petroleum ether and chloroform fractions of ethanolic extract of *H. subulatum* showed strong antibacterial activity against *E. coli*, *S. aureus*, *Streptococcus pneumonia* and *Bacillus subtilis*. That strong antibacterial activity might be due to the purification of five pyrrolizidine alkaloids from this plant [25]. The methaolic extract of aerial parts of *H. indicum* has broad spectrum antibacterial activity against *S. aureus*,

S. pneumonia, *Salmonella typhi*, *E. coli* and *Klebsiella pneumonia* [26]. The antibacterial significance of plant extracts is attributed mainly to the presence of terpenoids [27]. The sterols and triterpenoids such as β-sitosterol, stigmasterol, β-amyrin, friedelan-β-ol, cycloartenone, β-amyrin acetate and friedelin isolated from ethanol extract of the whole plant of *H. ellipticum* exhibited strong antibacterial activity against *E. coli*, *S. aureus* and *K. pneumonia* [28]. Filifolinol, one of the geranyl aromatic derivatives isolated from *H. sclerocarpum* and *H. filifolium* also showed significant antibacterial activity against *S. aureus*, *Bacillus cereus*, *B. subtilis* and *Micrococcus luteus* [29,30]. Another reported antibacterial potential was shown by the group of new 3 *H*-Spiro[1-benzofuran-2,1′-cyclohexane] derivatives such as 3′-hydroxy-2′,2′,6′-trimethyl-3*H*-spiro[1-benzofuran-2,1′-cyclohexane]-5-carboxylic acid, methyl 3′-acetyloxy-2′,2′,6′-trimethyl-3*H*-spiro[1-benzofuran-2,1′-cyclohexane]-5-carboxylate, methyl 3′-isopentanoyloxy-2′,2′,6′-trimethyl-3*H*-spiro[1-benzofuran-2,1′-cyclohexane]-5-carboxylate, and methyl 3′-benzoyloxy-2′,2′,6′-trimethyl-3*H*-spiro[1-benzofuran-2,1′-cyclohexane]-5-carboxylate isolated from the dichloromethane cuticle extract of *H. filifolium* against several gram positive and gram negative bacteria [31]. In addition to the genus *Heliotropium*, other plant species also exhibited antibacterial potential. The ethanolic extracts of *Curcuma longa* and *Alpinia galangal* displayed weak antibacterial activity against *S. aureus* and *S. typhi* and showed no inhibition against *B. subtilis*, *E. coli*, *P. aeruginosa* and *S. flexneri* [32]. Thus, from the above contributions, researchers have come to know that the identification, isolation and purification of different groups of organic compounds, mainly pyrrolizidine alkaloids, terpenoids and flavonoids, from *H. strigosum* should reveal that this plant has a perceptible future role in the field of antibacterial medicinal agents.

Different pathogenic fungi cause systemic infections of the skin, lungs, liver, mouth and blood [33–35]. Fungal attacks especially infect the skin and cause severe infections such as athlete's foot, tinea cruris and numerous others [36]. Only 10 antifungal drugs are permitted for the therapeutic management of invasive systemic fungal infections by the Food and Drug Administration (FDA) authority in United States of America [37]. Patients who have had pediatric lung transplantation are at serious risk of pulmonary fungal infection [33]. In the present study, the dichloromethane extract of whole plant material of *H. strigosum* demonstrated no antifungal activity and was found to be inactive against all the tested fungal strains. These results exposed the antifungal principles in a consistent manner, as established by different plant species of the family *Boraginaceae* and some other families. The methanolic extract of *Echium rauwolfii* and *E. horridum* showed no antifungal activity against *Aspergillus flavus* but were found to have weak activity against *C. albicans* [38]. The dichloromethane extract of *Cordia curassavica* [39] and *Cordia linnael* [40] showed equal antifungal activity to some extent against both *C. albicans* and *Clasdosporium cucumerinum*. The benzene extract of *Trichodesma amplexicaule* remained inactive against *Aspergillus niger* and *A. flavus* followed by chloroform extract with very low activity against these micro-organisms [41]. The ethyl acetate and n-butanol fractions of methanolic extract of *Onosma griffithii* reported no antifungal activity [42]. The ethyl alcohol and aqueous extracts of *Colendia procumbens* never showed antifungal activity against *C. albicans* [43]. No antifungal activity was displayed by the methanolic and aqueous extracts of *Trichodesma zeylanicum* and *Anchusa italic* [44]. Apart from the above consequences, different biological extracts and isolated bioactive constituents, mainly pyrrolizidine alkaloids and terpenoids from different *Heliotropium* species such as *H. indicum* [45], *H. ellipticum* [28,46] and *H. marifolium* [47], demonstrated significant antifungal activity against various pathogenic fungi. Our study reports for the first time the dichloromethane screening of *H. strigosum* for antifungal potential.

Due to the life threatening effects of cancer, it is known as a critical factors that increases the mortality rate worldwide. Cancer of the liver, lung, colon and stomach contribute to a major proportion of mortality cases all over the world [48]. In the present research work, the dichloromethane extract of *H. strigosum* shows positive cytotoxic activity with an LD_{50} of 462 μg/mL. The cytotoxic potential of this plant is extremely compatible with the previously reported developments in the field of antitumor drug discovery. The ethanolic, dichloromethane and n-hexane extracts of *H. subulatum* [49] and the methanolic extract of *H. indicum* [50] showed significant antineoplastic activity in the dose dependent manner. The ethanolic extracts of *Curcuma longa* and *Alpinia galangal* revealed strong cytotoxic potential with the LD_{50} of 33 μg/mL and 109 μg/mL, respectively [32]. The occurrence of cytotoxic activity was mainly due to the presence of different classes of organic compounds such as phenolic compounds (polyphenols), catechins and flavonoid constituents. A large number of polyphenols and flavonoids have been purified and isolated from different parts of *Bruguiera gymnorrhiza, Blumea lacera, Aegiceras corniculatum, Hygrophila auriculata* and *Hibiscus tiliaceous,* which might be responsible for their cytotoxic activity. In 2007, a scientific report from Bangladesh examined 32 extracts of 16 different Bangladehsi plant species for their cytotoxic potential. Among these tested extracts, the aqueous extracts possessed very low cytotoxic potential. This low antitumor potential of aqueous extracts is of great therapeutic significance because traditionally they are used in the medication of various ailments instead of cancer [51]. Another informative description of cytotoxic potential was reported in Brazil in which 60 species of different medicinal plants were screened to examine the cytotoxic activity. Only 10% of plant species showed better cytotoxicity with ED_{50} less than 1000 ppm [16]. In most of the reported statistical data about the cytotoxic potential of different medicinal plants, scientists used brine shrimp lethality bioassay instead of other scientific approaches because a progressive correlation existed between the toxicity of brine shrimp and human nasopharyngeal carcinoma [52].

In the developing countries, weeds are considered an important factor for environmental protection. Approximately 30,000 different species of weeds are present in the world, out of which a reported 1800 cause the loss of 9.7% of crop yields [53]. The presence of weeds reduced the agricultural productivity of crops that lead to massive economical loss among different regions of the world. In a recent study, the dichloromethane extract of *H. strigosum* demonstrated moderate phytotoxic activity at the higher tested concentration (1000 μg/mL) but showed low phytotoxic activity at the concentration of 10 and 100 μg/mL with the growth inhibition of 35% and 40%. The phytotoxic significances of this plant are followed by some other species of genus *Heliotropium* such as *H. dasycarpum* whose methanol and dichloromethane extract showed 100% inhibitory effect at the concentration of 1000 μg/mL, respectively [54]. Similar phytotoxic measurements were shown by ethanolic extract of *Curcuma longa* and *Alpinia galangal* [32]. The methanolic extract of *polygonatum verticillatum* exhibited significant phytotoxic activity at the tested doses of 5, 50 and 500 μg/mL [55]. A few scientific descriptions of allelopathic approaches of *H. indicum* [56] and *Chrysanthemum morifolium* [57] were also considered. The reduction of crops quantity and quality is given serious attention by the scientists who focus upon the discovery and development of newer weedicides because chemically synthetic weedicides cause harmful adverse effects, mainly the expansion of weedicide resistant populations, lowering the water and soil consumption and resulting in damaging effects on non-targeted organisms [53].

The destructive effects of free radicals can be prevented by using different organic and inorganic substances having low molecular weight. Some of the commonly used antioxidative agents are tocopherols, copper, vitamin C, zinc, thiols, iron and manganese [58]. The recent scientific studies also exposed the beneficial preventive effects of antioxidants in the treatment of cardiovascular diseases, ocular damage and certain type of cancers [59]. The consequences of our study shows that the dichloromethane extract of *H. strigosum* demonstrated very low radical scavenging activity, only up to 13%. Therefore, no antioxidant activity was shown by the tested extract and it was found to be inactive. However, some other species of genus *Heliotropium* showed excellent radical scavenging activity because of the presence of flavonoids. Flavonoids are the largest group of naturally occurring phenolic compounds and possessed some chemical and biological properties which are very helpful in the prevention of free radicals formation. Flavonoids are found to be ubiquitous in most of the plants growing in extreme conditions [60]. A new compound belonging to the group of flavanones named as Naringenin was identified and isolated from the resinous exudate of dichloromethane extract of *H. sclerocarpum* which displayed outstanding free radical scavenging activity [30]. In 2009, from the resinous exudates of dichloromethane extract of *H. taltalense*, three flavonoids, namely Naringenin, 3-*O*-methylgalangin and 7-*O*-methyleriodictiol were isolated and exhibited significant antioxidant activity [61]. The isolation of three new flavonoids, namely, 5,3′-dihydroxy-7,4′-dimethoxyflavanone,

5,4′-dihydroxy-7-methoxyflavanone and 4′-acetyl-5-hydroxy-7-methoxyflavanone from *H. glutinosum* was also reported [60]. From *H. sinuatum*, eight previously reported flavonoids along with one new compound 4-(3′,5′-dihydroxynonadecyl) phenol were isolated, which confirmed the antioxidant behavior of this plant [62]. All the above previous scientific reports confirmed that all these plants showed exceptional antioxidant potential. This gives scientists a new approach to identify, purify and isolate the flavonoids and other phenolic compounds from *H. strigosum* which lead towards the synthesis of new antioxidant agents in the world of medicines.

5. Conclusions

The dichloromethane screening of *Heliotropium strigosum* was done for the first time. The crude extract of this plant showed low antibacterial activity against two bacterial stains, one is gram positive and other is gram negative. There was no antifungal activity shown by the tested crude extract. The dichloromethane extract exhibited positive cytotoxic and moderate phytotoxic potential at the highest tested concentrations. No antioxidant behavior was exposed by this plant. In conclusion, scientists and pharmacologists should pay serious attention to the screening of this plant by using some other scientific bioassay methodologies which might serve as a source for the identification, purification and isolation of beneficial bioactive constituents that seems to be helpful in the synthesis of new therapeutic agents of desired interest. Therefore, in the future, *Heliotropium strigosum* will be used globally as a source of safer phytomedicines.

Acknowledgments: We shall be very thankful to the management of Faculty of Pharmacy, Bahauddin Zakariya University, Multan and International Center for Chemical and Biological Sciences, Hussain Ebrahim Jamal Research Institute of Chemistry for providing us the necessary resources to perform these studies.

Author Contributions: Bashir Ahmed Chaudhry and Muhammad Uzair conceived and designed the project. Muhammad Khurm collected the plant material, performed the experiments and wrote the manuscript. Khalid Hussain Janbaz analyze the results and made the necessary corrections.

References

1. Shanmugam, S.; Bhavani, P. Studies on the comparison of phytochemical constituents and antimicrobial activity of *Curcuma longa* varieties. *Int. J. Curr. Microbiol. Appl. Sci.* **2014**, *3*, 573–581.
2. Pranuthi, E.K.; Narendra, K.; Swathi, J.; Sowjanya, K.; Reddi, K.R.; Emmanuel, R.F.S.; Satya, A.K. Qualitative Assessment of Bioactive Compounds from a Very Rare Medicinal Plant *Ficus dalhousiae* Miq. *J. Pharmacogn. Phytochem.* **2014**, *3*, 57–61.
3. Nasir, E.; Ali, S. *Flora of West Pakistan*, 4th ed.; Feroz Sons Press: Karachi, Pakistan, 1974; p. 23.
4. Ghori, M.K.; Ghaffarı, M.A.; Hussaın, S.N.; Manzoor, M.; Azız, M.; Sarwer, W. Ethnopharmacological, phytochemical and pharmacognostic potential of genus *Heliotropıum* L. *Turk. J. Pharm. Sci.* **2016**, *13*, 143–168. [CrossRef]
5. Shinwari, M.I.; Khan, M.A. Folk use of medicinal herbs of Margalla hills national park, Islamabad. *J. Ethnopharmacol.* **2000**, *69*, 45–56. [CrossRef]
6. Bisset, N.G. *Max Wichtl's Herbal Drugs & Phytopharmaceuticals*; CRC Press: Boca Raton, FL, USA, 1994.
7. Thulin, M. *Flora of Somalia*; CRB Press: Harare, NY, USA, 1993; Volume 1.
8. Nagaraju, N.; Rao, K. A survey of plant crude drugs of Rayalaseema, Andhra Pradesh, India. *J. Ethnopharmacol.* **1990**, *29*, 137–158. [CrossRef]
9. Schmelzer, G.; Gurib-Fakim, A. *Plant Resources of Tropical Africa*; Backurys Publishers: Leiden, The Netherlands, 2008; Volume 11.
10. Ahmad, S.; Alam, K.; Wariss, H.; Anjum, S.; Mukhtar, M. Ethnobotanical studies of plant resources of Cholistan desert, Pakistan. *Int. J. Sci. Res.* **2014**, *3*, 1782–1788.
11. Watanabe, T.; Rajbhandari, K.R.; Malla, K.J.; Yahara, S. *A Hand Book of Medicinal Plants of Nepal*; Kobfai Publishing Project: Bangkok, Thailand, 2005; Volume 15.
12. Roeder, E.; Wiedenfeld, H. Pyrrolizidine alkaloids in medicinal plants of Mongolia, Nepal and Tibet. *Die Pharm. Int. J. Pharm. Sci.* **2009**, *64*, 699–716.

13. Mahmood, A.; Mahmood, A.; Shaheen, H.; Qureshi, R.A.; Sangi, Y.; Gilani, S.A. Ethno medicinal survey of plants from district Bhimber Azad Jammu and Kashmir, Pakistan. *J. Med. Plants Res.* **2011**, *5*, 2348–2360.
14. Pettit, R.K.; Weber, C.A.; Kean, M.J.; Hoffmann, H.; Pettit, G.R.; Tan, R.; Horton, M.L. Microplate Alamar blue assay for *Staphylococcus epidermidis* biofilm susceptibility testing. *Antimicrob. Agents Chemother.* **2005**, *49*, 2612–2617. [CrossRef] [PubMed]
15. Atta-ur-Rahman; Choudhary, M.I.; William, J.T. *Bioassay Techniques for Drug Development*; CRC Press: Reading, UK, 2001; pp. 8–23.
16. Alves, T.M.D.A.; Silva, A.F.; Brandao, M.; Grandi, T.S.M.; Smania, E.D.F.A.; Smania, J. Biological screening of Brazilian medicinal plants. *Mem. Inst. Oswaldo Cruz* **2000**, *95*, 367–373. [CrossRef] [PubMed]
17. Mayer, B.N.; Ferrigni, N.R.; Putnam, J.E.; Jacobsen, L.B.; Nicholas, P.E.; McLaughin, J.L. Brine Shrimp: A convenient general bioassay for active plant constituents. *Planta Med.* **1982**, *45*, 31–34. [CrossRef] [PubMed]
18. Atta-ur-Rehman. *Studies in Natural Product Chemistry*; Elsevier Science Publishers: Amsterdam, The Netherlands, 1991; Volume 9, pp. 383–409.
19. Rashid, R.; Farah, M.; Mirza, M.N. Biological screening of *Salvia cabulica*. *Pak. J. Bot.* **2009**, *41*, 1453–1462.
20. Uddin, N.; Siddiqui, B.S.; Begum, S.; Bhatti, H.A.; Khan, A.; Parveen, S.; Choudhary, M.I. Bioactive flavonoids from the leaves of *Lawsonia alba* (Henna). *Phytochem. Lett.* **2011**, *4*, 454–458. [CrossRef]
21. Sumner, J. *The Natural History of Medicinal Plants*; Timber Press: Portland, OR, USA, 2000; Volume 1.
22. Ullah, F.; Malik, S.; Ahmed, J. Antibiotic susceptibility pattern and ESBL prevalence in nosocomial *Escherichia coli* from urinary tract infections in Pakistan. *Afr. J. Biotechnol.* **2009**, *8*, 3921–3926.
23. Rafie, S.; MacDougall, C.; James, C.L. Cethromycin: A promising new ketolide antibiotic for respiratory infections. *Pharmacother.: J. Hum. Pharmacol. Drug Ther.* **2010**, *30*, 290–303. [CrossRef] [PubMed]
24. Angeh, J.E.; Huang, X.; Sattler, I.; Swan, G.E.; Dahse, H.; Härtl, A.; Eloff, J.N. Antimicrobial and anti-inflammatory activity of four known and one new triterpenoid from *Combretum imberbe* (Combretaceae). *J. Ethnopharmacol.* **2007**, *110*, 56–60. [CrossRef] [PubMed]
25. Singh, B.; Sahu, P.; Singh, S. Antimicrobial activity of pyrrolizidine alkaloids from *Heliotropium subulatum*. *Fitoterapia* **2002**, *73*, 153–155. [CrossRef]
26. Oluwatoyin, S.M.; Illeogbulam, N.G.; Joseph, A. Phytochemical and antimicrobial studies on the aerial parts of *Heliotropium indicum* Linn. *Ann. Biol. Res.* **2011**, *2*, 129–136.
27. Urzúa, A.; Rezende, M.C.; Mascayano, C.; Vásquez, L. A structure-activity study of antibacterial diterpenoids. *Molecules* **2008**, *13*, 882–891. [CrossRef] [PubMed]
28. Jain, S.; Singh, B.; Jain, R. Antimicrobial activity of triterpenoids from *Heliotropium ellipticum*. *Fitoterapia* **2001**, *72*, 666–668. [CrossRef]
29. Torres, R.; Villarroel, L.; Urzua, A.; Delle-Monache, F.; Delle-Monache, G.; Gacs-Baitz, E. Filifolinol, a rearranged geranyl aromatic derivative from the resinous exudate of *Heliotropium filifolium*. *Phytochemistry* **1994**, *36*, 249–250. [CrossRef]
30. Modak, B.; Salina, M.; Rodilla, J.; Torres, R. Study of the chemical composition of the resinous exudate isolated from *Heliotropium sclerocarpum* and evaluation of the antioxidant properties of the phenolic compounds and the resin. *Molecules* **2009**, *14*, 4625–4633. [CrossRef] [PubMed]
31. Urzúa, A.; Echeverría, J.; Rezende, M.C.; Wilkens, M. Antibacterial Properties of 3 H-Spiro [1-benzofuran-2, 1′-cyclohexane] Derivatives from *Heliotropium filifolium*. *Molecules* **2008**, *13*, 2385–2393. [CrossRef] [PubMed]
32. Khattak, S.; Shah, H.U.; Ahmad, W.; Ahmad, M. Biological effects of indigenous medicinal plants *Curcuma longa* and *Alpinia galanga*. *Fitoterapia* **2005**, *76*, 254–257. [CrossRef] [PubMed]
33. Danziger-Isakov, L.A.; Worley, S.; Arrigain, S.; Aurora, P.; Ballmann, M.; Boyer, D.; Conrad, C.; Eichler, I.; Elidemir, O.; Goldfarb, S. Increased mortality after pulmonary fungal infection within the first year after pediatric lung transplantation. *J. Heart Lung Transplant.* **2008**, *27*, 655–661. [CrossRef] [PubMed]
34. Fung, J.J. Fungal infection in liver transplantation. *Transpl. Infect. Dis.* **2002**, *4*, 18–23. [CrossRef] [PubMed]
35. Ker, C.C.; Hung, C.C.; Huang, S.Y.; Chen, M.; Hsieh, S.; Lin, C.; Chang, S.; Luh, K. Comparison of bone marrow studies with blood culture for etiological diagnosis of disseminated mycobacterial and fungal infection in patients with acquired immunodeficiency syndrome. *J. Microbiol. Immunol. Infect.* **2002**, *35*, 89–93. [PubMed]
36. Al-Sogair, S.; Moawad, M.; Al-Humaidan, Y. Fungal infection as a cause of skin disease in the eastern province of Saudi Arabia: Cutaneous candidosis. *Mycoses* **1991**, *34*, 429–431. [CrossRef] [PubMed]

37. Dismukes, W.E. Introduction to antifungal drugs. *Clin. Infect. Dis.* **2000**, *30*, 653–657. [CrossRef] [PubMed]
38. El-Shazly, A.; Abdel-All, M.; Tei, A.; Wink, M. Pyrrolizidine alkaloids from *Echium rauwolfii* and *Echium horridum* (*Boraginaceae*). *Z. Naturforschung. C J. Biosci.* **1999**, *54*, 295–300. [CrossRef]
39. Ioset, J.R.; Marston, A.; Gupta, M.P.; Hostettmann, K. Antifungal and larvicidal cordiaquinones from the roots of *Cordia curassavica*. *Phytochemistry* **2000**, *53*, 613–617. [CrossRef]
40. Ioset, J.R.; Marston, A.; Gupta, M.P.; Hostettmann, K. Antifungal and larvicidal meroterpenoid naphthoquinones and a naphthoxirene from the roots of *Cordia linnael*. *Phytochemistry* **1998**, *47*, 729–734. [CrossRef]
41. Singh, B.; Singh, S. Antimicrobial activity of terpenoids from *Trichodesma amplexicaule* Roth. *Phytother. Res.* **2003**, *17*, 814–816. [CrossRef] [PubMed]
42. Ahmad, B.; Ali, N.; Bashir, S.; Choudhary, M.I.; Azam, S.; Khan, I. Parasiticidal, antifungal and antibacterial activities of *Onosma griffithii* Vatke. *Afr. J. Biotechnol.* **2009**, *8*, 5084–5087.
43. Ramakrishnan, G.; Kothai, R.; Jaykar, B.; Rathnakumar, T.V. In vitro Antibacterial Activity of different extracts of Leaves of *Coldenia procumbens*. *Int. J. Pharm. Tech. Res.* **2011**, *3*, 1000–1004.
44. Bahraminejad, S. In vitro and in vivo antifungal activities of Iranian plant species against *Pythium aphanidermatum*. *Ann. Biol. Res.* **2012**, *3*, 2134–2143.
45. Rao, P.R.; Nammi, S.; Raju, A.D.V. Studies on the antimicrobial activity of *Heliotropium indicum* Linn. *J. Nat. Rem.* **2002**, *2*, 195–198.
46. Jain, S.C.; Sharma, R. Antimicrobial activity of pyrrolizidine alkaloids from *Heliotropium ellipticum*. *Chem. Pharm. Bull.* **1987**, *35*, 3487–3489. [CrossRef] [PubMed]
47. Singh, B.; Dubey, M. Estimation of triterpenoids from *Heliotropium marifolium* Koen. ex Retz. in vivo and in vitro. I. Antimicrobial screening. *Phytother. Res.* **2001**, *15*, 231–234. [CrossRef] [PubMed]
48. Das, S.; Das, M.K.; Mazumder, P.M.; Das, S.; Basu, S.P. Cytotoxic activity of methanolic extract of *Berberis aristata* DC. on colon cancer. *Glob. J. Pharmacol.* **2009**, *3*, 137–140.
49. Singh, B.; Sahu, P.; Jain, S.; Singh, S. Antineoplastic and antiviral screening of pyrrolizidine alkaloids from *Heliotropium subulatum*. *Pharm. Biol.* **2002**, *40*, 581–586. [CrossRef]
50. Rahman, M.A.; Mia, M.A.; Shahid, I.Z. Pharmacological and phytochemical screen activities of roots of *Heliotropium indicum* Linn. *Pharmacologyonline* **2011**, *1*, 185–192.
51. Uddin, S.J.; Grice, I.D.; Tiralongo, E. Cytotoxic effects of Bangladeshi medicinal plant extracts. *Evid. Based Complement. Altern. Med.* **2011**, *2011*, 1–7. [CrossRef] [PubMed]
52. Ateeq, R.; Mannan, A.; Inayatullah, S.; Akhtar, M.Z.; Qayyum, M.; Mirza, B. Biological evaluation of wild thyme (*Thymus serpyllum*). *Pharm. Biol.* **2009**, *47*, 628–633.
53. Li, Y.; Sun, Z.; Zhuang, X.; Xu, L.; Chen, S.; Li, M. Research progress on microbial herbicides. *Crop Prot.* **2003**, *22*, 247–252. [CrossRef]
54. Ghaffari, M.A.; Bano, S.; Hayat, K. Antimicrobial and Phytotoxic Effects of the Plant *Heliotropium Dasycarpum* L. *Int. J. Pharm. Biol. Sci.* **2013**, *4*, 339–345.
55. Saeed, M.; Khan, H.; Khan, M.A.; Simjee, S.U.; Muhammad, N.; Khan, S.A. Phytotoxic, insecticidal and leishmanicidal activities of aerial parts of *Polygonatum verticillatum*. *Afr. J. Biotechnol.* **2010**, *9*, 1241–1244.
56. Mongelli, E.; Desmarchelier, C.; Coussio, J.; Ciccia, G. The potential effects of allelopathic mechanisms on plant species diversity and distribution determined by the wheat rootlet growth inhibition bioassay in South American plants. *Rev. Chil. Hist. Nat.* **1997**, *70*, 83–89.
57. Beninger, C.W.; Hall, J.C. Allelopathic activity of luteolin 7-*O*-β-glucuronide isolated from *Chrysanthemum morifolium* L. *Biochem. Sys. Ecol.* **2005**, *33*, 103–111. [CrossRef]
58. Machlin, L.J.; Bendich, A. Free radical tissue damage: Protective role of antioxidant nutrients. *FASEB J.* **1987**, *1*, 441–445. [PubMed]
59. Stanner, S.A.; Hughes, J.; Kelly, C.N.M.; Buttriss, J. A review of the epidemiological evidence for the 'antioxidant hypothesis'. *Public Health Nutr.* **2004**, *7*, 407–422. [CrossRef] [PubMed]
60. Modak, B.; Rojas, M.; Torres, R.; Rodilla, J.; Luebert, F. Antioxidant activity of a new aromatic geranyl derivative of the resinous exudates from *Heliotropium glutinosum* Phil. *Molecules* **2007**, *12*, 1057–1063. [CrossRef] [PubMed]

61. Modak, B.; Rojas, M.; Torres, R. Chemical analysis of the resinous exudate isolated from *Heliotropium taltalense* and evaluation of the antioxidant activity of the phenolics components and the resin in homogeneous and heterogeneous systems. *Molecules* **2009**, *14*, 1980–1989. [CrossRef] [PubMed]
62. Modak, B.; Torres, R.; Lissi, E.; Monache, F.D. Antioxidant capacity of flavonoids and a new arylphenol of the resinous exudate from *Heliotropium sinuatum*. *Nat. Prod. Res.* **2003**, *17*, 403–407. [CrossRef] [PubMed]

Permissions

All chapters in this book were first published by MDPI; hereby published with permission under the Creative Commons Attribution License or equivalent. Every chapter published in this book has been scrutinized by our experts. Their significance has been extensively debated. The topics covered herein carry significant findings which will fuel the growth of the discipline. They may even be implemented as practical applications or may be referred to as a beginning point for another development.

The contributors of this book come from diverse backgrounds, making this book a truly international effort. This book will bring forth new frontiers with its revolutionizing research information and detailed analysis of the nascent developments around the world.

We would like to thank all the contributing authors for lending their expertise to make the book truly unique. They have played a crucial role in the development of this book. Without their invaluable contributions this book wouldn't have been possible. They have made vital efforts to compile up to date information on the varied aspects of this subject to make this book a valuable addition to the collection of many professionals and students.

This book was conceptualized with the vision of imparting up-to-date information and advanced data in this field. To ensure the same, a matchless editorial board was set up. Every individual on the board went through rigorous rounds of assessment to prove their worth. After which they invested a large part of their time researching and compiling the most relevant data for our readers.

The editorial board has been involved in producing this book since its inception. They have spent rigorous hours researching and exploring the diverse topics which have resulted in the successful publishing of this book. They have passed on their knowledge of decades through this book. To expedite this challenging task, the publisher supported the team at every step. A small team of assistant editors was also appointed to further simplify the editing procedure and attain best results for the readers.

Apart from the editorial board, the designing team has also invested a significant amount of their time in understanding the subject and creating the most relevant covers. They scrutinized every image to scout for the most suitable representation of the subject and create an appropriate cover for the book.

The publishing team has been an ardent support to the editorial, designing and production team. Their endless efforts to recruit the best for this project, has resulted in the accomplishment of this book. They are a veteran in the field of academics and their pool of knowledge is as vast as their experience in printing. Their expertise and guidance has proved useful at every step. Their uncompromising quality standards have made this book an exceptional effort. Their encouragement from time to time has been an inspiration for everyone.

The publisher and the editorial board hope that this book will prove to be a valuable piece of knowledge for researchers, students, practitioners and scholars across the globe.

List of Contributors

Huai-Ching Tai
School of Medicine, Fu-Jen Catholic University, New Taipei City 242, Taiwan
Department of Urology, Fu-Jen Catholic University Hospital, New Taipei City 242, Taiwan

Tzong-Huei Lee and Ming-Shian Lee
Institute of Fisheries Science, National Taiwan University, Taipei 106, Taiwan

Chih-Hsin Tang
Chinese Medicine Research Center, China Medical University, Taichung 404, Taiwan
Department of Pharmacology, School of Medicine, China Medical University, Taichung 404, Taiwan
Department of Biotechnology, College of Health Science, Asia University, Taichung 413, Taiwan

Lei-Po Chen and Wei-Cheng Chen
Department of Orthopaedics, MacKay Memorial Hospital, Taipei 104, Taiwan
Ph.D. Degree Program of Biomedical Science and Engineering, National Chiao Tung University, Hsinchu 300, Taiwan

Pei-Chi Chen and Chih-Yang Lin
Department of Medicine, Mackay Medical College, New Taipei City 252, Taiwan

Chih-Wen Chi
Department of Medical Research, MacKay Memorial Hospital, New Taipei City 251, Taiwan

Yu-Jen Chen
Department of Medical Research, MacKay Memorial Hospital, New Taipei City 251, Taiwan
Department of Radiation Oncology, MacKay Memorial Hospital, Taipei 104, Taiwan

Cheng-Ta Lai
Division of Colon and Rectal Surgery, Department of Surgery, MacKay Memorial Hospital, Taipei 104, Taiwan

Shiou-Sheng Chen
Division of Urology, Taipei City Hospital HepingFuyou Branch, Taipei 100, Taiwan
Commission for General Education, National United University, Miaoli 360, Taiwan

Kuang-Wen Liao
Ph.D. Degree Program of Biomedical Science and Engineering, National Chiao Tung University, Hsinchu 300, Taiwan
Institute of Molecular Medicine and Bioengineering, National Chiao Tung University, Hsinchu 300, Taiwan
Department of Biotechnology and Bioindustry Sciences, National Cheng Kung University, Tainan 300, Taiwan

Chien-Hsing Lee
Department of Pharmacology, Graduate Institute of Medicine, College of Medicine, Kaohsiung Medical University, Kaohsiung 807, Taiwan
Department of Medical Research, Kaohsiung Medical University Hospital, Kaohsiung 807, Taiwan

Shih-Wei Wang
Department of Medicine, Mackay Medical College, New Taipei City 252, Taiwan
Graduate Institute of Natural Products, College of Pharmacy, Kaohsiung Medical University, Kaohsiung 807, Taiwan

Chidi Edenta
Department of Biochemistry, Renaissance University, Ugbawka, Enugu State 402212, Nigeria

Stanley I. R. Okoduwa
Directorate of Research and Development, Nigerian Institute of Leather and Science Technology, Zaria, Kaduna State 810221, Nigeria
Infohealth Awareness Unit, SIRONigeria Global Limited, Abuja, Federal Capital Territory 900288, Nigeria

Oche Okpe
Department of Biochemistry, Federal University of Agriculture, Makurdi, Benue State 970101, Nigeria

Ming-Fang Cheng
Department of Pathology, Tri-Service General Hospital, National Defense Medical Center, Taipei 10086, Taiwan
Division of Histology and Clinical Pathology, Hualian Army Forces General Hospital, Hualien 97144, Taiwan

Chun-Shu Lin
Department of Radiation Oncology, Tri-Service General Hospital, National Defense Medical Center, Taipei 10086, Taiwan

Yu-Hsin Chen and Ching-Feng Weng
Department of Life Science and Institute of Biotechnology, National Dong Hwa University, Hualien 97401, Taiwan
Graduate Institute of Marine Biotechnology, National Dong Hwa University, Pingtung 94450, Taiwan

Ping-Jyun Sung
Department of Life Science and Institute of Biotechnology, National Dong Hwa University, Hualien 97401, Taiwan
Graduate Institute of Marine Biotechnology, National Dong Hwa University, Pingtung 94450, Taiwan
National Museum of Marine Biology and Aquarium, Pingtung 94450, Taiwan

Shian-Ren Lin and Yi-Wen Tong
Department of Life Science and Institute of Biotechnology, National Dong Hwa University, Hualien 97401, Taiwan

Prosper T. Kinda, Samson Guenné, Moussa Compaoré and Martin Kiendrebeogo
Laboratoire de Biochimie et Chimie Appliquées, Université Ouaga I-Pr Joseph KI-ZERBO, 03 PB 7021 Ouagadougou 03, Burkina Faso

Patrice Zerbo
Laboratoire de Biologie et écologie végétale, Université Ouaga I-Pr Joseph KI-ZERBO, 03 BP 7021 Ouagadougou 03, Burkina Faso

Alin Ciobica
"Alexandru Ioan Cuza" University of Iasi, Faculty of Biology, Department of Research, Carol I Avenue, No. 20A, Iasi 700505, Romania

Marthe Aimée Tchuente Tchuenmogne, Silvère Augustin Ngouela and Etienne Tsamo
Laboratory of Natural Products and Organic Synthesis, Department of Organic Chemistry, Faculty of Science, University of Yaoundé 1, Yaoundé, Cameroon

Thierry Ngouana Kammalac, Rufin Marie Toghueo Kouipou and Fabrice Fekam Boyom
Antimicrobial & Biocontrol Agents Unit, Laboratory for Phytobiochemistry and Medicinal Plants Studies, Department of Biochemistry, Faculty of Science, University of Yaoundé I, Yaoundé, Cameroon

Sebastian Gohlke and Norbert Sewald
Chemistry Department, Organic and Bioorganic Chemistry, Bielefeld University, D-33501 Bielefeld, Germany

Abdulselam Aslan
Faculty of Engineering, Department of Industrial Engineering, Giresun University, 28200 Giresun, Turkey

Ana Isabel Neto
Azorean Biodiversity Group, Centre for Ecology, Evolution and Environmental Changes (CE3C), Department of Biology, University of Azores, 9501-801 Ponta Delgada, Portugal

Muslum Kuzu
Faculty of Pharmacy, Department of Basic Pharmaceutical Sciences, Agrı Ibrahim Cecen University, 04100 Agri, Turkey

Veysel Comakli and Ramazan Demirdag
School of Health, Department of Nutrition and Dietetics, Agrı Ibrahim Cecen University, 04100 Agri, Turkey

Bruno Ndjakou Lenta
Department of Chemistry, Higher Teacher Training College, University of Yaoundé 1, Yaoundé, Cameroon

Fernando Bastos Presa, Maxsuell Lucas Mendes Marques and Hugo Alexandre Oliveira Rocha
Departamento de Bioquímica, Universidade Federal do Rio Grande do Norte, Natal 59078-970, Rio Grande do Norte, Brazil
Programa de Pós-graduação emCiências da Saúde, Universidade Federal do Rio Grande do Norte, Natal 59078-970, Rio Grande do Norte, Brazil

Rony Lucas Silva Viana and Leonardo Thiago Duarte Barreto Nobre
Departamento de Bioquímica, Universidade Federal do Rio Grande do Norte, Natal 59078-970, Rio Grande do Norte, Brazil

Leandro Silva Costa
Instituto Federal de Educação, Ciência, e Tecnologia do Rio Grande do Norte (IFRN), Ceara-Mirim 59900-000, Rio Grande do Norte, Brazil

Mohammad A. Al-Tamimi
Deptartment of Nutrition and Food Technology, An-Najah National University, Nablus 415, Palestine

Bob Rastall
Department of Food and Nutritional Sciences, The University of Reading, Whiteknights, Reading RG6 6AP, UK

Ibrahim M. Abu-Reidah
Deptartment of Nutrition and Food Technology, An-Najah National University, PO Box 7, Nablus 415, Palestine
Deptartment of Chemistry, An-Najah National University, PO Box 7, Nablus 415, Palestine

Lisete Paiva
Biotechnology Centre of Azores (CBA), University of Azores, 9501-801 Ponta Delgada, Portugal

Ashutosh Pathak and Anupam Dikshit
Biological Product Lab, Department of Botany, University of Allahabad, Allahabad 211002, India

Elisabete Lima and José Baptista
Biotechnology Centre of Azores (CBA), University of Azores, 9501-801 Ponta Delgada, Portugal
Research Center for Agricultural Technology (CITA-A), University of Azores, 9501-801 Ponta Delgada, Portugal

Vincent Ouedraogo and Martin Kiendrebeogo
Laboratoire de Biochimie & Chimie Appliquées, Université Ouaga 1 Pr. Joseph KI-ZERBO, Ouagadougou, 03 BP 7021, Burkina Faso

Olaoye S. Balogun, Olukayode S. Ajayi and Olayinka S. Lawal
Department of Chemistry, Obafemi Awolowo University, Ile-Ife 220005, Nigeria

Dalip Kumar Upreti
Lichenology Laboratory, CSIR-National Botanical Research Institute, Rana Pratap Marg, Lucknow 226001, India

Liang-Mou Kuo
Graduate Institute of Clinical Medical Sciences, College of Medicine, Chang Gung University, Taoyuan 333, Taiwan
Department of General Surgery, Chang Gung Memorial Hospital, Chiayi 613, Taiwan

Po-Jen Chen
Graduate Institute of Natural Products, College of Medicine, Chang Gung University, Taoyuan 333, Taiwan
Chinese Herbal Medicine Research Team, Healthy Aging Research Center, Chang Gung University, Taoyuan 333, Taiwan

Ping-Jyun Sung
Graduate Institute of Marine Biology, National Dong Hwa University, Pingtung 944, Taiwan
National Museum of Marine Biology and Aquarium, Pingtung 944, Taiwan
Chinese Medicine Research and Development Center, China Medical University Hospital, Taichung 404, Taiwan
Graduate Institute of Natural Products, Kaohsiung Medical University, Kaohsiung 807, Taiwan
Department of Marine Biotechnology and Resources, National Sun Yat-sen University, Kaohsiung 804, Taiwan

Yu-Chia Chang
National Museum of Marine Biology and Aquarium, Pingtung 944, Taiwan
Doctoral Degree Program in Marine Biotechnology, National Sun Yat-sen University & Academia Sinica, Kaohsiung 804, Taiwan

Chun-Ting Ho and Yi-Hsiu Wu
Graduate Institute of Natural Products, College of Medicine, Chang Gung University, Taoyuan 333, Taiwan

Tsong-Long Hwang
Graduate Institute of Natural Products, College of Medicine, Chang Gung University, Taoyuan 333, Taiwan
Chinese Herbal Medicine Research Team, Healthy Aging Research Center, Chang Gung University, Taoyuan 333, Taiwan
Research Center for Chinese Herbal Medicine, Research Center for Food and Cosmetic Safety, Graduate Institute of Health Industry Technology, College of Human Ecology, Chang Gung University of Science and Technology, Taoyuan 333, Taiwan
Department of Anaesthesiology, Chang Gung Memorial Hospital, Taoyuan 333, Taiwan

Nara O. dos Santos, Renata C. Pascon, Marcelo A. Vallim and Patricia Sartorelli
Instituto de Ciências Ambientais, Químicas e Farmacêuticas, Universidade Federal de São Paulo, Diadema 09972-270, SP, Brazil

Carlos R. Figueiredo
Disciplina de Biologia Celular, Departamento de Micro, Imuno e Parasitologia, Universidade Federal de São Paulo, Sao Paulo 04021-001, SP, Brazil

Marisi G. Soares
Instituto de Química, Universidade Federal de Alfenas, Alfenas 37130-000, MG, Brazil

João Henrique G. Lago
Instituto de Ciências Ambientais, Químicas e Farmacêuticas, Universidade Federal de São Paulo, Diadema 09972-270, SP, Brazil
Centro de Ciências Naturais e Humanas, Universidade Federal do ABC, Santo Andre 09210-180, SP, Brazil

Shih-Wei Wang
Graduate Institute of Natural Products, College of Pharmacy, Kaohsiung Medical University, Kaohsiung 807, Taiwan
Department of Medicine, Mackay Medical College, New Taipei City 252, Taiwan

Bai-Luh Wei
Department of Life Science, National Taitung University, Taitung 950, Taiwan

Jihoon Lee, So Jeong Nam, Yun Ju Kang, Youjin Han, Kwangik Choi, Mihwa Kwon and Im-Sook Song
College of Pharmacy and Research Institute of Pharmaceutical Sciences, Kyungpook National University, Daegu 41566, Korea

Min-Koo Choi and Young A. Choi
College of Pharmacy, Dankook University, Cheon-an 31116, Korea

Dongjoo Lee
College of Pharmacy, Ajou University, Suwon 16499, Korea

Xiaogang Wang
Tongji School of Pharmacy, Huazhong University of Science and Technology, Wuhan 430030, Hubei, China

Raphael Dubois, Caitlyn Young, Eric J. Lien and James D. Adams
Department of Pharmacology and Pharmaceutical Sciences, School of Pharmacy, University of Southern California, Los Angeles, CA 90899-9121, USA

Hsin-Hsien Yu
Institute of Clinical Medicine, College of Medicine, National Cheng Kung University, Tainan 701, Taiwan
Division of General Surgery, Department of Surgery, Wan Fang Hospital, Taipei Medical University, Taipei 116, Taiwan

Edward Chengchuan KO
School of Dentistry, College of Dental Medicine, Kaohsiung Medical University, Kaohsiung 807, Taiwan
Division of Oral and Maxillofacial Surgery, Kaohsiung Medical University Hospital, Kaohsiung 807, Taiwan
Department of FUJISOFT Cartilage and Bone Regeneration, Tissue Engineering, The University of Tokyo, Tokyo 113-0033, Japan

Chia-Lun Chang
Department of Hemato-Oncology, Wan Fang Hospital, Taipei Medical University, Taipei 116, Taiwan
Department of Internal Medicine, School of Medicine, College of Medicine, Taipei Medical University, Taipei 11031, Taiwan

Kevin Sheng-Po Yuan
Department of Otorhinolaryngology, Wan Fang Hospital, Taipei Medical University, Taipei 116, Taiwan

Alexander T. H. Wu
Ph.D. Program for Translational Medicine, Taipei Medical University, Taipei 11031, Taiwan

Yan-Shen Shan
Institute of Clinical Medicine, College of Medicine, National Cheng Kung University, Tainan 701, Taiwan
Department of Surgery, National Cheng Kung University Hospital, College of Medicine, National Cheng Kung University, Tainan 701, Taiwan

Yan-Shen Shan
Institute of Clinical Medicine, College of Medicine, National Cheng Kung University, Tainan 701, Taiwan
Department of Surgery, National Cheng Kung University Hospital, College of Medicine, National Cheng Kung University, Tainan 701, Taiwan

Szu-Yuan Wu
Department of Internal Medicine, School of Medicine, College of Medicine, Taipei Medical University, Taipei 11031, Taiwan
Department of Radiation Oncology, Wan Fang Hospital, Taipei Medical University, Taipei 116, Taiwan

Javier Rodríguez Villanueva
Biomedical Sciences Department, Pharmacy and Pharmaceutical Technology Unit, Faculty of Pharmacy, University of Alcalá, Ctra. de Madrid-Barcelona (Autovía A2) Km. 33,600, 28805 Alcalá de Henares, Madrid, Spain

Jorge Martín Esteban
Phytotherapy Faculty, University of Barcelona, Gran Via de les Corts Catalanes, 585, 08007 Barcelona, Spain

Laura Rodríguez Villanueva
Faculty of Pharmacy, University of Alcalá, Ctra. de Madrid-Barcelona (Autovía A2) Km. 33,600 28805 Alcalá de Henares, Madrid, Spain

Szu-Yin Yu and Chien-Jung Su
Graduate Institute of Natural Products, College of Pharmacy, Kaohsiung Medical University, Kaohsiung 807, Taiwan

Tsong-Long Hwang
Graduate Institute of Natural Products, College of Medicine, and Chinese Herbal Medicine Research Team, Healthy Aging Research Center, Chang Gung University, Taoyuan 333, Taiwan
Research Center for Chinese Herbal Medicine, Research Center for Food and Cosmetic Safety, and Graduate Institute of Health Industry Technology, College of Human Ecology, Chang Gung University of Science and Technology, Taoyuan 333, Taiwan
Department of Anesthesiology, Chang Gung Memorial Hospital, Taoyuan 333, Taiwan

Shih-Wei Wang
Graduate Institute of Natural Products, College of Pharmacy, Kaohsiung Medical University, Kaohsiung 807, Taiwan
Department of Medicine, Mackay Medical College, New Taipei City 252, Taiwan

Bai-Luh Wei
Department of Life Science, National Taitung University, Taitung 950, Taiwan

Fang-Rong Chang
Graduate Institute of Natural Products, College of Pharmacy, Kaohsiung Medical University, Kaohsiung 807, Taiwan
National Research Institute of Chinese Medicine, Ministry of Health and Welfare, Taipei 112, Taiwan

Yuan-Bin Cheng
Graduate Institute of Natural Products, College of Pharmacy, Kaohsiung Medical University, Kaohsiung 807, Taiwan
Department of Medical Research, Kaohsiung Medical University Hospital, Kaohsiung 807, Taiwan

Olubukola Sinbad Olorunnisola, Olumide Samuel Fadahunsi and Peter Adegbola
Department of Biochemistry, Faculty of Basic Medical Sciences, Ladoke Akintola University of Technology, Ogbomoso, PMB 4000, Oyo State, Nigeria

Benqi Teng
School of Life Sciences, University of Technology Sydney, NSW 2007, Australia
Department of Obstetrics, The Third Affiliated Hospital of Sun Yat-sen University, 600 Tianhe Road, Guangzhou 510630, China

Jie Peng
School of Life Sciences, University of Technology Sydney, NSW 2007, Australia
Department of Gynaecology and Obstetrics, Suzhou Wuzhong People's Hospital, Suzhou 215128, China

Madeleine Ong and Xianqin Qu
School of Life Sciences, University of Technology Sydney, NSW 2007, Australia

Muhammad Khurm, Bashir A. Chaudhry and Muhammad Uzair
Faculty of Pharmacy, Natural Product Chemistry Unit, Bahauddin Zakariya University, Multan 60800, Pakistan

Khalid H. Janbaz
Akson College of Pharmacy, Mirpur University of Science and Technology, Mirpur 10250, Pakistan

Index

www.ingramcontent.com/pod-product-compliance
Lightning Source LLC
LaVergne TN
LVHW080926210926
848485LV00004B/739

9781639897964